Neuromorphic Circuits

A constructive approach

Online at: https://doi.org/10.1088/978-0-7503-5097-6

About the Series

The series in Physics and Engineering in Medicine and Biology will allow the Institute of Physics and Engineering in Medicine (IPEM) to enhance its mission to 'advance physics and engineering applied to medicine and biology for the public good'.

It is focused on key areas including, but not limited to:
- clinical engineering
- diagnostic radiology
- informatics and computing
- magnetic resonance imaging
- nuclear medicine
- physiological measurement
- radiation protection
- radiotherapy
- rehabilitation engineering
- ultrasound and non-ionising radiation.

A number of IPEM–IOP titles are being published as part of the EUTEMPE Network Series for Medical Physics Experts.

A full list of titles published in this series can be found here: https://iopscience.iop.org/bookListInfo/physics-engineering-medicine-biology-series.

Neuromorphic Circuits

A constructive approach

Edited by
Alice C Parker
Ming Hsieh Department of Electrical and Computer Engineering—Systems University of Southern California (United States), Systems University of Southern California, Los Angeles, CA, USA

Rick Cattell
Independent Consultant

IOP Publishing, Bristol, UK

ISBN   978-0-7503-5097-6 (ebook)
ISBN   978-0-7503-5095-2 (print)
ISBN   978-0-7503-5098-3 (myPrint)
ISBN   978-0-7503-5096-9 (mobi)

DOI   10.1088/978-0-7503-5097-6

Version: 20231101

IOP ebooks

British Library Cataloguing-in-Publication Data: A catalogue record for this book is available from the British Library.

Published by IOP Publishing, wholly owned by The Institute of Physics, London

IOP Publishing, No.2 The Distillery, Glassfields, Avon Street, Bristol, BS2 0GR, UK

US Office: IOP Publishing, Inc., 190 North Independence Mall West, Suite 601, Philadelphia, PA 19106, USA

This book is dedicated to my son Joseph Cline Bebel and to my late co-author Rick (Roderic G G) Cattell. This book would not have made it to press without their input and assistance. Rick Cattell passed away September 25, 2022.

Contents

Preface   xv

Acknowledgements   xvii

Editor biographies   xviii

List of contributors   xx

Contributor biographies   xxi

Acronyms   xxvi

1   Introduction   1-1
     Alice C Parker, Rick Cattell, Rami Alzahrani, Chih-Chieh Hsu,
     Yilda Irizarry-Valle, Jon Joshi, Rebecca Lee, Pezhman Mamdouh,
     Jason Mahvash and Ko-Chung Tseng

1.1 Introduction to neurons and to the brain   1-1
1.2 The axon initial segment—the spiking circuit   1-10
1.3 The synapse   1-11
     1.3.1 Electrical synapses   1-16
     1.3.2 AMPA and NMDA channels and receptors   1-17
1.4 Dendritic computation   1-17
     1.4.1 Dendritic spikes   1-18
     1.4.2 Dendritic plasticity   1-23
1.5 Variability in neural behavior   1-24
     1.5.1 Biological neural variability   1-26
     1.5.2 Background   1-28
     1.5.3 Synaptic variability   1-30
     1.5.4 Ion-channel variability   1-30
     1.5.5 Spontaneous firing   1-31
1.6 Structural plasticity   1-32
1.7 Astrocytes   1-34
     1.7.1 Astrocyte glutamate   1-38
     1.7.2 Astrocytes' role in binding information   1-39
     1.7.3 Astrocytes contribute to a wide range of biological processes   1-40
     1.7.4 Calcium waves: a coding mechanism in astrocytes   1-41
     1.7.5 Patterns of astrocytic calcium waves   1-42
     1.7.6 Intercellular propagation of calcium waves in astrocytes   1-43
     1.7.7 Integration of synaptic information   1-44
     1.7.8 Retrograde signaling   1-45
     1.7.9 Homeostatic plasticity   1-45

1.8   The retina   1-47
       1.8.1 The outer retina   1-48
       1.8.2 The inner retina   1-51
1.9   The neural code   1-55
       1.9.1 The axon initial segment definition   1-56
       1.9.2 Voltage gated ion channels at the AIS   1-56
       1.9.3 Dynamical neural modulation and signal processing at the AIS   1-58
       1.9.4 Bursting through calcium ion channels   1-59
       1.9.5 Astrocytes roles in neural signaling and synaptic strengthening 1-60
1.10   Chapter conclusions and future thoughts   1-61
1.11   Exercises   1-62
       References   1-62

2   Introduction to neuromorphic circuits   2-1
       Alice C Parker and Rick Cattell

2.1   The history of neuromorphic circuits   2-1
2.2   Complexities of modeling the brain   2-5
       2.2.1 Introduction to the toughest challenges for artificial brains   2-5
       2.2.2 Reliability and fault tolerance in biological neurons   2-15
       2.2.3 Other neuromorphic system and circuit surveys   2-16
2.3   Chapter conclusion   2-17
2.4   Book outline   2-17
2.5   Exercises   2-17
       References   2-17

3   Approach to neuromorphic circuits   3-1
       Alice C Parker

3.1   Introduction   3-1
3.2   Introduction to electronic modeling of neurons   3-5
       3.2.1 *RC* (resistance–capacitance) time constants   3-7
       3.2.2 Basic neural models   3-8
3.3   Basic analog circuits   3-12
       3.3.1 Why analog circuits?   3-15
3.4   Chapter summary   3-16
3.5   Exercises   3-16
       References   3-16

4 Mathematical models   **4-1**

Alice C Parker, Yilda Irizarry-Valle, Rebecca Lee
and Suraj Chakravarthi Raja

4.1 Izhikevich's spiking model   4-1

    4.1.1 Izhikevich's spiking patterns   4-2

    4.1.2 Mathematics of Izhikevich's spiking model   4-5

4.2 Leaky integrate-and-fire spiking model   4-7

4.3 The Hodgkin–Huxley model 1952   4-8

4.4 Other spiking models   4-11

4.5 Astrocyte mathematical models   4-12

4.6 Chapter summmary   4-15

4.7 Exercises   4-15

    References   4-16

5 The axon and the spiking mechanism   **5-1**

Chih-Chieh Hsu and Alice C Parker

5.1 Introduction   5-1

5.2 Farquhar and Hasler's spiking circuit   5-2

5.3 Hsu's spiking circuit   5-8

    5.3.1 The regular-spiking circuit   5-9

5.4 Variations in Hsu's axon initial segment   5-12

5.5 Modeling axonal propagation   5-14

5.6 Chapter summary   5-14

5.7 Exercises   5-15

    References   5-16

6 Neural input circuits—the synapse   **6-1**

Chih-Chieh Hsu, Jon Joshi and Alice C Parker

6.1 Single-transistor synapse circuit   6-1

6.2 Indiveri's synapses   6-2

6.3 The BioRC synapses   6-5

    6.3.1 Variations in BioRC excitatory synapses to control strengths   6-6

6.4 Spike timing dependent plasticity (STDP)   6-14

    6.4.1 Joshi's STDP circuit   6-16

    6.4.2 Yue's STDP circuit   6-18

6.5 The silent synapse   6-19

6.6 Chapter summary   6-19

6.7 Exercises   6-20

    References   6-20

7   The passive dendritic arbor   **7-1**
     Chih-Chieh Hsu and Alice C Parker

7.1   Elias' passive dendritic model   7-1
7.2   Passive voltage addition in the dendritic arbor   7-1
      7.2.1 Hsu's average-amplify circuit   7-3
7.3   Hsu's computations in the dendritic arbor   7-3
      7.3.1 Shunting inhibition   7-4
      7.3.2 Spatiotemporal signal processing in passive dendrites   7-7
      7.3.3 Temporal integration window effect   7-10
      7.3.4 Temporal summation for sequence detection   7-12
7.4   Chapter summary   7-15
7.5   Exercises   7-15
      References   7-15

8   Dendritic spiking and dendritic plasticity   **8-1**
     Chih-Chieh Hsu and Alice C Parker

8.1   Introduction   8-1
      8.1.1 Excitation and inhibition integration   8-2
8.2   Active dendrites: dendritic spiking   8-6
      8.2.1 Neuromorphic circuit implementation   8-6
      8.2.2 Spatio-temporal processing in active dendrites   8-10
8.3   Dendritic spike-enhanced precise AP spike timing   8-12
      8.3.1 Effect of dendritic spike on AP spike timing   8-16
      8.3.2 Effect of synaptic activation level on AP spike timing   8-19
      8.3.3 Effect of input synchronization on AP spike timing   8-20
      8.3.4 Down-regulated dendritic excitability   8-24
      8.3.5 Up-regulated dendritic excitability   8-27
8.4   Back-propagating action potential activated calcium spike   8-29
8.5   Back-propagating action potential characterization   8-31
8.6   Other neuromorphic circuits for dendritic computations   8-32
      8.6.1 Farquhar and Hasler's dendritic arbor   8-33
      8.6.2 Hynna, Arthur and Boahen's dendritic computations   8-34
      8.6.3 Wang and Liu's dendritic computations   8-37
      8.6.4 Comparison summary   8-38
8.7   Chapter summary   8-39
8.8   Exercises   8-39
      References   8-39

9   Variable neural behavior   **9-1**
Jason Mahvash, Kun Yue and Alice C Parker

9.1   Introduction   9-1
      9.1.1 Ion-channel variability in the Hodgkin–Huxley model   9-2
      9.1.2 Ion-channel variability in the integrate-and-fire model   9-3
9.2   Circuit implementation of intrinsic variability   9-4
9.3   Neurotransmitter-release variability in the synapse circuit   9-5
9.4   Ion-channel variability in the axon hillock circuit   9-13
9.5   Chaotic signal generation   9-18
      9.5.1 Introduction   9-18
      9.5.2 Chaotic map   9-19
9.6   Random pulse generation (RPG) noise generator   9-20
      9.6.1 Random pulse generator device   9-22
      9.6.2 Discrete noise signals   9-22
      9.6.3 Continuous noise signals   9-24
      9.6.4 Probability and distribution   9-24
9.7   Chapter summary   9-26
      References   9-26

10   Learning and strengthening   **10-1**
Jon Joshi, Kun Yue, Eric Evans, Dena Giovinazzo and Alice C Parker

10.1 Structural plasticity   10-1
      10.1.1 Approach to neuromorphic network restructuring   10-2
              using synapse claiming
10.2 The blank slate cortical column   10-7
      10.2.1 Learning without forgetting   10-7
      10.2.2 Related research on dopamine   10-7
      10.2.3 Architecture of the blank slate cortical column   10-8
      10.2.4 Blank slate training approach   10-10
      10.2.5 Training the blank slate neuromorphic network   10-12
      10.2.6 The neural code in the blank slate   10-14
      10.2.7 Adding pain signals to the inputs   10-14
      10.2.8 Future blank slate investigations   10-16
10.3 The PRONON programmable neuron   10-17
10.4 Chapter summary   10-17
      References   10-18

11   Astrocytes   **11-1**
Jon Joshi, Yilda Irizarry-Valle, Rebecca Lee and Alice C Parker

11.1   Introduction   11-1
11.2   The tripartite synapse   11-2
11.3   Experimental tripartite communication network   11-4
11.4   Neural phase synchrony   11-6
       11.4.1 Circuit implementation   11-9
11.5   Retrograde signaling   11-21
       11.5.1 The retrograde messenger (RGM) generation circuit   11-23
       11.5.2 The retrograde (RG) excitatory synapse circuit   11-25
       11.5.3 The astrocyte circuit   11-26
11.6   Self-repair by RGM-mediated synaptic plasticity   11-30
11.7   Chapter summary   11-33
       References   11-33

12   The retina   **12-1**
Ko-Chung Tseng and Alice C Parker

12.1   Related retinal neuromorphic research   12-1
       12.1.1 Neuromorphic designs of the retina in silicon circuits   12-2
       12.1.2 Neuromorphic models of motion detection in the   12-3
               visual system
       12.1.3 Implantable artificial retinas   12-3
12.2   Comparison of Tseng's research to state of the art   12-4
12.3   The outer retina design   12-4
       12.3.1 The photoreceptor circuit and testing results   12-6
       12.3.2 Horizontal cell design   12-10
       12.3.3 The outer retina network and testing results   12-11
       12.3.4 Glutamate reuptake   12-13
       12.3.5 Contrast enhancement   12-15
       12.3.6 Center-surround property   12-18
       12.3.7 Edge detection   12-20
12.4   The inner retina design   12-20
       12.4.1 On-type BC design   12-20
       12.4.2 A directionally-selective neuromorphic circuit   12-22
       12.4.3 A neuromorphic circuit that computes differential motion 12-31
       12.4.4 Retinal pathways   12-48
12.5   Chapter summary   12-56
       References   12-57

13   The neural code   13-1
Rami Alzahrani and Alice C Parker

13.1 Introduction to dynamic neuronal coding circuits   13-2
13.2 Dynamic neuronal coding circuit implementations   13-3
13.3 Various dynamic spiking and bursting patterns   13-5
    13.3.1 Various spiking patterns using dynamic neuronal encoding   13-6
    circuits
    13.3.2 Various bursting patterns using dynamic neuronal encoding   13-8
    circuits
    13.3.3 Other spiking patterns using dynamic neuronal encoding   13-9
    circuits
    13.3.4 The working principles of the AIS modulation   13-9
13.4 Chapter summary   13-12
References   13-12

14   Other neural codes   14-1
Rebecca K Lee and Alice C Parker

14.1 Lee's dendritic morphology and plasticity   14-1
    14.1.1 Motivation   14-1
    14.1.2 Neuron circuit with multiple dendrites   14-2
    14.1.3 Background: dendrite-specific AP shapes   14-4
    14.1.4 A neuron circuit with input-specific spiking   14-5
    14.1.5 Astrocyte-mediated repair   14-11
    14.1.6 Summary   14-19
14.2 Cauwenberghs' Izhikevich spiking circuit   14-19
14.3 Chapter summary   14-22
14.4 Exercises   14-22
References   14-22

15   Circuits with nanotechnologies   15-1
Kun Yue, Jon Joshi, Chih-Chieh Hsu, Rebecca K Lee and Alice C Parker

15.1 Introduction   15-1
15.2 Carbon nanotube (CNT) neuromorphic circuits   15-1
15.3 Molybdenum disulfide neuromorphic circuits   15-5
    15.3.1 Introduction and background   15-5
    15.3.2 The molybdenum disulfide FET   15-8
    15.3.3 Neuromorphic circuit models   15-9
    15.3.4 Network with astrocytes   15-12
    15.3.5 MoS_2 FET neuromorphic network conclusion   15-13

15.4 Other BioRC nanotechnological neuromorphic circuits   15-14
    15.4.1 Hybrid carbon nanotube/silicon neuromorphic circuits   15-14
    15.4.2 Magnetic analog memristor/silicon neuromorphic circuits   15-14
15.5 Future neuromorphic nanotechnologies   15-15
15.6 Chapter summary   15-16
    References   15-17

16   Advanced topics   16-1

Chih-Chieh Hsu, Yilda Irizarry-Valle, Ko-Chung Tseng, Pezhman Mamdouh and Alice C Parker

16.1 Sound localization in birds   16-1
16.2 Burst potentiation possibilities   16-4
16.3 A depressing synapse   16-7
16.4 Border ownership   16-9
    16.4.1 Border-ownership background   16-10
    16.4.2 Discussion of border-ownership algorithms   16-12
    16.4.3 The proposed border-ownership neuron   16-13
    16.4.4 Contour detection using nonlinear dendritic computation   16-15
    16.4.5 Proposed border-ownership neural network   16-21
16.5 Ultra-low-power dendritic computations   16-23
16.6 Chapter summary   16-23
    References   16-23

17   Neuromorphic systems   17-1

Rick Cattell, Michael Boemler-Rudolph Mercury and Alice C Parker

17.1 Introduction   17-1
17.2 IBM's true north   17-2
17.3 Intel's Loihi   17-2
17.4 BrainChip's Akida   17-3
17.5 Manchester's SpiNNaker   17-4
17.6 BrainScaleS   17-5
17.7 Further reading   17-5
17.8 Conclusions   17-6
17.9 Exercises   17-6
    References   17-6

18   Epilogue   18-1

Alice C Parker and Rick Cattell   18-1
    References

Preface

Neuromorphic electronic circuits, circuits that model biological neurons with electronics, provide an underlying circuit approach for constructing models of neurons and networks of neurons for the human brain and nervous system as well as for other animals, including the microscopic worm, *Caenorhabditis elegans* (*C elegans*) with its 302 neurons. These models are useful for demonstrating neural behavior, including behaviors invoked by brain disorders. Neuromorphic circuits are also of value when demonstrating memory and learning. The ultimate application of neuromorphic circuits is electronic systems with brain-like behavior, including robots, diagnostic systems and autonomous vehicles.

These models aim at low-power and low-cost design, both urgent priorities when constructing circuits containing millions to billions of neurons. These priorities force consideration of nanotechnologies as well as CMOS (complementary metal-oxide semiconductor) transistors to achieve ultra-low powered, scaled systems with upwards of a billion neurons. Further efficiencies are afforded by implementing these neural systems in hardware (as opposed to software) and using analog circuits wherever possible. This text focuses on neuromorphic analog circuits, with a brief discussion of nanotechnologies, to achieve the end goals of minimum power and massive scale, much like the human brain.

This text is the result of an evolving course at the University of Southern California on CMOS/Nano Neuromorphic Circuits, taught at the graduate level in the Electrical and Computer Engineering Department and cross-listed with the Biomedical Engineering Department. Many of the course lectures draw on dissertations produced as part of the BioRC Biomimetic Real-time Cortex. While the text contains the material covered in course lectures, it also includes much depth not covered in the course. Students are expected to have undergraduate background in digital circuits, some knowledge of VLSI design and interest in neuroscience, with senior or graduate standing in electrical and computer engineering. Motivated students with biological backgrounds have excelled in the course, where readings from the literature and laboratory circuit simulation exercises comprise major activities in the course.

The text begins chapter 1 with an introduction to human neuroscience necessary for the first six chapters of the text. Chapter 2 summarizes a short history of neuromorphic circuits and presents an extended discussion of the complexities and challenges of building an artificial brain with analog neuromorphic circuits. Chapter 3 contains original material, drawn from class lectures, on the approach to neuromorphic circuits taken from Parker's BioRC project. A review of relevant mathematical models of neural behavior is the topic of chapter 4. Basic neural circuits modeling neurons and synapses connecting neurons are covered in chapters 5, 6, and 8. Chapters 8–14 contain more advanced neuromorphic circuits, much of which is contained in BioRC dissertations. Chapter 15 contains a collection of BioRC approaches to nanotechnologies. Advanced topics are introduced in chapter 16. Large scale digital hardware and software neuromorphic systems are introduced in chapter 17.

BioRC dissertation authors have coauthored chapters drawn from their dissertations. Much of the disseration material was not published in archival journals, so the text provides the opportunity for publication. We are grateful for former PhD students' participation in this book.

Alice C Parker
July 2022
Rancho Palos Verdes, CA

Rick Cattell
July 2022
Tiburon, CA

Acknowledgements

Alice Parker would like to acknowledge funding provided by NSF Grant 0726815 and DARPA Seedling Contract W911NF-18-2-0264 that supported BioRC research described in this text, as well as funding provided by the USC WiSE Women in Science and Engineering program and the Viterbi School of Engineering. Numerous students suffered through drafts of the text when enrolled in EE 582, CMOS/Nano Neuromorphic Circuits or took Directed Research EE 590 at the University of Southern California. Cover and chapter heading artwork were provided by Khushnood Irani. Students assisting with draft versions included Vrit Raval, Deeksha Kiran, Tanaya Banerjee, Wei Zhao, Meera Ramprasad, Chirag Renoji, Jaya Sampath Vayalapalli, Aruna Manjunath and Neeraja Rane. Faculty collaborators included Tansu Celikel, Bartlett Mel, Chongwu Zhou, Han Wang, Francisco Valero-Cuevas, Peter Beerel, and John Choma. Figure assistance was provided by Lisa Huang. Original figures were provided by Evan Clark.

Editor biographies

Alice C Parker

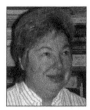

Alice C Parker received the BSEE and PhD degrees from North Carolina State University and an MSEE from Stanford University. Dr Parker is a Professor Emerita and former Dean's Professor of Electrical Engineering at the University of Southern California. She has served the university as Vice Provost for Research and Graduate Studies and Dean of Graduate Studies. She was previously on the faculty at Carnegie Mellon University.

Dr Parker has been involved in digital system synthesis research since 1975. Her current research activities are developing electronic neural circuits using nano-technology models of circuit elements, the preliminary steps necessary to construct a synthetic brain. She and her colleagues produced a synapse containing a carbon nanotube transistor. She was elected a Fellow of the IEEE for her contributions to design automation in the areas of high-level synthesis, hardware description languages and design representation. Dr Parker has been honored with an NSF Faculty Award for Women Scientists and Engineers.

Dr Parker is a winner of a Viterbi teaching award, an award from South Central Scholars in appreciation her work in mentoring talented but underrepresented college-bound scholars in the USC University Park neighborhood, an IEEE-USA Award for Distinguished Literary Contributions and a mentoring award given by ASEE. Other awards include Engineer's Council Distinguished Engineering Educator Award 2021, WiSE Architects of Enduring Change Award 2020, Orange County Engineers Council Distinguished Engineer Award 2018, and NCSU ECE Hall of Fame Award 2017.

R G G 'Rick' Cattell

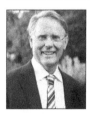

R G G 'Rick' Cattell passed away September 25, 2022. He was most recently an independent consultant in database systems. He previously worked as a Distinguished Engineer at Sun Microsystems, most recently on open source database systems and distributed database scaling. Dr Cattell served for 20+ years at Sun Microsystems in management and senior technical roles, and for 10 years in research at Xerox PARC and at Carnegie Mellon University. Dr Cattell was best known for his contributions in database and server software, including database scalability, enterprise Java, object/relational mapping, object-oriented databases, and database interfaces. He is the author of several dozen papers, five books, and eight U.S. patents. At Sun he instigated the Enterprise Java, Java DB, and Java Blend projects, and was a contributor to a number of Java APIs and products. He previously developed the Cedar DBMS at Xerox PARC, the Sun Simplify database GUI, and SunSoft's

CORBA-database integration. He was a co-founder of SQL Access (a predecessor to ODBC), the founder and chair of the Object Data Management Group (ODMG), the co-creator of JDBC, the author of the world's first book on object/relational and object databases, a recipient of the ACM Outstanding PhD Dissertation Award, and an ACM Fellow.

List of contributors

Rami Alzahrani
Electrical and Computer Engineering, King Abdulaziz University, Saudi Arabia

Rick Cattell
Independent Consultant

Eric Evans
FPGA/ASIC Design Engineer, Boeing Satellite Systems, El Segundo, USA

Dena Giovinazzo
Electrical Engineer, NASA's Jet Propulsion Laboratory, Pasadena, USA

Chih-Chieh Hsu
Senior Engineer in Hardware Technology, Apple,USA

Yilda Irizarry-Valle
Aerospace and Defense Engineer

Jon Joshi
Founder and CEO of Eduvance, Mumbai, India

Rebecca K Lee
Advanced Micro Devices, North Hollywood, USA

Pezhman Mamdouh
Google, California, USA

Jason Mahvash
Senior Technical Program Manager, Amazon Prime Video, California, USA

Michael Boemler-Rudolph Mercury
Director of Applied Engineering, Exploration Institute, Wyoming, USA

Alice C Parker
University of Southern California, Los Angeles, USA

Suraj Chakravarthi Raja
University of Southern California, Los Angeles, USA

Ko-Chung Tseng
ASIC Design Manager, Chigma Technology, Santa Clara, USA

Kun Yue
Nvidia, California, USA

Contributor biographies

Rami A Alzahrani

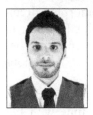

Rami A Alzahrani is an accomplished electrical engineer and academic born in Jeddah, Saudi Arabia. He earned his PhD in Electrical Engineering—Electrophysics and Electronics from the University of Southern California (USC) in 2022. During his time at USC, Dr Alzahrani also worked as a graduate teaching assistant in the electrical and industrial engineering departments, where he taught various advanced courses in electrical and industrial engineering.

Dr Alzahrani's expertise and field of research focused on neuromorphic artificial intelligence (AI) electronic systems and AI-related drone projects. Currently, Dr Alzahrani serves as an assistant professor in the Electrical and Computer Engineering Department and is a member of the ABET and NCAAA accreditation group at King Abdulaziz University in Saudi Arabia.

Eric William Evans

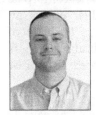

Eric William Evans received a BSCE from California State University Fullerton and an MSEE from the University of Southern California. Eric's graduate research included the development of a transistor-based inhibitory interneuron signal routing network utilizing variable spike frequency axon hillock and spike frequency selective synapse circuits. While at USC, Eric also developed the framework for synaptic communications between the BioRC cortical blank slate neuromorphic circuit and a sub-cortical bioinspired tendon-driven limb system. Eric is currently an FPGA/ASIC design engineer for Boeing Satellite Systems in El Segundo, California.

Dena Giovinazzo

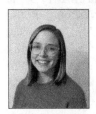

Dena Giovinazzo received her BSEE from the University of California, Santa Cruz and her MSEE from the University of Southern California. She is an Electrical Engineer at NASA's Jet Propulsion Laboratory. Her research interests include analog and mixed signal IC design in radiation environments. Dena won the JPL Discovery award in 2021 for her work on the Nancy Grace Roman Space Telescope's Coronagraph Instrument.

Chih-Chieh Hsu

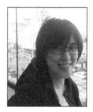

Chih-Chieh Hsu received her PhD in electrical engineering and MS in biomedical engineering from the University of Southern California. Her research and thesis focuses on neuromorphic circuit design and simulation in nanotechnology. As a Senior Engineer in Hardware Technology at Apple, Chih-Chieh is currently responsible for developing neural engine system-on-chip (SoC) solutions that have a tangible impact to the world.

In addition to her work at Apple, Chih-Chieh is a devoted mother of a four-year-old daughter. She balances her busy career with spending quality time with her family and enjoys exploring new places and activities with her daughter. Chih-Chieh is committed to inspiring her daughter to pursue her own passions and interests as she grows up.

Yilda Irizarry-Valle

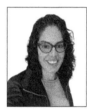

Yilda Irizarry-Valle obtained her PhD in electrical engineering from the University of Southern California, in 2016. She has a bachelor's and a master's degree in electrical engineering from the University of Puerto Rico-Mayaguez. Her doctoral thesis was in neuromorphic engineering, specifically studying glial cells and their effects on neuronal synchrony. She has several publications in the field of neuromorphic engineering that involves mimicking brain behaviors in CMOS VLSI. Prior to her PhD she was awarded the GEM fellowship and interned during two summers at FermiLab, the most prestigious US National Lab in particle physics. During her summer internships she participated on projects that led to research publications with high citations in the field of particle physics.

Yilda Irizarry-Valle currently works for the aerospace and defense Industry. She is a subject matter expert in the fields of model-based systems engineering and digital engineering. Dr Yilda Irizarry-Valle during her free time contributes to support STEM activities through mentoring of engineers. Dr Yilda Irizarry-Valle has won several awards in her studies and career. She was conferred the Viterbi School of Engineering fellowship during her first year at USC, in 2010. Dr Yilda Irizarry-Valle received a best paper award for her publication 'Astrocyte on Neuronal Phase Synchrony in CMOS' at the Network and Systems Applications ISCAS Conference, in 2014. Dr Yilda Irizarry-Valle received a notable distinction as a stellar teaching assistant at USC, in 2015. Dr Yilda Irizarry-Valle was hired by Northrop Grumman to be part of their selective Future Technical Leadership program, in 2016. Dr Yilda Irizarry-Valle received the GEM Alumni Emerging Leadership Award for her contributions in the Aerospace and Defense Industry, in 2019. Dr Yilda Irizarry worked as a Sr Manager and Scientist for L3 Harris between 2020 and 2022. Dr Yilda Irizarry-Valle currently works as an aerospace and defense engineer and supports multiple programs in aerospace and defense.

Jonathan Joshi

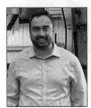

Jonathan Joshi received his BEng from University of Mumbai and MSEE and PhD degrees from the University of Southern California. Dr Joshi is the Founder and CEO of Eduvance, an educational technology and digital capability building company based out of Mumbai. He has over ten years of experience in electronics engineering, education and technology strategy.

He has published several papers in the field of VLSI design and IoT and is the recipient of a conference best paper award. He holds multiple patents in the field of memory systems design, IoT and educational technology. He consults with multiple industry leading companies in the domains of Industry 4.0 and digital capability building.

On the teaching front he is an award winning teaching assistant having won awards during his time in the United States. He is also a visiting faculty at various engineering colleges in India and abroad.

Rebecca K Lee

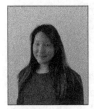

Rebecca K Lee is at Advanced Micro Devices in North Hollywood, CA. Previously she was employed by Northrup Grumman Corporation, and received her PhD in electrical engineering from University of Southern California.

Mohammad Mahvash

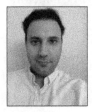

Mohammad Mahvash is Senior Technical Program Manager, Amazon Prime Video, and received his PhD in electrical engineering from University of Southern California.

Pezhman Mamdouh

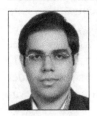

Pezhman Mamdouh received his PhD in electrical engineering from University of Southern California.

Michael Boemler-Rudolph Mercury

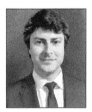

Michael Boemler-Rudolph Mercury holds a Master of Science (2010) and a Bachelor of Science (2008) in astronautical engineering from the University of California. He worked for nine years at NASA's Jet Propulsion Laboratory (JPL) as an imaging spectroscopy systems engineer, advanced concepts systems engineer, study manager, and system analyst/tool developer. He was the lead systems engineer on two winning proposals (MISE, EMIT) which brought in over $100M to the lab. He also spearheaded the detailed design, led trade studies, and formulated the requirements for the Mapping Imaging Spectrometer for Europa (MISE). He received multiple awards at JPL, including the Voyager Award for systems engineering excellence.

He is currently the Director of Applied Engineering at Exploration Institute, where he leads the Advanced Projects Research and Development Group (APRDG). He supports Exploration Institute as a systems engineer and i2i Facilitator, and leads research and development work in neuromorphic algorithms and applications. He is the principal investigator on multiple NASA and DoD contracts developing neuromorphic systems for commercial and government applications including the demonstration of the first online learning using neuomorphic hardware in space.

Suraj Chakravarthi Raja

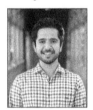

Suraj Chakravarthi Raja is an electrical engineer and neuroroboticist. He received his PhD in electrical engineering—systems, MS in electrical engineering, and MS in computer engineering from the University of Southern California. A native of Chennai, India, Suraj received a bachelor's degree in electronics and communication engineering from SRM University. His doctoral dissertation brought together neuromorphic computing, FPGA acceleration of real-time control algorithms, and sensorimotor neuroscience to enable mammal-like movement in tendon-driven robots. He was the recipient of the 2019 Research Enhancement Fellowship from the USC Graduate School for his work.

Ko-Chung Tseng

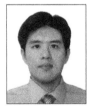

Ko-Chung Tseng is currently an ASIC Design Manager at Chigma Technology where he has been working on DSP circuit and system design. Prior to joining Chigma Technology, he worked for SanDisk and Marvel Storage Group. He received his PhD degree in electrical engineering from USC in 2012. During his PhD coursework, he held a research assistant (RA) position under Professor Alice C Parker at USC BioRC Lab. Meanwhile, he was teaching assistant (TA) in VLSI and ASIC design classes at USC.

He also received two MS degrees in electrical engineering and computer science at USC in 2005 and 2009, respectively. He completed his BS degree in communication engineering from National Chiao Tung University in Taiwan.

His research interests include neuromorphic circuit design, digital circuit design, computational algorithms, memory design, and computer architecture.

Kun Yue

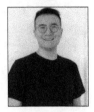

Kun Yue received his PhD in electrical engineering from the University of Southern California. He is employed by Invidia Corporation.

Acronyms

2-AG	2-Arachidonoylglycerol
ACh	Acetylcholine
AER	Address event representation
AMPA	α-amino-3-hydroxy-5-methyl-4-isoxazolepropionic acid receptor
AMPAR	AMPA receptor
AP	Action potential
AIS	Axon initial segment
ASIC	Application-specific integrated circuit
ATP	Adenosine triphosphate
BAC	firing back-propagating AP-activated spike
BEF	Ballistic enhancement factor
BioRC	Biomimetic real-time cortex
BC	Bipolar cell
BO	Border ownership
BSP	Branch strength potentiation
CB1R	Cannabinoid type 1 receptor
CNT	Carbon nanotube
CNTFET	Carbon nanotube field effect transistor
CPU	Central processing unit
CF/CP	Centrifugal/centripetal
CI-AMPAR	Calcium impermeable AMPAR
CS1	Class-1 spikes
CMOS	Complementary metal-oxide semiconductor
CICR	calcium-induced calcium release
CNS	Central nervous system
CP-AMPAR	Calcium permeable AMPAR
CX43	Connexin
cFL	Contralateral maps for the forelimb
cHL	Contralateral maps for the hindlimb
CUBA	Current based
DAP	Depolarization after potential
DSE	Depolarization-induced suppression of excitation
DSGCs	Direction-selective ganglion cells
DS	Direction selectivity
ED	Edge detection
e-SP	Synaptic potentiation through an RGM-mediated pathway
EAAT1 and EAAT2	Excitatory amino acid type 1 & 2
EPSC	Excitatory post-synaptic current
EPSP	Excitatory post-synaptic potential
FPGA	Field programmable gate array
FLOPs	Floating point operations
GABA	Gamma aminobutyric acid
$GABA_A$ and $GABA_B$	GABA receptors
GALS	Globally asynchronous locally synchronous
GC	Ganglion cells
GATs GABA	transporters
Glu	Glutamate

GT	Gliotransmitter
HVA	High-voltage-activated
HICANN	High input count neural network
HH	Hodgkin–Huxley model
HC	Horizontal cell
H chip	Horizontal cell network chip
IAF	Integrate and fire
INT	Integrator spikes
INRC	Intel Neuromorphic research community
IRDS	International Roadmap for Devices and Systems
ITRS	International Technology Roadmap for Semiconductors
iGluRs	Ionotropic glutamatate receptors
IP3	Insositol 1,3,4 triphosphate
IP3R	IP3 receptor
IPSP	Inhibitory post-synaptic potential
L-EPSP	Light-evoked EPSP
LPF	Low pass filter
LTP	Long-term potentiation
LTD	Long-term depression
mAChR	Metabatropic acetylcholine receptor
mESPC	Miniature excitatory post-synaptic currents
mGluR	Metabotropic glutamate receptor
MIX	Mixed mode
MOS	Metal oxide semiconductor
MOSFET	Metal oxide semiconductor field effect transistor
MoS2	Molybdenum diSulfide
nAChR	Nicotinic acetylcholine receptors
NMDA	N-methyl-D-aspartate
NMDAR	NMDA receptor
NMOS	n-channel metal-oxide semiconductor
NOI	Nanotube-on-insulator
NT	Neurotransmitter
OECT	Organic electrochemical transistor
OSC	Subthreshold oscillation
OMS	Object-motion sensitivity
PS-DAP	Phasic spike with depolarization after potential
P chip	Photoreceptor network chip
PDE	Partial differential equation
PS	Phasic spikes
PLC	Phospholipase C
PMOS	p-channel metal-oxide semiconductor
POSD	Post-synaptic differentiation
PRESD	Pre-synaptic differentiation
PEs	Processing unit
PRONON	PROgrammable NeurON
PSP	Postsynaptic potential
RF	Receptive field
RG	Retrograde
RGM	Retrograde messenger
RPG	Random pulse generator

RS	Regular spikes
RS-DAP	Regular spikes with depolarization after potentials
RRP	Relative refractory period
RG	Retrograde
RGM	Retrograde messenger
RW	Random walk
SAC	starburst amacrine cell
SERCA	Sarco-endoplasmic reticulum CA++-ATPase
SIC	Slow inward current
SB	Single burst per stimulus
SNN	Spiking neural network
SNR	Signal-to-noise ratio
SOC	Slow outward current
SoC	System-on-chip
SPAD	Single-photon avalanche diode
SRAM	Statice random access memory
STDP	Synaptic timing-dependent plasticity
STP	Short-term potentiation
TB	Tonic bursts
TRP/TRPL	Transient receptor potential-like channel
TMD	Transition metal dichalcogenide
TMDFET	Transition metal dichalcogenide FET
VLSI	Very large scale integration

IOP Publishing

Neuromorphic Circuits
A constructive approach
Alice C Parker and Rick Cattell

Chapter 1

Introduction

**Alice C Parker, Rick Cattell, Rami Alzahrani, Chih-Chieh Hsu,
Yilda Irizarry-Valle, Jon Joshi, Rebecca Lee, Pezhman Mamdouh,
Jason Mahvash and Ko-Chung Tseng**

This text covers analog circuits modeling brain neurons, analog *neuromorphic* circuits. The first chapter introduces basic neuroscience and highlights the complexities of the biological brain, setting the stage for the chapter that follows, which begins the coverage of neuromorphic circuits. This first chapter introduces neurons and other brain cells, beginning with the axon initial segment, the spiking circuit. The chapter continues with the synapse and neural dendrites. Variable neural behavior is introduced, and astrocytes, another brain cell, are presented. The retina of the eye, considered part of the brain, is discussed in chapter 1, and the neural code, the information presented in the spiking and bursting patterns of the brain, is also introduced.

1.1 Introduction to neurons and to the brain

Understanding the brain is an ongoing, daunting task. Modeling the brain with electronic circuits relies on this ever-evolving knowledge and is itself a challenging task, with researchers implementing multiple approaches. It is not even clear the level of detail of neuroscience knowledge which must be incorporated to produce human-brain-like behavior.

Parker's and Cattell's favorite poem[1] describing brain research is the following:

> **THE BLIND MEN AND THE ELEPHANT**
> A HINDOO(*sic*) FABLE

---

[1] From *The poems of John Godfrey Saxe*, 1872, by John Godfrey Saxe. The poem is reprinted here exactly as published in 1872 based on a parable. Early versions of this parable date to 500 BC. Information from Wikipedia https://en.wikipedia.org/wiki/Blind_men_and_an_elephant

doi:10.1088/978-0-7503-5097-6ch1

I.

IT was six men of Indostan
To learning much inclined,
Who went to see the Elephant
(Though all of them were blind),
That each by observation
Might satisfy his mind.

II.

The First approached the Elephant,
And happening to fall
Against his broad and sturdy side,
At once began to bawl:
'God bless me!—but the Elephant
Is very like a wall!'

III.

The Second, feeling of the tusk,
Cried: 'Ho!—what have we here
So very round and smooth and sharp?
To me 't is mighty clear
This wonder of an Elephant
Is very like a spear!'

IV.

The Third approached the animal,
And happening to take
The squirming trunk within his hands,
Thus boldly up and spake:
"I see," quoth he, "the Elephant
Is very like a snake!"

V.

The Fourth reached out his eager hand,
And felt about the knee.
"What most this wondrous beast is like
Is mighty plain," quoth he;
"'T is clear enough the Elephant
Is very like a tree!"

VI.

The Fifth, who chanced to touch the ear,
Said: "E'en the blindest man

Can tell what this resembles most;
Deny the fact who can,
This marvel of an Elephant
Is very like a fan!"

VII.

The Sixth no sooner had begun
About the beast to grope,
Than, seizing on the swinging tail
That fell within his scope,
"I see," quoth he, "the Elephant
Is very like a rope!"

VIII.

And so these men of Indostan
Disputed loud and long,
Each in his own opinion
Exceeding stiff and strong,
Though each was partly in the right,
And all were in the wrong!

MORAL.

So, oft in theologic wars
The disputants, I ween,
Rail on in utter ignorance
Of what each other mean,
And prate about an Elephant
Not one of them has seen!

We think we are all like metaphorical blind men, trying to understand the elephant. Everything we write here about the brain is limited, is not quite true, is not exact, and what is true is understood better each passing day. The brain is indeed like a computer, but thoughts and memory are intertwined, unlike the traditional compute engine. Moreover, the brain consumes only a few watts of power, unlike modern deep-learning systems. Finally, the brain learns incrementally, bottom-up, not by top-down training all at one time[2]. These thoughts drive our book about neuromorphic circuits. Neuromorphic analog electronics capture size and low-power goals, as well as mix processing and memory, and hence are the substrate on which our neuromorphic text rests.

---

[2] By bottom-up we mean that individual synapses and small numbers of synapses are strengthened in a single learning step. In top-down learning, the entire neural network is strengthened/weakened in a single step.

We write this textbook not to communicate facts but to describe approaches and encourage further investigation. The text assumes an electrical engineering background with some knowledge of digital electronics and basic digital architecture. Analog circuit design is helpful but not a requirement for reading and understanding the text.

Interest in the brain, and in neuromorphic circuits, electronic circuits that model the brain, has increased dramatically in the last two decades. Much like the interest in outer space in the last half of the twentieth century, the brain is now the final frontier. Modeling the brain and neurons in the brain with electronics is massively difficult, and progress historically had been slow. Neuroscience, the science of the brain and neurons is exploding[3]. While there were several waves of interest that foretold the final emergence of artificial intelligence as a useful tool for solving practical problems like face recognition, voice recognition, speech recognition and human identification, there had been fewer waves of interest in artificial neuron hardware apart from the interest in artificial neural networks that began with a coarse, simplified model of biological neurons and the biological brain. Now, however, new technologies, new circuits and new architectures have been fused into structures that are increasingly brain-like, more neuromorphic. The latest Mercedes-Benz concept car, the Vision EQXX, uses a neuromorphic chip from California-based artificial-intelligence developer *BrainChip* to create systems based on the company's *Akida* hardware and software, for example.

The focus of this text is analog circuits modeling brain neurons, in contrast to computer models that simulate neural behavior using conventional (or at least digital) multiprocessors. Autonomous vehicle navigation, identity determination, robotic manufacturing, and medical diagnostics are all engineering challenges that can benefit from technological solutions with specialized analog neuromorphic hardware replacing software simulations or digital hardware. A further motivation for creating artificial brain structures is neural prostheses, integrated circuits and systems that connect to the human brain to enhance or repair it. While other challenging engineering problems are being solved to interface biological and artificial neurons, understanding the technological requirements and possibilities for isolated artificial brain structures could accelerate the hope that such prostheses could become a reality. Analog circuits offer the promise of scalability and low power, partly due to the efficiency of analog computation. More discussion of the utility of analog circuits is found in chapter 3.

Before the text begins its detailed coverage of analog neural electronics, there is discussion in chapter 2 of why electronic models of the brain (and the neurons that make up the brain) are complex and require an entire text. In order to motivate this discussion, the present chapter will begin by presenting a very small window into the structure and behavior of biological neurons, and into the structure and function of the brain, the anatomy and physiology, as it were. We should note that everything we say about biological neurons in general is contradicted somewhere in some

---

[3] It is possible that progress in neuromorphic systems was delayed in the past due to science and technology not being sufficiently developed to provide a basis on which to build artificial brains.

studies, and/or in some species. Not all neurons have the same anatomy and physiology. Our brief diversion into biology is intended to present a summary of what is presently understood in general about the biological neuron, and that knowledge is growing and changing daily.

Each section of this chapter covers aspects of neuroscience that are relevant to some of the following chapters describing neuromorphic circuits, and will reference those chapters. Each subsequent neuroscience section in this chapter is designed to be read before, and in conjunction with the neuromorphic chapters referred to in the neuroscience section.

This text focuses on circuits modeling the neurons in the human cerebral cortex, although the structures modeled could be modified easily to model other animals' neurons, and peripheral as well as central neurons. There are about 100 billion neurons (single-cell structures) in the human brain (which includes the retina), along with various *glial* (glue) cells that support the neurons as well as provide supplementary processing. The astrocyte, a type of star-shaped glial cell, appears to be the main glial cell that processes information. Neurons connect with each other primarily as if they were arcs in a directed graph, as shown in figure 1.8, although other connections between neurons can occur[4]. Specialized structures called *synapses* connect the neurons to each other. In the cortex, where much learning and reasoning occurs, each neuron is connected to up to 100 000 synapses (inputs), and the *axons* (output) each connect to up to 10 000 more neurons through synapses. Neurons signal each other with small voltage spikes (about 100 mV) while the voltages interior to the neural cells (generally called the membrane potentials) are lower, and sometimes negative, especially when the neuron is quiescent (not spiking). Astrocytes connect with each other and with neurons in several different ways that will be discussed later in the text, first in section 1.7 and later in chapter 13.

This text covers circuits modeling the *central nervous system* (CNS), the brain and the spinal cord. Neurons outside the CNS, in the body, are *peripheral neurons*, and form the peripheral nervous system (PNS). Peripheral neurons can be further classified into *sensory neurons* that respond to outside stimulation like touch and *motor neurons* that send signals to muscles from the CNS. *Afferent neurons* convey information to the CNS. *Efferent neurons* convey information from the CNS to the body. This text focuses on cortical neuron emulation, specifically the *pyramidal neurons* in the *cerebral cortex* for two reasons. First, the cortex (including the hippocampus) is the primary brain region where cognitive tasks[5], such as information processing, learning and memory formation, occur[6]. Second, pyramidal neurons, one of the well-studied types of principal neurons in the cortex, have unique dendritic structures and elaborate dendritic properties including nonlinear integration, spiking behavior and *plasticity* that are believed to be essential for

---

[4] In particular, gap junctions connect neuron cell bodies (somas), axons and dendrites to similar structures in other neurons.

[5] Cognitive processing refers to the brain's ability to process, store and take action on information.

[6] Very little study has involved neuromorphic neurons modeling hippocampal neurons, unfortunately, since the hippocampus involves memory.

neural information processing and learning. Even though pyramidal neurons in different cortical layers are not exactly identical, they share similar fundamental mechanisms in the dendritic domain such as synaptic integration, and excitability, as well as *plasticity* [1]. Synaptic integration can involve superlinear addition of postsynaptic potentials that are very close together. Neurons can spike with single spikes or *bursts* with clusters of spikes, with rates determined by patterns of synaptic inputs. Plasticity refers to change of neuronal physiology (behavior) and/or anatomy (structure) in response to events: strengthening or weakening responses, and making connections or breaking connections. More details about nonlinearity, spiking and plasticity are given later in this section and later in the chapter.

The cerebral cortex contains a wrinkled surface of neurons that is six neurons deep, and covers connections (called white matter). It is actually separated into right and left portions joined by specialized white matter called the *corpus callosum*. The cortex not only performs reasoning but processes sensory information from the eyes and ears, and performs movement planning, and sends movement information to the muscles.

There can be multiple synapses connected to a neuron and dendrites connecting these synapses within a neuron, but usually only one axon. Ions like sodium, calcium, potassium and chloride contribute to the electrical transmission in neurons because they are charged particles. Ion flow into or out of neurons is through *ion channels* that are voltage or *ligand* (chemically) gated, meaning that they open either when the surrounding cell voltage is high enough, or when a ligand is present near enough to the channel to attach to *receptors* that open the channel, as shown in figure 1.1. Chemicals called *neurotransmitters* are used to signal between neurons at synapses.

A sketch of a synapse is shown in figure 1.2. Here. the axon ends in a terminal, and the synapse spans the gap between the axon and the postsynaptic neuron. The spike potential causes calcium channels to open and calcium ions to flow into the axonal terminal in the dendritic spine. This causes vesicles to form, capture

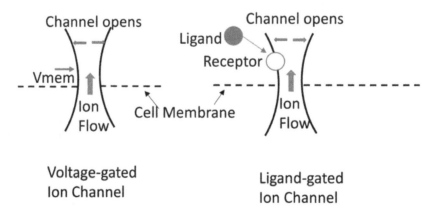

Figure 1.1. Voltage-gated and ligand-gated ion channels in neurons. Cell interiors are above cell exteriors in the figure.

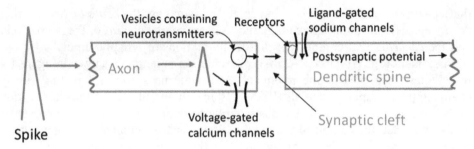

Figure 1.2. Sketch of a synapse showing ion channels.

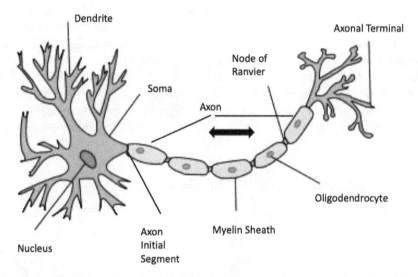

Figure 1.3. A neuron cartoon with basic structures. This File:Neuron Hand-tuned.svg image has been obtained by the authors from the Wikimedia website where it was made available under a CC BY-SA 3.0 licence. https://creativecommons.org/licenses/by-sa/3.0/deed.en. It is included within this book on that basis. It is attributed to Quasar Jarosz.

neurotransmitters (NTs), and move to the terminal membrane, where they open. NTs move across the synapse in the synaptic cleft and attaches to receptors in the postsynaptic neuron. These receptors open ligand-gated sodium channels, and the potential inside the postsynaptic neuron rises.

Figure 1.3 shows a single neuron, with *soma* (cell body), *axon* (the fibers carrying the output signal, and the *axon initial segment* where spikes to other neurons are thought to originate[7]. The figure shows the *oligodendrocytes* (another *glial* cell type)

---

[7] With advances in measurement techniques,it is currently believed that spikes primarily originate in the *Axon Initial Segment* (AIS), downstream from where the axon originates in the *axon hillock*, although spikes could originate as far downstream as the *nodes of Ranvier*, according to other sources. For the purposes of this text, we will assume that the axon hillock and axon initial segment are connected, and electronic circuits model the region where they both are found. Not shown in this figure are the synapses connecting to other neurons.

that enwrap the axon to insulate and speed the signaling, the *nodes of Ranvier* that act as repeaters to restore spike magnitude and shape, the *nucleus* of the neuron cell, and the *dendrites* that compute nonlinear summations of synaptic inputs.

First, fast, large (100 mV, 1–2 ms) spikes (action potentials), shown in figure 1.4 travel down the presynaptic axon and arrive at the synapses, creating slowly changing postsynaptic potentials (PSPs) <10 mV in amplitude, >10 ms in duration in the postsynaptic neuron. These postsynaptic potentials are combined in nonlinear ways, and when the combined potential (voltage) is large enough, or rising rapidly enough, the neuron emits a voltage spike at the *axon initial segment* that travels down the axon to the next neurons connected through synapses, and stimulates the attached synapses. The starting voltage for the beginning of the action potential is the *resting potential.* Voltage inside the neuron rises steadily until it reaches a threshold. When it reaches threshold, there is a positive spike that rises very quickly and then it falls, in this case, to less than resting potential with *hyperpolarization,* or *undershoot* (in electronic terms) when the spike falls.

A more-detailed cartoon of a pyramidal neuron is shown in figure 1.5. In this figure, the *dendritic arbor* is shown and labeled as *apical* (like tree branches), and other dendrites are labeled as *basal,* that are near the soma (like tree roots). Apical dendrites typically have less impact on neural spiking than basal dendrites for an

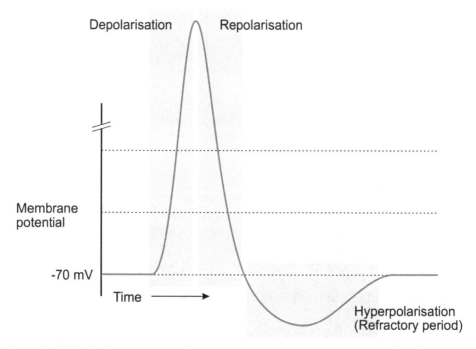

Figure 1.4. Schematic of an action potential, including depolarization, repolarization, and hyperpolarization phases. This File:Action potential schematic.svg has been obtained by the authors from the Wikimedia website https://commons.wikimedia.org/wiki/File:Action_potential_schematic.svg, where it is stated to have been released into the public domain. It is included within this book on that basis.

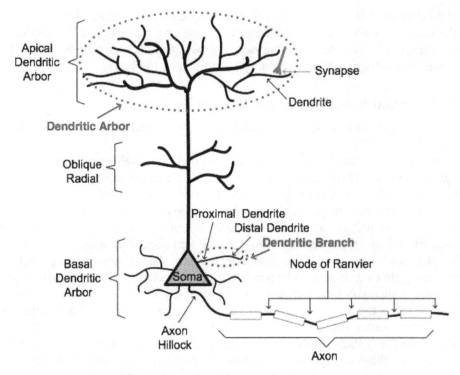

Figure 1.5. Details of a pyramidal neuron. The axon hillock shown is just upstream from the axon initial segment (not shown), the site of spike origination. Reproduced from [2].

equivalent synaptic strength. Along the dendritic trunk, *oblique radial* dendrites are shown. A *dendritic branch* is shown, with *proximal* (near) and *distal* dendritic locations noted. The *axon* that stretches from the soma to downstream (postsynaptic) neurons completes the sketch. *Nodes of Ranvier* along the axon refresh the spike signal, acting as repeaters. *Tufts*, not shown, are clusters of dendritic branches, usually in the apical dendritic arbor.

Synaptic plasticity refers to the changing strengths of synapses, manifest in either the presynptic or postsynaptic side, or both. *Structural plasticity* refers to the ability of the nervous system to add or delete synapses, connecting/disconnecting neurons from each other, and in some cases awaken dormant synapses of postsynaptic neurons, called *silent synapses*. Dendrites can also change their ability to transmit signals, another form of plasticity. *Intrinsic plasticity* is the modification of a neuron's electrical properties by changes in the properties of its ion channels. Intrinsic plasticity can affect how inputs from synapses are integrated, how signals within the neuron propagate in all directions, how spikes are generated, and how synaptic plasticity is modulated (*meta-plasticity*). This text does not cover details of neuromorphic circuits implementing intrinsic plasticity, leaving it open for future investigations[8].

---

[8] Scholarpedia contains discussion of intrinsic plasticity and meta-plasticity.

This chapter continues with sections providing more neuroscience information. In order to organize the neuroscience coverage in the text, it is grouped into sections in this chapter. The remainder of the neuroscience sections can be read just before reading each corresponding neuromorphic chapter in the book.

1.2 The axon initial segment—the spiking circuit

This section supports the material found in chapter 5, and should be read prior to reading that chapter.

Neurons 'fire' when they send an electrical signal to a neighboring neuron. A flow diagram shows the sequence of events that occurs when a neuron spikes (figure 1.6). The location of onset of firing is believed to be the *Axon Initial Segment* although traditionally the spike origination was believed to be the nearby *axon hillock*[9]. Spikes can vary enormously in patterns and frequencies, but less so in amplitude. Spikes are caused by sodium ions entering the neural cell, and potassium ions exiting the cell. The presence of calcium ions can affect spike shapes and spiking patterns. Neuromorphic circuits related to spiking are introduced in chapter 5. Much more detail about the axon initial segment is given in section 1.9.

Figure 1.7 shows how the spiking of a neuron occurs. Sodium Na^+ and potassium K^+ ion flows cause a voltage spike to occur. When the voltage inside (intracellular) is higher than the voltage outside (extracellular) the difference is positive; the difference between these voltages is also called the *membrane potential*. The membrane potential either reaches a threshold voltage that causes a spike or the rate of increase

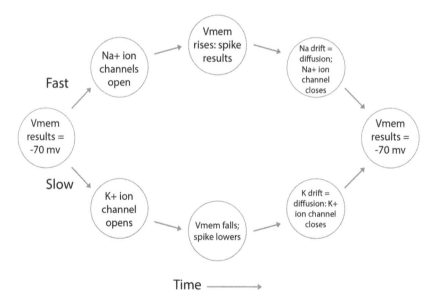

Figure 1.6. Flow diagram illustrating the spiking sequence in the neuron.

<hr />

[9] Earlier BioRC research referred to the spiking circuit as the axon hillock.

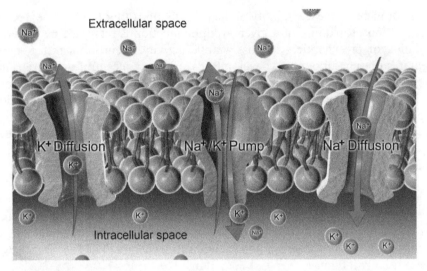

Figure 1.7. How the spiking of a neuron occurs. Reproduced from [4]. CC BY 3.0.

of the voltage is sufficient to cause a spike. The voltage causes the sodium and potassium channels to open and the ions to diffuse through the channels depending on their relative concentrations inside and outside the neuron. Sodium diffuses into the neuron, raising the membrane potential, and potassium diffuses out of the neuron. Since the potassium ions are larger, the flow out is slower, so the membrane potential rises due to the sodium influx and subsequently falls due to the potassium outflux. Molecular structures called *pumps* move the ions back to their original locations, preserving *homeostasis*, or steady state, a stable equilibrium of physiological processes. *Hyperpolarization*, or undershoot, is caused by the potassium ion channels moving more charge out of the neuron at some point than the sodium channels move in. The ion pumps restore the *resting potential* of the cell (usually slightly negative) by moving charges back to their resting balance. An input spike arriving from a presynaptic (sending) neuron travels down the axon to the synapse of the presynaptic neuron. At this point, usually there is a chemical, a neurotransmitter, that will be emitted from the presynaptic (sending) side and move from the presynaptic to the postsynaptic (receiving) neuron. This will cause a voltage rise (the membrane potential) inside the receiving neuron. Voltage responses of the synapses impinging on the postsynaptic neuron are combined nonlinearly. When the membrane potential reaches a threshold, the neuron generates another spike that travels to the next synapse. The detailed operation of the synapse is described in the next section.

1.3 The synapse

This section supports the material found in chapter 6, and should be read prior to reading that chapter.

The biological synapse is complex, with controllable *neurotransmitters* (sometimes called transmitters in the neuroscience literature) which are chemicals that can decrease or increase the excitability of the postsynaptic (after the synapse) receptors. The activation probability of a given synaptic junction is regulated by the amount and timing of presynaptic and postsynaptic activity. Neurotransmitters must be present in sufficient amounts to develop PSPs, and the concentration of transmitters released can affect the height and duration of the PSP, a voltage in the neural cell body [4]. Action potentials impinging on the same synaptic cleft (the space between the presynaptic neuron and the postsynaptic neuron) can result in *temporal summation* (summing over time) of the resulting PSPs, increasing the likelihood of the postsynaptic neuron eventually firing, and one or more spikes traveling to another neuron.

In the human cortex, there are about 80% *excitatory* synapses (with a positive voltage response) and 20% *inhibitory* synapses (with a negative voltage response). Excitatory synapses contribute to neuron potential for firing. Inhibitory synapses either lower the probability of firing or veto the possibility of firing. Simpler neurons that control the flow of information between neurons are called *interneurons*, and they are usually inhibitory.

Inhibitory synapses play an important role in neuronal behavior. For example, the local inhibitory *interneuron* circuit controls the development of the columnar architecture during a critical period in the primary visual cortex [5]. There are two types of inhibition: *hyperpolarizing* inhibition and *shunting* inhibition. The former generates a hyperpolarizing (negative, opposite to depolarizing or positive) potential, or in other words, adds a relatively negative potential to the resting potential. The latter type of inhibition, shunting, vetoes any upstream excitatory synapses, but has no effect on downstream excitatory synapses. Further demonstrations of these two types of inhibition in neuromorphic circuits are discussed in chapters 1, 3 and 7.

The synaptic cleft (part of the synapse) is the *interstitial* space between the presynaptic (sending) neuron and the postsynaptic (receiving) neuron. *Neurotransmitters*, the chemicals signaling between neurons, are sent between neurons through the synaptic cleft. Neurotransmitters fall into several categories:

- Excitatory neurotransmitters like glutamate, aspartate and serotonin that raise the internal voltage of a neuron,
- Inhibitory neurotransmitters like GABA, glycine and serotonin that lower the internal voltage of a neuron, and
- Modulatory neurotransmitters like dopamine, acetylcholine, and serotonin that act to raise or lower probabilities of firing in a more subtle way.

Synaptic *vesicles* contain neurotransmitters. When an action potential arrives at the presynaptic *axon terminal* of the synapse, the positive voltage (potential) opens voltage-gated calcium channels in the presynaptic neuron's axonal terminal. Positive calcium ions flowing into the axon terminal keep the vesicles near the membrane at the synapse, and neurotransmitter transporters carry the neurotransmitters to the synapse cleft, the space between the presynaptic and postsynaptic neurons. Receptors on the postsynaptic side of the synapse attach to the neurotransmitters, and open ion channels that bring in charged ions into the postsynaptic density of the synapse on the dendritic spine. G proteins in the axon terminal can also travel through the cleft and bind to receptors (acting as a secondary messenger).

Positive ions flow when the synapse is *excitatory*, causing an excitatory post-synaptic potential, *EPSP*, *depolarizing* the postsynaptic density and negative ions flow when the synapse is *inhibitory*, *hyperpolarizing* the potential, causing an *IPSP* (inhibitory postsynaptic potential). Inhibitory synapses can *shunt* the potential back to the *resting potential*, essentially preventing the postsynaptic neuron from firing if the synapse is in an appropriate place close to the axon hillock or axon initial segment. Thus inhibitory synapses can block excitatory synapses from having an effect on the postsynaptic neuron. Inhibitory synapses can *mutually inhibit* neurons from firing, so that the stronger neuron of the neurons firing inhibits the weaker neuron. This mechanism is shown in figure 1.8. Inhibitory neurons also can select pathways, acting as a gating function on neural transmission.

As this chapter has presented, figure 1.9 [6] shows a cartoon of a typical neural synapse. The sending neuron is yellow and the receiving neuron is green. At the synapse, when a spike arrives on the presynaptic side, voltage-gated calcium channels open on the presynaptic side bringing in Ca^{2+}. Calcium causes vesicles to move to the cell wall and to open, releasing neurotransmitters. The neuro-tranmitters attach to receptors on the surface of the receiving neuron, causing the pink ion channels (ligand-gated ion channels) to open, and positive or negative ions

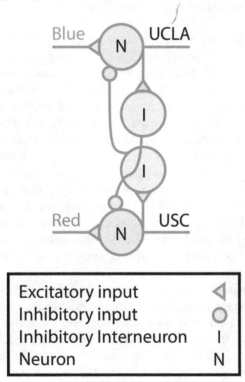

Figure 1.8. Mutual inhibition between neurons. If a strong blue input is presented and a weak red, the UCLA neuron fires, for example.

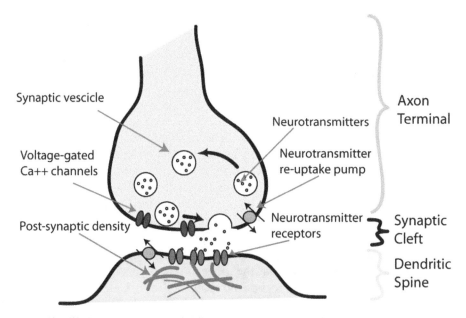

Figure 1.9. Simplified synapse cartoon. This File:Synapse Illustration unlabeled.svg image has been obtained by the authors from the Wikimedia website where it was made available under a CC BY-SA 3.0 licence. It is included within this book on that basis. It is attributed to Looie496.

to rush in, raising or lowering the voltage inside the receiving cell. This PSP is summed nonlinearly with other PSPs from other synapses on the same postsynaptic neuron. If the potential is high enough or rises quickly enough, output action potentials (spikes) are formed in the postsynaptic neuron's AIS (axon initial segment) that can back-propagate passively to its dendrites and synapses. Action potentials primarily travel down the axon to stimulate other neurons.

The biological inhibitory synapse has a complex structure [4, 7]. Inhibitory synapses can also be shunting, effectively vetoing depolarization caused by excitatory postsynaptic potentials, or hyperpolarizing, subtracting potential from the dendrite. The modulation of quantity of neurotransmitters released at the presynaptic terminal affects the actions of the receptors on the postsynaptic side that control ligand-gated ion channels, resulting in a variation in hyperpolarizing potentials across the cell membrane. The rate that neurotransmitters are reuptaken into the presynaptic terminal also affects synaptic behavior by controlling the decrease in postsynaptic potential.

Synapses vary their strengths (plasticity) with learning. Changes in synaptic strength are also thought to underlie learning and storage of new memories. Sleep can up-regulate strong synapses and down-regulate weak ones. A short article on sleep and the brain can be found in [8] and a much longer article is in [9]. A synapse can strengthen its *presynaptic* side (the sending neuron) through *facilitation* or its *postsynaptic* side through *potentiation*. Facilitation adds neurotransmitters to the presynaptic side, and potentiation adds receptors or more positive ions to increase the membrane potential to the postsynaptic side. Synapses can also be weakened through lowering neurotransmitters, receptors or membrane potential to either side of the synapse. Plasticity can be short term, lasting tens of milliseconds to a fraction of a minute, or long term, lasting minutes to hours.

postsynaptic changes include strengthening the synaptic response (*long-term potentiation (LTP)*) a form of strengthening possibly due to a *burst* stimulus of spikes (that could be caused by *dendritic spiking*[10]) in the presynaptic (sending) neuron, called *burst potentiation*, opening NMDA channels (section 1.3.2) and introducing CA ions to increase the membrane potential, enlarging the post side of the synapse or the dendritic spine, making the synapse stronger with more receptors, and *spike-timing dependent plasticity* (STDP) [10–12]. Thus, a strong presynaptic spiking with a cluster of spikes (a burst of spikes) can cause significant strengthening of the postsynaptic neuron, resulting in burst potentiation.

With STDP, a synapse is strengthened (long-term potentiation *LTP*) when the presynaptic action potential at a particular synapse precedes the postsynaptic action potential (the output of the neuron containing the synapse). A synapse is weakened (*LTD*) when the postsynaptic action potential precedes the presynaptic action potential. Thus, neurons modify their synaptic connections to adapt to changes in sensory input. The ability of many neurons to modulate the strengths of their synaptic connections has been shown to depend on the relative timing of pre- and postsynaptic action potentials (APs). STDP has become an attractive model for learning at the single-cell level [10]. The temporal order of presynaptic and postsynaptic firing is a critically important aspect of STDP. The synapse is thought to be strengthened by APs back-propagating along the dendrites along with depolarization caused by a previous AP impinging on a synapse. With the back-propagation absent, the previous AP weakens the future synaptic response.

Weakening the synaptic response (*long-term depression, LTD*) also can be due to strong stimulation or persistent weak stimulation. Synapses can also depress their responses (called a *depressing synapse*) in the face of repeated rapid stimulation. Figure 1.10 shows the response of a depressing synapse.

Some synapses are called *silent synapses* because they do not respond to presynaptic release of neurotransmitters. These synapses either have ineffective AMPA channels or the AMPA channels are missing. NMDA channels are present, and when activated by rising potentials and chemical signals due to other activity, AMPA channels form or awaken, and the synapses become active. Sometimes neurotransmitters are present in the synapse, but receptors in the postsynaptic side of the synapse are missing or encapsulated in vesicles. When the synapse is awakened, vesicles containing receptors move to the membrane and AMPA ion channels open when transmitters arrive. AMPA and NMDA channels are described more in section 1.3.2. Kandel [14] found that *silent synapses* could be awakened by proteins that result from DNA expression of RNA that synthesizes proteins. The proteins travel to the silent synapse and act somewhat like prions, self-duplicating to maintain synaptic strength.

---

[10] Introduced later in this chapter.

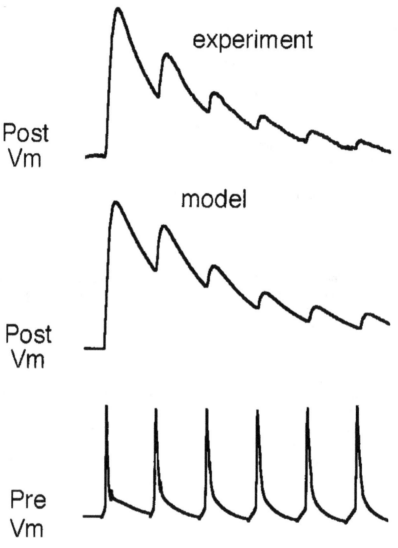

Figure 1.10. The response of a depressing synapse to repeated stimulation, taken from part of figure 1 in [13], copyright 1997, National Academy of Sciences, USA. The mathematical model and experimental postsynaptic EPSPs are shown, along with the experimental presynptic spikes.

1.3.1 Electrical synapses

Electrical synapses are reciprocal pathways for ionic current and small organic molecules [15]. They allow the adjacent neurons to have direct communication between their diffused membranes through channels called *gap junctions*. Electrical synapses allow faster synaptic transmission for APs compared to chemical synapses; they also help to synchronize entire groups of neurons. Electrical synapses are now being intensively examined in mammals [15].

1.3.2 AMPA and NMDA channels and receptors

Two major ion channels in the brain, both opened to the flow of positive ions with the neurotransmitter *glutamate* (also called a ligand), are the *AMPA* channel and the N-methyl-D-aspartate *NMDA* channel. The receptors for glutamate that open the channels are called *AMPAR* and *NMDAR*. AMPA channels form when enough receptors are present and open when enough glutamate is present. NMDA channels are more complex; they open when glutamate is present and the membrane potential (voltage inside the neuron) is high enough to remove a magnesium ion block that prevents the channel from opening. AMPA channels primarily support the flow of sodium and potassium ions; NMDA channels also support the flow of calcium ions that are involved in strengthening connections between neurons, hence learning. Hebbian learning involves strengthening synapses when voltage rise at the synapse of a presynaptic neuron causes the postsynaptic neuron of that synapse to fire. It is often said that neurons that fire together, wire together. NMDA channels can be seen as coincidence detectors, an important function demonstrated about 30 years ago [11] that has a key role in LTP and LTD, as well as in other cognitive functions through which they exhibit the Hebbian nature of synaptic plasticity [4]. The receptor is composed of three main subunits: GluN1, GluN2, and GluN3. For the complete activation of the NMDAR, each subunit needs to be bound by transmitters. Glutamate transmitters bind the GluN2 subunit, while either glycine or D-serine binds GluN1 and GluN3 subunits.

Synaptic plasticity is enabled by the ability of neurons to sense information from both presynaptic and postsynaptic sides of the synapse. NMDA channels are able to sense activity from both sides through a series of cascade events. Initially, the NMDA channel at the postsynaptic membrane is unable to open, even when glutamate release from the presynaptic synapse debinds the receptor, due to its inherent magnesium block that opposes the influx of sodium and Ca^{2+} ions into the cell. The magnesium block can be expelled from the NMDA channel if there is enough depolarization at the postsynaptic membrane. This depolarization can be achieved through AMPA (amino-3-hydroxy-5- methyl-4-isoxazolepropionic) channels. The AMPA channel (possibly at other synapses) is able to open upon sensing a considerable level of glutamate. Activation of AMPAR allows sodium ions to rush into the postsynaptic cell, causing temporal summation of EPSPs to depolarize the membrane, so that the magnesium block is removed from the NMDA channel by a process known as electrostatic repulsion. The coincidence-detection nature of the NMDA channel is the result of two simultaneous events, the presynaptic release of transmitters binding the receptor and the postsynaptic depolarization by EPSPs.

This concludes the basic material found in chapter 1 and the reader can continue reading chapters 2–6, returning to section 1.4 before reading further chapters.

1.4 Dendritic computation

Dendritic computation refers to the computation as a neuron processes its inputs' spatio-temporal information, depending on *where* the synapses are formed and *when* the synapses are activated in the dendrites[11]. Over the past two to three decades, neurobiologists and neuroscientists have devoted intense effort to explore how dendritic computations affect the learning process in mammals. They have found that dendrites, as part of a neuron, are not merely responsible for transporting the synaptic inputs from the generation sites to the soma and axon where the neuronal output AP is initiated. Indeed, there are complex nonlinear computations taking place in the dendrites, such as location-dependent integration, and dendrites transmit strong sometimes regenerative signals that are known as *dendritic spikes*.

Dendrites in the pyramidal neurons are complex computational units that combine synaptic potentials, often in nonlinear ways. Dendrites' electrical properties such as membrane potential amplitude, potential half-width, rise time, propagation strength, and excitability change with their physiological properties such as the thickness of the dendrites, the location of the dendrites (proximal/distal[12]), (basal/apical[13]), and the ion channel density in the dendrites [16–18]. Therefore one challenge to modeling neurons is the complexity of the individual neuron, including location-dependent and spatio-temporal dendritic computation, dendritic spike mechanisms, and dendritic plasticity. For example, Sjöström and Häusser found that unsuccessful back-propagating action potential (bAP) invasion into the distal dendritic branches in neocortical pyramidal neurons results in LTP in the proximal synapses but LTD in the distal synapses [19]. Thus synaptic plasticity not only depends on pre/postsynaptic neuronal activity but also depends on the synapse locations in the dendrite and the excitability of the dendrite.

Experiments on the basal dendrites in pyramidal rat neurons show that the recorded somatic response varies with the stimulation location and the stimulation strength [20], as shown in figure 1.11. The findings also support a two-layer model, such that each thin dendritic branch acts as the first-layer sigmoidal subunit (each synaptic output is summed with nearby synaptic outputs and the sum takes the form of a sigmoid) and the soma acts as the second-layer summation unit [21]. The interaction between excitation and inhibition is also highly nonlinear and asymmetric. Studies have shown that the location of the inhibitory synaptic input is a critical factor for signal integration. Where a synapse is activated is a key factor in dendritic computations, particularly for inhibitory synapses. The shunting inhibitory synapse only vetoes its upstream (further from the soma on the same branch) excitatory synapses, as shown in figure 1.12. Multiple dendritic inputs on thin dendritic branches tend to saturate the voltage response.

1.4.1 Dendritic spikes

As the text mentioned earlier, dendrites are not simply funnels; their active[14] properties enrich the computational capacity within an individual neuron.

---

[11] This section supports the neuroscience material found in chapters 7 and 8, and should be read prior to reading those chapters.

[12] Near/far.

[13] Where the synapses are clustered with respect to the soma.

[14] Active denotes mechanisms that result in superlinear mechanisms. In this case, PSPs result in *dendritic spikes*.

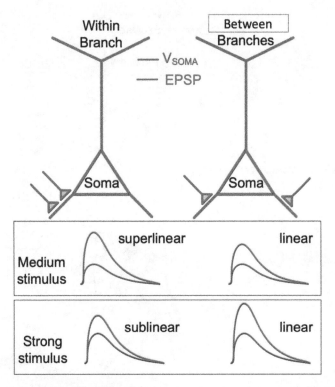

Figure 1.11. Nonlinear summation in the pyramidal neuron's basal dendrites. Nonlinear summation depends on input location and strength in the thin basal dendrites. Medium synaptic inputs on the same dendritic branch tend to sum superlinearly (left) while those on different branches sum linearly (right). Strong synaptic inputs on the same dendritic branch, on the other hand, sum sublinearly. The blue trace is the unitary EPSP and the red trace is the resultant somatic potential. Note that excitatory synapses are indicated as triangles. Figure adapted from Polsky *et al* [20], copyright (2004), with permission from Springer Nature.

Dendritic spikes are a result of the nonlinear amplification of spatio-temporally clustered synaptic inputs, and hence these local dendritic spikes can be viewed as input-feature detectors. Many studies have shown that active conductances in dendrites can amplify the PSP and evoke a local dendritic spike that propagates more effectively than PSP alone [18, 23]. *Ariavet al* [24] shows that active dendritic spiking enriches the computational capacity within individual neurons, such as precise signal transformation, that is essential for neural temporal coding. Losonczy *et al* [25] also have observed that with a strong propagating dendritic spike induced by branch strength potentiation (BSP), a mechanism for dendritic plasticity, a neuron can produce a precisely-timed AP spike.

Furthermore, dendritic spikes can mediate synaptic plasticity and they can even evoke LTP and LTD without somatic spiking [26, 27]. Learning rules suggest that spike-timing-dependent plasticity (STDP) depends on dendritic synapse location [19, 28, 29]. Sjöström and Häusser found that the same EPSP-AP pairing protocol

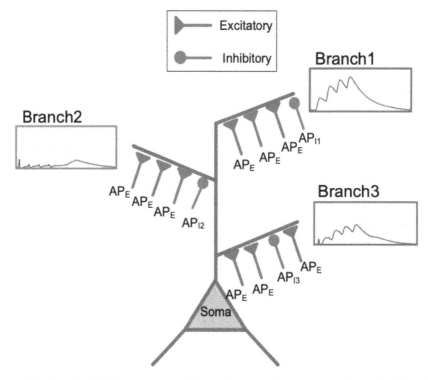

Figure 1.12. Shunting inhibitory synapses vetoing upstream excitatory synapses. Rperoduced from [2].

generates LTP at proximal (nearby) L5–L5[15] synaptic connections and LTD at distal (far) L2/3 to L5 synaptic connections. They further discovered dendritic depolarization (rise in voltage) or dendritic spikes can promote bAP efficacy, and therefore mediate the polarity of the plasticity along the apical dendrite.

Compared to the small EPSPs, dendritic spikes have a faster rise, larger amplitude and sometimes prolonged duration depending on the type of dendritic spike. Due to these aforementioned properties, dendritic spikes can propagate along the dendritic trunk to the soma more effectively compared to PSPs alone, and therefore can initiate APs shown in figure 1.13 [30]. Note that the dendritic spikes do not propagate actively, so that the rapid rise in the dendrites is attenuated and spread when the spike reaches the soma, as shown in figure 1.13.

Figure 1.14 shows the results of dendritic spiking causing neural spiking. Spatio-temporal (occuring nearby and within a small time interval) clustered input activation causes dendritic spikes. These spikes propagate more robustly than the PSP alone, and can cause the neuron to spike [23, 30].

There are three major types of dendritic spikes found in the cortical pyramidal neurons: calcium spikes, sodium spikes, and NMDA spikes [23], as shown in figure 1.15:

---

[15] L refers to the neuron layer in the cortex.

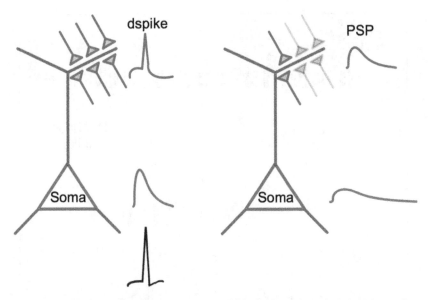

Figure 1.13. Active dendritic spike propagates more effectively from the apical dendrite to the soma in pyramidal neuron. Dendritic spike (*dspike*, left) that propagates robustly with less attenuation than *PSP* (right) alone results in larger somatic potential and therefore can initiate an action potential at the axon hillock. The blue trace is the dendritic potential, and the red trace is the resultant somatic potential. Reproduced from [2].

- Calcium (Ca^{2+}) spikes are generated in the apical dendrites, where a high density of voltage-gated calcium channels reside [31, 32]. They have larger amplitude and a more plateau-shape potential than other dendritric spikes. They can induce burst firing in the cortical pyramidal neuron and their thresholds can be lowered by the bAP [33–35]. Evidence also suggests that calcium spikes mediate STDP based on synapses' location on the dendrite [19, 29].
- Sodium (Na^+) spikes appear in most of the regions in the dendrites [18, 34]. They are fast rising and short in duration. They can evoke precisely-timed and reliable APs in the neuron [24, 36]. Remy *et al* found that sodium dendritic spikes can prevent synaptic plasticity on a particular branch that spiked because of unsuccessful bAP invasion [37].
- NMDA (*N*-methyl-D-aspartate) spikes are found in the thin basal and tuft dendrites [18, 38, 39]. They have relatively smaller amplitude but sharper rising slope and prolonged plateau. Because the plateau potential of these spikes can last between twenty and up to hundreds of milliseconds, and they can occur close to the soma, they can propagate spikes to the soma more effectively than sodium spikes. NMDA spikes can be triggered by bursting inputs and can cause bursting neuronal output. They are a reliable source to propagate bursts through the cortical network [40].

bAP-activated calcium spikes (BAC firing) in the distal dendrite is a mechanism that enhances coincidence detection among different cortical layers in pyramidal neurons. Larkum *et al* found that apical supra-threshold stimulation initiates

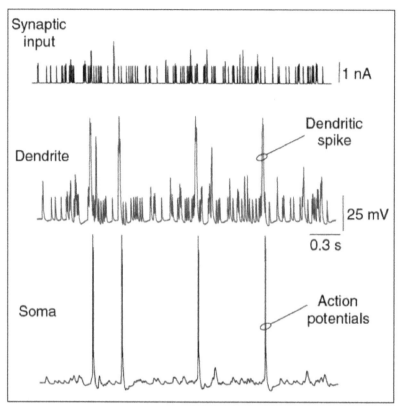

Figure 1.14. Dendritic spiking causing neural spiking (figure from [30], copyright (2008), with permission from Elsevier).

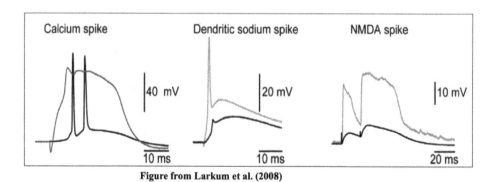

Figure from Larkum et al. (2008)

Figure 1.15. Dendritric spike types (from [23], copyright (2008), with permission from Elsevier): EPSP-like current injection to the apical dendrite results in the generation of a Ca^{2+} spike (blue trace, left) that evokes a short burst of APs at the soma. A similar current injection to a basal dendrite can evoke a local Na^+ spike (orange trace, middle) that is strongly attenuated towards the soma. Focal, extracellular synaptic stimulation to the basal dendrites can evoke an NMDA receptor mediated regenerative dendritic spike (NMDA spike, orange trace, right) that is less attenuated towards the soma as compared to a subthreshold EPSP.

calcium spikes and hence can trigger action potentials [32]. They also found that apical subthreshold stimulation preceded with somatic stimulation can initiate calcium spikes that then cause a neuron to fire. They concluded that the bAP lowers the threshold of calcium spikes; this mechanism is referred to as *back-propagating* AP-activated calcium spike (*BAC* firing).

1.4.2 Dendritic plasticity

Neural plasticity is believed to be an essential mechanism underlying learning and memory formation. Dendritic plasticity in particular appears to support learning.

Besides their impact on synaptic plasticity, dendritic spikes also modulate the excitability of the dendrites, which is referred to as *dendritic plasticity*. There have been research findings suggesting that synaptic plasticity and dendritic plasticity are cooperative and the dendrites can regulate Hebbian learning without the presence of postsynaptic spikes [19, 23, 41]. We discuss two forms of dendritic plasticity in the following sections: *short-term plasticity 'Local and global resets on dendritic excitability'* and *long-term plasticity 'Branch strength potentiation'*.

1.4.2.1 Local and global resets on dendritic excitability
Remy *et al* found that the pyramidal neuron's output is mediated by dendritic sodium spike depression in that neuron's basal dendrites [37]. The experimental results have shown that if a dendritic sodium spike fails to trigger an AP output, that dendritic spike will suppress subsequent *local* dendritic sodium spikes restricted to that particular branch for a time period ranging from hundreds of milliseconds to a few seconds. On the other hand, if an AP is generated at the soma, and it back-propagates efficiently to the dendritic arbor, it will cause a *global* suppression of excitability in a wide range of the dendritic arbor, suppressing dendritic sodium spikes. Therefore, they concluded that local and global *reset* mechanisms that decrease the excitability of the dendrites are highly activity-dependent. Figure 1.16

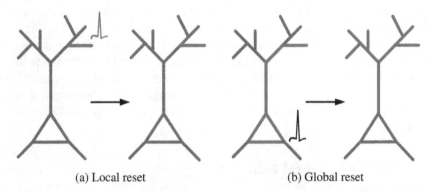

(a) Local reset   (b) Global reset

Figure 1.16. The effect of local and global reset on the dendritic excitability. (a) A dendritic sodium spike that fails to trigger an action potential will only reset that local branch's excitability (shown in blue). (b) If an action potential is generated at the neuron's output, the back-propagating AP will reset the global dendritic arbor's excitability (shown in blue). Reproduced from [2].

illustrates the effects of these two types of feedback on excitability of the dendrites. The computational implication of their findings is that this *reset* mechanism establishes a limit on the number of input patterns that can be stored with dendritic sodium spikes as well as how frequently the patterns can be recalled, approximately one pattern per second if the neuron spikes.

1.4.2.2 Branch strength potentiation

Losonczy *et al* found that the coupling of local calcium dendritic spikes to the soma can be modified in a branch-specific manner that leads to *BSP*, a form of dendritic plasticity [25]. Dendrites have elaborate morphology as each dendrite branches out to thinner ones going backwards towards the synapse. They identified two distinct populations of dendrites in the hippocampal CA1 pyramidal neurons: 78% in the entire dendritic arbor are considered 'weak' terminal branches in coupling strength and the rest, 22%, are considered 'strong' (ten-fold stronger) primary branches. They also discovered that the dendritic branch coupling strength is highly hierarchically structured; more (75%) proximal (primary) branches can initiate strong spikes and less (18%) distal (terminal) branches can initiate strong spikes.

Losonczy *et al* further defined BSP associated with calcium spikes as a mechanism where the excitability of a dendritic branch increases or strengthens under the circumstances when repetitive stimuli are coupled with bAP or a high level of acetylcholine (ACh) activation (during exploratory behavior). They proposed that BSP represents a mechanism for memory formation of uniquely correlated inputs and its interaction with synaptic plasticity can increase the time information is stored. More discussion of this is found in [42].

Two cases that demonstrate how BSP enhances feature detection are described as follows. In the hippocampus, CA1 pyramidal neurons receive inputs from CA3 neurons that represent some sequence feature. Under the assumption that no potentiation of dendritic branch occurs (the branch coupling strength is equal among the entire dendritic arbor), imprecisely-timed AP output is observed at the CA1 pyramidal neuron's output when subsequent correlated inputs are applied as shown in figure 1.17(a). In contrast, if branch coupling strength is hierarchically structured throughout the dendritic arbor as Losonczy *et al* suggested, precise and time-invariant output AP is observed when subsequent correlated inputs are applied as shown in figure 1.17(b). For example, when a stimulus (coming from CA3 neurons) on the weak daughter (distal) branch is correlated with high acetylcholine level or bAPs, a spike propagation to the strong parent (proximal) branch is enhanced and robustly developed that then causes a precisely-timed output AP in the CA1 neuron.

1.5 Variability in neural behavior

Variability is a prominent feature of biological behavior, playing a central role in the behavior of the neurons in the nervous system[16]. While the purpose of such

---

[16] This section supports the material found in chapter 9, and should be read prior to reading that chapter.

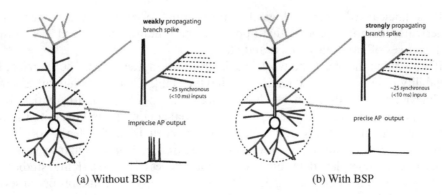

(a) Without BSP   (b) With BSP

Figure 1.17. The effect of BSP mechanism on spike timing in CA1 pyramidal neuron. (a) When branch strength does not change (without BSP), imprecise output spikes are observed given the same input sequence feature from CA3 pyramidal neurons. (b) With BSP, precise output spikes are observed when primed by the same inputs in (a). The dendritic branch receiving these inputs is potentiated in (b) (shown in red), and hence the local spike can propagate to the soma and trigger precisely-timed APs at the CA1 neuron. Strong branches are shown in red. Figure from Losonczy *et al* [25].

variability is not completely understood, studies to be described in this section indicate that variability might offer distinct advantages. Variability in synaptic and ion-channel behavior could lead to structural plasticity and other forms of learning by causing a postsynaptic neuron to fire. This firing could cause active synapses to be strengthened (STDP), so that subsequently the neuron could fire even with typical synapse or ion-channel behavior in the axon hillock. In terms of system behavior, variability in synaptic or ion-channel behavior could assist in moving a neural network from a local minimum.

At the neuronal level, variability could enhance sensitivity to weak signals, a phenomenon that is known as *stochastic resonance* [43]. Also variability could play a constructive role leading to increased reliability of neuronal firing in single neurons [44]. Inputs with low variability or without variability produce imprecise spike trains, whereas inputs with high variability coming from synaptic variability produce spike trains with reproducible timing. At the network level, variability could halt infinite looping behavior with positive feedback in a neural network such as those thought to occur in obsessive-compulsive disorder. Examples of stochastic resonance in neuromorphic circuits are found in [45].

Variability exists even in the best-understood biological systems; therefore it would be impossible to predict deterministic individual behavior of biological neurons. There are a number of systems from single neurons and synapses to invertebrate and vertebrate animals including humans that generate variable output despite no variations in input at all [46]. At the neuronal level, researchers typically deal with this variability in laboratory studies. They do multiple measurements at different times and plot the results. Trial-to-trial variability is observed by many researchers studying biological neural networks [47, 48].

It is unclear whether biological neurons are noisy or whether there is an underlying, unknown process that appears to be random. In this text, we consider both sources of variability, noise and chaos.

If we assume the neural network is a deterministic system, then one source of this variability might be *chaos* (chaotic behavior) [49]. Chaotic behavior is highly nonlinear behavior that can be characterized with nonlinear mathematics. If the system's dynamics are highly sensitive to the initial conditions and the initial state of the neural circuitry varies at the beginning of each trial, this leads to different neuronal and behavioral responses; some researchers believe synapse variability arises from a complex deterministic chaotic process [50, 51]. King studied the diversity of nonlinear characteristics of the neuron and synapse and proposed several chaotic models for neural processes [49].

Another source of variability could be noise, which behaves in a stochastic manner. There is evidence that shows the source of this variability is noisy behavior on the part of a neural mechanism [52, 53]. Any telecommunication system that is transferring and processing information is noisy. Noise is in fact a random or irregular signal that interferes with or obscures a main signal that contains information. The biological nervous system is no exception and, like other systems, is noisy when receiving signals in the sensory neurons, processing information in the CNS or sending information to the motor neurons.

Some neuroscience researchers classify variability as *sensory, motor* or *cellular variability* [47]. Others call cellular variability *intrinsic variability* [54]. We classify variability in the nervous system as extrinsic or intrinsic if it is outside or inside the CNS. Therefore sensory variability and motor variability are in the *extrinsic variability* category because they refer to variability outside the CNS.

Inside the CNS, the two main mechanisms that possess intrinsic variability are the neuron firing mechanism (the spiking mechanism) and the synapse. Neurons communicate with each other by generating a stream of action potentials (spikes). Action potentials are triggered when signals combining from several synapses result in enough positive ions inside the neuron to bring the membrane potential up to the threshold voltage. However, intrinsic variability could cause some neurons to fire even when the membrane potential is not above the threshold or even fire when there is no signal coming from synapses. Also, conversely, intrinsic variability might prevent a neuron from firing even when the membrane voltage is above the threshold. Therefore intrinsic variability plays an important role in neuronal behavior.

1.5.1 Biological neural variability

Variability in a single-neuron response and its consequences for neural networks have been under scrutiny for many decades. In 1964, the random-walk (RW) model was introduced to model the stochastic discharge of neurons that was measured experimentally. Carelli claimed that the irregularities found in the membrane potential of bursting neurons are related to nonlinear and chaotic properties of the cells [55]. Faisal reviewed the sources of noise in the nervous system and showed how noise contributes to trial-to-trial variability [47].

The effects of intrinsic variability in the ion channels of the neuronal membranes have been studied for a long time, with pioneering studies by Pecher [56], Fatt and Katz [57, 58], and numerous others. Ion-channel variability has important effects on its information processing capabilities, changing action potential dynamics, enhancing signal detection, altering the spike-timing reliability and affecting the tuning properties of the cell [59–62].

Knight in 1972 pioneered the study of the effect of noise on the dynamics of a simple spiking neuron using the integrate-and-fire (IAF) model [63]. The noise model he studied was a simplified model in which the threshold is drawn randomly after each spike. Gerstner extended these results and studied both slow noise models and fast-escape-rate noise models [64]. Fourcaud and Brunel completed previous works by studying the impact of synaptic variability on the dynamics of the firing probability of a spiking neuron using the IAF model [65].

Several authors investigated advantages of the variability in single-neuron and neural networks. Mainen and Sejnowski studied reliability of spike timing in rat neocortical slices [44]. They applied two types of inputs to the neuron, inputs with low noise or without noise and inputs with high noise. The timing of spikes drifted from one trial to the next. By comparing the trial-to-trial results for two types of inputs, they demonstrated that the precision of spike timing depends on the level of noise in the input; the more noise in the input, the more precise timing of the output spiking. Inputs with high noise generate spike trains with reproducible timing. Mainen and Sejnowski used cortical neurons in their study, but this argument also applies to synaptic transmission in sensory pathways [66]. Reliability of spike timing was studied by Cecchi, *et al* using the leaky IAF model [67]. Overall, several researchers demonstrate this phenomenon in theory, simulation and experiments [68–70]. These research findings have encouraged BioRC researchers to examine spike timing characteristics with neurotransmitter-release variability in the BioRC neuromorphic circuit simulations, as discussed in chapter 9. More references to neural variability are found in [45].

At the network level, neuronal networks that have formed in the presence of noise will be more robust and explore more states that will facilitate learning and adaptation to the changing demands of a dynamic environment [47]. Manwani and Koch [71] provide arguments that indicate variability is helpful, while others suggest that unreliability in transmission in the cortex due to variability is an energy-saving feature, and multiple pathways increase the reliability.

The next section describes different sources of variability in the nervous system. We briefly review sensory variability and motor variability from the extrinsic variability category and then we focus on two main sources of intrinsic variability: synaptic variability and ion-channel variability. Ion-channel variability causing spontaneous firing and ion-channel variability in the Hodgkin–Huxley model and the IAF model are also reviewed in the 'Variability' chapter.

Chapter 9 describes electronic circuits that model intrinsic variability at the circuit level. We focus on two main sources of intrinsic variability at the circuit level, neurotransmitter-release variability in the synapse circuit and ion-channel variability in the axon hillock circuit. We also cover an electronic circuit designed to capture noise generated by photons in chapter 9.

1.5.2 Background

At the biochemical and biophysical level there are many stochastic processes[17] in neurons. These include protein production and degradation, the opening and closing of ion channels, the fusing of synaptic vesicles and the diffusion and binding of signaling molecules to receptors. Combination of all stochastic elements could be a big source of randomness in the nervous system, however, by averaging large numbers of such stochastic elements, the randomness of individual elements could be eliminated.

One source of extrinsic variability is variability in the sensory system. Variability in the sensory system is mainly in the form of noise; therefore, we use noise as a source of sensory variability. External sensory stimuli are intrinsically noisy because they are coming from a noisy environment. In the auditory system, noise exists in the input in the form of random collisions of air molecules against the eardrum or of Brownian motion of cochlear components that imposes a limit on the auditory system [72].

In the visual system, photoreceptors receive photons at a rate governed by a Poisson process. Similar to the auditory system, this noise limits contrast sensitivity in vision. This impact is reduced at low light levels when the number of photons arriving at the photoreceptors is less [73].

In the olfactory and gustatory systems, chemical sensing is affected by thermodynamic noise because molecules arrive at the receptor at random rates owing to diffusion and because receptor proteins are limited in their ability to accurately count the number of signaling molecules [74, 75].

As shown in figure 1.18(a), in the sensory transduction and amplification stage, a sensory signal is converted into a chemical signal (in the visual, olfactory and gustatory systems) or a mechanical signal (in the auditory system) and then is amplified and is converted into an electrical signal. Noise in later stages is a combination of sensory noise plus noise during the amplification process (transducer noise). Therefore, signals that are weaker than the noise cannot be distinguished from noise after amplification [76].

When we talk about noise in a system consisting of multiple stages, we can show mathematically that reducing noise in the first stage is more important than at other stages. For example in telecommunication systems, at the receiver side, the first stage is the *LNA* (low noise amplifier) that has better noise performance than other stages in the receiver. Therefore, to reduce noise in the nervous system, organisms often pay a high metabolic and structural price at the first stage (the sensory stage). For example, a fly's photoreceptors account for 10% of its resting metabolic consumption and its eye's optics make up over 20% of the flight payload [77].

---

[17] Or at least processes that appear to be stochastic, but may not be completely understood.

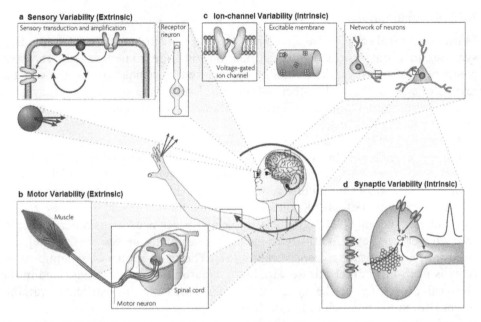

Figure 1.18. Overview of variability in the nervous system. Reprinted from [47], copyright (2008), with permission from Springer Nature.

Another source of extrinsic variability is variability in the motor system. We consider noise as the only source of motor variability. As shown in figure 1.18b, motor neurons receive signals from the CNS and convert them into mechanical forces in the muscle fibers. The number of muscle fibers that are innervated from a single neuron is proportional to the force. In addition, when the whole-muscle force increases, the firing rates of the active motor neurons increase, such that those that innervate a small number of muscle fibers have the highest firing rate.

The human skeletal muscle produces a force that has variability. The variability is proportional to the average force that is produced by that muscle. Whole-muscle force is determined by the number of active motor neurons and the firing rates of these neurons. The motor neuron that innervates the most fibers will have the lowest firing rate. Therefore, any variability in the force that is generated by the muscle fibers that are innervated by this motor neuron will contribute the most to whole-muscle force variability.

Human motor behavior from eye movements to hand trajectories is in such a way as to eliminate or reduce the effects of motor noise by optimal control. However, it is still unclear how much of the observed trial-to-trial movement variability is because of motor variability and how much is due to other sources of variability in the motor system [78, 79].

In the following sections, we focus on two dominant sources of intrinsic variability, synaptic variability and ion-channel variability.

1.5.3 Synaptic variability

Many neocortical cells receive an intense synaptic bombardment from thousands of synapses, that contains meaningful information and noise from other cells. The main component of the synaptic variability experienced by a neuron originates in the myriad of synapses made by other cells onto it. Every spike arriving at this synapse contributes a random amount of charge to the cell. Neuroscientists usually call this *synaptic background noise*.

During synaptic processing of presynaptic action potentials, there are several steps that generate variability such as the spontaneous opening of intracellular Ca^{2+} channels, synaptic Ca^{2+} channel noise, spontaneous fusion of a vesicle release pathway, spontaneous fusion of a vesicle with the membrane, and neurotransmitter-release variability [80–84]. Koch demonstrated that chemical synapses release transmitters randomly [85]. Variability in the number of neurotransmitter molecules released per vesicle ($\sim$2000) arises owing to variations in vesicle size [86] and vesicular neurotransmitter concentration [87]. The main source of synaptic variability is neurotransmitter release variability. Neurotransmitters are involved in the chemical processing of the synapse. We will focus on this particular variable mechanism in the research described here.

In chapter 9, we model the amplitude of neurotransmitter release variability at the circuit level. In particular, a Gaussian noise or chaotic signal is added to the potential at the output of a synapse circuit to model the neurotransmitter release variation in an unpredictable manner. Variation in neurotransmitter concentration in the synaptic cleft causes a change in the peak PSP of the synapse. We will talk about modeling neurotransmitter release variability at the circuit level in that chapter.

1.5.4 Ion-channel variability

One main source of intrinsic variability is ion-channel variability. Nervous systems use the action potential (spike) to send information along axons to other synapses and neurons. The action potential is generated in the neuron by voltage-gated ion channels whose gating behavior is subject to thermodynamic fluctuations. The reliability of the spike is an important requirement for encoding, transmitting and computing neural information. The precision of spike arrival times is on the order of 1–10 ms in many species [88], and cortical neurons have specialized to detect coincident arrival of spikes on millisecond timescales [89].

Both Na^+ and K^+ ion channels are involved in the production of an action potential. Both Na^+ and K^+ channels are opened by depolarizing the membrane, but they respond independently and sequentially. Na^+ channels open before K^+ channels. Each Na^+ channel has two gates, an activation gate and an inactivation gate at either end of the channel. In order to have diffusion through the Na^+ channel, both activation and inactivation gates must be open. At step one (resting state) the activation gate is closed and the inactivation gate is open. At step two (depolarization) a stimulus opens the activation gates on some of the Na^+ channels. That allows more Na^+ ions to diffuse into the cell. At step three, depolarization opens the activation gates on most Na^+ channels, while the K^+ channels activation gates remain closed. Na^+ ions inside the cell make the inside of the membrane positive with respect to the outside. Once the threshold is crossed, a positive feedback cycle rapidly increases the membrane potential. At step four, the inactivation gates on most Na^+ channels close and the activation gates on most K^+ channels open, causing the membrane potential to come back toward the resting potential.

As mentioned above, the AP is generated by voltage-gated ion channels whose gating behavior is subject to thermodynamic fluctuations. The Na^+ and K^+ channels open and close in a stochastic fashion, following the laws of probability. However, distinct from tossing a coin or a die, the probability of finding the channel closed or open is not a fixed number but can be modified by some external stimulus, such as the voltage. This stochastic behavior produces random ionic current changes that cause variability in the responses, called ion-channel variability. It is unclear whether ion channels are stochastic or whether there is an underlying, unknown process that appears to be random. One source of ion-channel variability might be chaos.

Impact of variability depends on the way in which the spike trains may carry information, the frequency (rate) coding or the temporal coding. In rate coding, the average number of spikes per time period (the firing rate) is important and carries information, while the variations in frequency are noise or some chaotic signal. The firing rate is related to the stimulus intensity, i.e., the firing rate increases with increasing stimulus intensity. In rate coding, we can use statistical averages of many inputs to find the information and then ion channel variability does not have big impact on the information. Temporal coding employs the timing of the spikes or the particular ordering of interspike intervals. Variability in spiking with temporal coding is assumed to convey information. In this case, because ion channel variability causes jitter in interspike intervals, it has a big impact on the information.

Ion-channel variability has impact on the propagation and the initiation of APs, can introduce uncertainty into threshold properties of APs and can cause jitter in interspike intervals of repetitive firing. Neuroscientists showed that ion-channel variability can generate variability in the AP threshold at nodes of Ranvier [90]. Also, ion-channel variability in the dendrite and in the soma produces membrane potential fluctuations that are large enough to affect AP timing. Variability in the AP initiation in membrane patches might be because of ion-channel variability [91].

1.5.5 Spontaneous firing

The strength of the ion channel variability is proportional to the axonal input resistance and it depends inversely on axon diameter ($D^{-\frac{3}{2}}$). In axons less than 0.3 μm diameter, the input resistance is large enough that opening of just a single Na^+ channel could generate an AP in the absence of any other inputs. In this case, the neuron fires without any input from any synapses. This firing mechanism is called spontaneous firing. In this chapter, we model spontaneous firing at the circuit level.

Spontaneous APs become exponentially more frequent as axon diameter decreases. Therefore, for axons below 0.08–0.10 μm, the rate of spontaneous firing

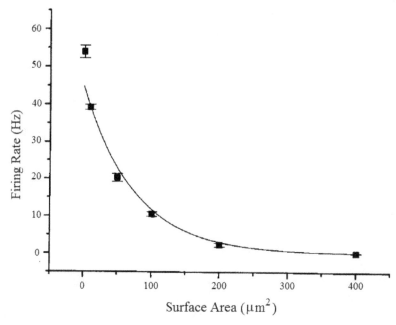

Figure 1.19. Spontaneous firing rate as a function of membrane surface area. Reprinted from [93] with permission from Elsevier, copyright 1996 The Biophysical Society.

is too high, which makes axons useless for communication. This lower limit matches the smallest diameters of axons across species. Therefore, ion-channel variability sets the lower limit for the diameter of excitable cell bodies to 3 μm [92]. Figure 1.19 shows spontaneous firing rate as a function of axon area.

1.6 Structural plasticity

This section supports the material found in Chapter 10, and should be read prior to reading that chapter.

Plasticity refers to the ability of neurons and neural networks to be altered over time. The text introduced synaptic plasticity earlier, in section 1.3. Structural plasticity refers to the changes in connectivity between neurons over time, a subject surveyed excellently in [94].

Changes in the human cortex are believed to play an important role in learning and memory. While synaptic plasticity (LTP/LTD) is an important mechanism supporting memory and learning, the addition of new synaptic connections, new synapses, and incorporation of synapses recruited from other purposes are mechanisms that are also believed to be required. *Synaptogenesis* [95, 96] is the process by which new synapses are formed. This involves the growth of a neuronal axon that forms an *axodendritic contact* with the dendritic structures of another neuron. It has been observed that these connections are formed locally [96] and demonstrate structural plasticity both *in vitro* (in a Petri dish or test tube) and *in vivo* (in a living organism).

The fundamental aspect behind the formation of a new synapse is the formation of an axodendritic contact. The general belief had been that axons perform active roles, whereas dendrites are relatively passive, probably a carryover from studies concerning the formation of the neuromuscular junction, where the targets (muscles) are rather stationary [97]. However, dendrites also extend growth cones displaying elongation and bifurcation. Furthermore, research [98] reveals that numerous synapses formed are located on newly grown dendritic growth cones and filopodia. These observations lead to the conclusion that many of the new synapses occurring during this period are initiated by dendritic growth. As early as 2002, Trachtenberg *et al* [99] suggested that sensory experience drives the formation and elimination of synapses and that these changes might underlie structural plasticity. *In vitro* studies show that high-frequency synaptic stimulation leading to local synaptic LTP has been shown to induce the extension of numerous dendritic filopodia, some of which make axodendritic contacts to create new synapses [100, 101]. High frequency stimulation *in vitro* could be unrealistic as many neurons fire at lower frequencies. Experiments performed *in vivo* using external stimuli received from neurons rather than probe stimuli [102] show that previously connected neurons can form new synapses along the same dendritic arbors due to growth of new dendritic spines, showing an increase in synaptic strength with formation of new synapses. Paola *et al* [103] suggest that structural plasticity of axonal branches and synaptic boutons at the ends of the axonal branches contribute to the remodeling of biological neural circuits.

Synapses form by a process known as *synaptogenesis* [95]. This involves the formation of an axodendritic contact (a contact between an axon terminal and a dendrite of nearby neurons) followed by a series of events. As reviewed in [96], after an axodendritic contact is formed there is activity from the axonal side that triggers the uptake of synaptic vesicles. This process is called presynaptic differentiation (PRESD). PRESD then triggers the dendritic (postsynaptic) side to recruit receptors for the neurotransmitter contained in the synapses, thus completing the synapse. This mechanism forms a part of postsynaptic differentiation (POSD). There is speculation in the findings that say PRESD triggers POSD in the formation of a synapse. Another school of thought says that POSD is independent of PRESD as dendrites are active elements as well [96]. BioRC synapse circuits have been modeled to include neurotransmitter and receptor concentrations in synapses that can be used to model PRESD and POSD [104].

To summarize the neural mechanisms under investigation, increase in neural activity causes axonal growth. Increase in local synaptic efficacy leads to growth of a dendritic spine and, on formation of an axodendritic contact, synaptogenesis occurs that involves PRESD triggering POSD. The case where POSD is triggered independently is not considered, as this is an effect that is being investigated and can be modeled if needed.

Research has suggested structural changes that lead to the addition or subtraction of synapses between previously connected pre- and postsynaptic units [102]. In addition to weight changes, learning could involve alterations to the connection network, whereby previously unconnected units become connected and vice versa.

Wiring changes require structural plasticity. In this learning mode, the storage capacity lies in the neuron's ability to connect (form synapses) with other postsynaptic neurons. Weight and wiring changes are not mutually exclusive (wiring plasticity can even be viewed as a special case of weight plasticity), and current research is investigating how neurons and their synapses might be engaged in both forms of learning [94].

At many synapses, the induction of spike-timing-dependent LTP/LTD requires activation of the NMDA glutamate receptors (NMDARs) [12]. In some cases, LTD induction was also shown to require the activation of calcium channels. A straightforward explanation for the temporally-asymmetric STDP is that the relative timing of glutamate binding to NMDARs and the spiking of the postsynaptic bAP determine the Ca^{2+} level required for either LTP or LTD; Pre-post spiking (presynaptic firing first) leads to the opening of NMDA channels via depolarization-induced removal of the Mg^{2+} block [11], resulting in a high-level Ca^{2+} influx, whereas post-pre spiking (postsynaptic spiking first) leads to a low-level sustained Ca^{2+} rise by the opening of voltage-dependent Ca^{2+} channels (VDCCs) and/or limited NMDAR activation. These cellular mechanisms, among others, underlie induction of STDP [10]. Astrocytes are involved in generation of new synapses, a topic of future research and discussion.

1.7 Astrocytes

Two decades ago the discovery of a new form of bidirectional communication between astrocytes, a subtype of glial cells, and neurons turned attention to astrocytes[18]. Recent evidence has shed light on biological mechanisms through which astrocytes receive, integrate and transmit information to establish astrocyte-neuron and astrocyte–astrocyte communication. Astrocytes participate in the modulation of sleep *homeostasis*, the formation of synapses, and control of synaptic strength. It is due to their role in many higher-level functions in the brain that astrocytes are now being considered computational units that work together with neurons in major brain communication processes, as shown in figure 1.20.

In recent years, neuroscientists have found significance evidence that astrocytes contribute to neural processing. While astrocytes were known to provide nutritional support for neurons, their roles are now known to be much broader. Direct and diffuse communications between neurons and astrocytes influence not only neural behavior [106, 107], but also neural circuit structure. Astrocytes are involved in complex signaling with neurons; astrocyte-neuronal signaling is observed to be a complex bidirectional communication [108–110]. Astrocytes respond to neurotransmitters, detect the flow of ions in and out of neighboring neurons, protein signals, and release gliotransmitters and ions that can affect neural behavior. This signaling, involving both positive and negative feedback, is complex and not fully understood. Studies have shown that astrocytes modulate synaptic transmission and plasticity mechanisms through the regulation of neurotransmitters and

---

[18] This section supports the material found in chapter 13, and should be read prior to reading that chapter.

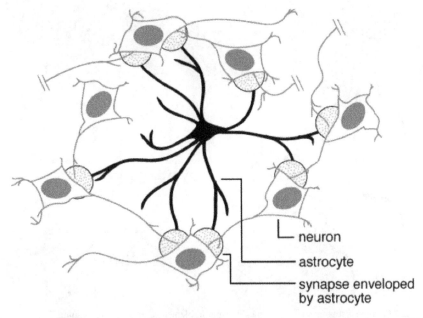

neuron

astrocyte

synapse enveloped
by astrocyte

Figure 1.20. An astrocyte forming tripartite synapses with a group of neurons (figure taken from [105] with permission from SAGE). The astrocyte is represented by many long thin branches. Neurons are surrounding the astrocyte.

gliotransmitter concentrations (transmitters released from glial cells) [108, 111, 112]. By uptaking or releasing glutamate and other chemicals such as GABA, D-serine, and ATP in the synaptic cleft, astrocytes can fine-tune neuronal excitability and behavior. Astrocytes have been implicated in synaptic plasticity, synaptogenesis [113], and homeostatic functions [114, 115]. Through Ca^{2+} signaling, astrocytes also provide a form of communication between neurons that are not directly connected through synapses. Astrocytes allow the activity of a neuron to have far-reaching effects on neurons that are not in its immediate vicinity. This type of global communication is not realizable by neuron-only networks, where communication only occurs between connected neurons. Note that *synapse 1* affects both *synapse 1* and *synapse 2* via the astrocyte. Figure 1.21 shows a schematic cartoon that demonstrates a high-level view of one of the astrocyte-neuron mechanisms that we emulate using the BioRC neural circuits with CMOS circuits. The cartoon shows two synapses as part of an astrocytic *microdomain*, a small local region of an astrocyte process (arm) communicating with several neurons, and integrating their interaction, in this case at the synapses [108][19]. We show the sequence of events to explain how the BioRC network behaves. Increase in synaptic activity releases glutamate into the synaptic cleft (1). Some of the glutamate in the cleft is taken up by the astrocyte (2) to cause elevation of Ca^{2+} concentrations [108]. These Ca^{2+} elevations cause glutamate to be released by the astrocyte at the postsynaptic site

---

[19] Neuroscientists often model these microdomains as single *compartments*.

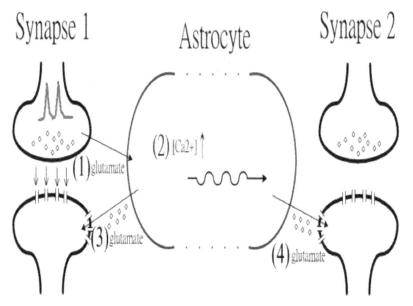

Figure 1.21. Cartoon showing astrocytic mechanisms implemented (Credit: Ko-Chung Tseng). Copyright 2011 IEEE. Reprinted, with permission, from [116].

of Synapse 1 and at other postsynaptic sites (e.g. Synapse 2) in the microdomain (4). This increases the PSP at Synapse 2, thus increasing the probability of firing.

One location where astrocytes communicate with synapses is called a *tripartite synapse* [108, 109], a complex location with many chemical processes. The tripartite synapse is the main computational unit, consisting of three terminals, the presynaptic neuron, the postsynaptic neuron and the astrocytic process. Since all terminals are able to release/uptake transmitters, all of them can have influence on each other.

Neural activity at the synapse leads to release of glutamate that is taken up by the astrocyte. Local increase in glutamate leads to increase in Ca^{2+} concentration in the astrocyte that causes the astrocyte to release a group of chemicals called *gliotransmitters* [110], including glutamate, adnosine triphosphate (ATP) and D-serine. Glutamate and D-serine are believed to play an excitatory role at the synapse, whereas ATP plays a regulating role. Glutamate release can increase the synapse's excitability, leading to a higher PSP when APs impinge on it. This can cause the neuron to fire with fewer EPSPs from stimulated synapses combining in the dendritic arbor.

Since one astrocyte is connected to over 100 000 synapses [108], astrocytes are capable of monitoring wide-ranging neuronal communication through their long thin processes. This endows the astrocyte with the ability to potentially coordinate a massive amount of neuronal information between a spatial distributed group of neurons. The most widely-accepted astrocytic mechanism is the monitoring of glutamate released by synapses. The glutamate released by synapses and up taken by the astrocyte causes calcium (Ca^{2+}) waves that spread across the astrocyte.

These waves lead to release of glutamate at other synaptic locations in the microdomain. Current research [108, 110] discusses the possible case where glutamate released by the astrocyte increases neural excitability due to increase of glutamate at these synaptic locations. Astrocytes contiguously tile the entire CNS in a non-overlapping fashion.

Also, astrocytes are known to exert modulatory properties on receptors located at the *extrasynaptic* side of neurons away from the synapse, while neurons, through the spillover of transmitters, could reach and modulate receptors in the outer membrane of the astrocyte.

There is a wide variety of receptors by which astrocytes sense activity at tripartite synapses, such as purinergic receptors, AMPA receptors (AMPARs), metabotropic glutamate receptors (mGluRs), GABA receptors (GABARs), nicotinic acetylcholine receptors (nAChRs), and muscarinic receptors (mAChRs), among others [117, 118]. By means of these receptors, astrocytes uptake neurotransmitters such as glutamate, D-serine, GABA, and ATP and then, according to astrocytic calcium levels, may also release transmitters back to neurons. Some of these receptors are modeled in neuromorphic circuits presented in the text and will be discussed later in the text.

Intracellular and intercellular astrocyte Ca^{2+} waves and oscillations have been reported, with communication between astrocytes thought to occur via *gap junctions*, connections between the membranes of astrocytes [107]. Calcium waves in the *intracellular* (within a cell) space of the astrocyte represent the encoding mechanism that carries the information regarding the communication to be established with the surrounding synapses. It is now well established that the properties of intracellular calcium can be modulated by neurotransmitters released from nearby neurons. Subsection 1.7.4 is dedicated to the discussion of astrocytic calcium waves and their ability to encode and modulate synaptic information. Nonlinearity in the intracellular astrocyte Ca^{2+} processing has been reported (e.g. [119]), suggesting a neuromorphic circuit implementation of intracellular Ca^{2+} processing in the *cytosol* might be complex.

Astrocytes provide neurons with a form of long-range communication. Through Ca^{2+} signaling in astrocytes, neurons that are not directly connected to each other through synapses can influence each other. Ca^{2+} signaling behavior depends on the intensity of neural activity [120]. The types of Ca^{2+} signaling include microdomain, intracellular, and intercellular signaling. When activity is low, astrocytic stimulation is low and Ca^{2+} levels increase only slightly in spatially-localized regions adjacent to active synapses. These regions are called *microdomains*. When neural activity is higher, Ca^{2+} in the microdomain is higher and it can start a wave of Ca^{2+} through a regenerative process called calcium-induced-calcium-release (CICR) [121]. During CICR, initial elevations of intracellular Ca^{2+} trigger the formation of inositol 1,4,5-trisphosphate (IP3). IP3 then activates IP3 receptors (IP3R), inducing the release of Ca^{2+} inside the astrocyte from the endoplasmic reticulum. The released Ca^{2+} can then form more IP3 which activates neighboring IP3Rs and releases more Ca^{2+} from internal stores in a regenerative process. Through calcium-induced calcium release (CICR), oscillating Ca^{2+} waves are produced that can spread out intracellularly to other parts of the astrocyte. Gliotransmitters are then released at synapses outside of the initial microdomain due to the propagating calcium wave. This mechanism allows a neuron to affect the activity of other neurons that are not in direct synaptic contact. Territories formed by astrocytes have been found to be in contact with more than 100 000 synapses. Thus astrocytes provide neurons with a form of global, indirect communication. This is in contrast with communication via synapses, which is a type of local communication between neurons that are in direct contact. Ca^{2+} waves can also propagate intercellularly between astrocytes through gap junctions, increasing the area of influence. This type of communication requires even higher levels of neuronal activity.

It is necessary to clearly draw the distinctions between astrocyte cells and neurons. Astrocytes are chemically excitable cells with a very slow response in the form of analog graded potentials, and they do not fire APs. They have shown ability to encode synaptic information through intracellular calcium waves by complex nonlinear processes that involve a wide variety of chemicals and the activation of many different receptors. Yet, although they are slow compared to neurons, they do contribute to neuronal processing and have influence over the message transmitted across groups of neurons.

It is well known that astrocytes are particularly efficient in the uptake of glutamate due to their excitatory amino acids such as EAAT1 and EAAT2 [122]. They are indeed, by far, more efficient than neurons. Although neurons have their own uptake mechanism, their transporters face the opposition of a higher electrochemical gradient and constant variations in the membrane potential [122–124]. The astrocyte's efficacy in the uptake of glutamate contributes to maintaining the balance in the extracellular space and prevent excitotoxicity and possible pathological conditions. In the absence of astrocytes, an uncontrollable amount of glutamate in the extracellular space would lead to the saturation of synapses and the eventual loss of synaptic connections [125, 126]. Undoubtedly, the uptake mechanism of astrocytes represents an important synapse regulator. Other astrocyte neuroscience information can be found in [127].

1.7.1 Astrocyte glutamate

Astrocyte uptake of glutamate limits the calcium entry into neurons through NMDA channels, and contributes to support a healthy neuronal environment by the prevention of neurodegenerative diseases. Without an uptake mechanism, such as the astrocyte uptake, and under an excessive release of glutamate into the extracellular space, neurons become vulnerable to the influx of calcium ions by the overstimulation of neuronal NMDA channels. An imbalance of calcium in the cell is highly undesirable and associated with neuronal death by toxicity [128]. Without the astrocyte uptake mechanism, presynaptic neurons would disconnect their synapses from the postsynaptic neurons when a large amount of neurotransmitters was released into the synaptic cleft [125].

Studies have shown that astrocytic release of glutamate, binding extrasynaptic NMDAR located at the postsynaptic membrane, leads to the induction of excitatory currents with slow kinetics and large amplitudes into the neurons, capable of

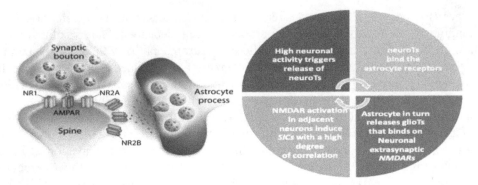

Figure 1.22. The left side of the figure shows a tripartite synapse, where an astrocytic process stimulates subunits of the NMDA channel (figure taken from [108], copyright 2006 the American Physiological Society). The right side shows flow diagram describing the main steps in the activation by the astrocyte of the extrasynaptic NMDA channels.

inducing synchronized neuronal activity [129]. These currents are known as *slow inward currents* (SICs).

The relevance of astrocytic induction of SICs lies in the role they could potentially play in the coordination of neuronal activity. Two aspects of SICs appear to be important for the induction of synchronized activity: (1) SICs activate NMDAR with a high degree of correlation on synapses of adjacent neurons, and (2) their amplitudes are overwhelmingly larger than typical EPSCs; the ratio is one to five, with SICs about five times larger than EPSCs on average. Their slow decay time constants allow for a time window through which synchronization of neuronal activity remains active. The SIC decay is significantly slower compared to EPSCs, i.e. about 60 times [129]. The activation of an NMDAR extrasynaptic receptor by the astrocyte is summarized by the steps in figure 1.22. The release of glutamate transmitters from surrounding neurons, sensed by the astrocyte, induces intracellular calcium waves in the astrocytic microdomain. These calcium waves in turn stimulate the release of transmitters back to the synapse, and such transmitters bind and activate extrasynaptic NMDA channels, causing the induction of SIC events at the postsynaptic side of the synapse. Fellin presents comprehensive biological detail on this mechanism.

1.7.2 Astrocytes' role in binding information

The implication of the role of astrocytes in the coordination of massive neuronal activity is undergoing research that could dramatically impact our understanding of cognitive functions [130], as well as neurodegenerative diseases such as epilepsy [131]. A very important consideration is that a single astrocyte in rodents is capable of reaching between 20 000 and 100 000 synapses, while in humans a protoplasmic astrocyte can contact between 270 000 and two million synapses [132]. More important is that astrocytes in the brain do not usually work as single units; they form an astrocytic syncytium, i.e. a network of astrocytes connected by gap junctions, while a single astrocyte has about 235 gap junctions that connect it to other astrocytes [133]. Astrocytes rely on neurons to access sensory information. The binding of information refers to the process where independent features of an object are encoded in the brain through different neuronal paths with different axonal delays [134]. It remains unknown how these paths are combined and this is known as the binding problem [135]. The astrocentric hypothesis proposed by Robertson [136] considers the astrocyte as the missing link in the binding of information, where independent information is consolidated. The basis for this hypothesis is the ability of astrocytes to integrate neuronal information. Binding of information is important for conscious processing, where synchrony of activity is considered to be a fundamental process. Pereira and Augusto Furlan conjectured that astrocytic calcium waves carry the content of perceptual conscious processes [137]. He proposed a model of brain mental functions that combines the role of large-scale calcium waves in a network of astrocytes with signals that modulate neuronal networks [130]. In his model, large-scale calcium waves are produced through neuronal synchronized events [137]. These neuronal synchronized events can be potentially activated by astrocytes through the induction of SICs into extrasynaptic NMDA receptors as observed in experiments [129].

1.7.3 Astrocytes contribute to a wide range of biological processes

Recent publications have shown that astrocytes, like neurons, integrate, process information, and discriminate between synapses [138, 139]. The ability of astrocytes to discriminate synaptic information was experimentally shown by Araque *et al* [140]. His experiment shows that glutamatergic axons from the *alveus* area of the hippocampus do not elicit calcium waves in astrocytes; however astrocytes respond to cholinergic axons from the alveus and to glutamatergic axons from the *Schaffer collateral* areas[20]. In another study, Perea and Araque [141] experimentally demonstrated the ability of astrocytes to integrate synaptic information by the simultaneous stimulation of both pathways. The authors reasoned that if astrocytes have the ability to integrate synaptic information, then that should elicit a nonlinear calcium wave when both pathways are stimulated simultaneously. In agreement with this reasoning, the authors have shown synaptic integration experimentally by the nonlinear response of astrocytic calcium waves. In the hippocampus area, astrocytes selectively discriminate between glutamatergic synapses from different pathways, and appear to distinguish pathways with the same type of neurotransmitters.

In another role, astrocytes control neuronal inhibition in the barrel cortex of rats by means of $GABA_A$ and $GABA_B$ receptors [142]. Two of the principal GABA transporters (GATs) are known to exist preferentially in astrocytes. Astrocytes also play a role in tonic inhibition, a form of feedback which is important in the balance between inhibition and excitation, by complex feedback that consists of the uptake of glutamate from a network of neurons and the release of GABA back to the network [143]. In the thalamus, astrocytes act as a gatekeeper controlling the

---

[20] The Schaffer collateral areas are areas of the hippocampus where neurons in regions CA1 and CA3 connect.

spillover of GABA transmitters to other extrasynaptic sides and thus prevent the formation of seizures [144], through the Glu/GABA exchange mechanism due to its negative feedback nature.

Heja [143] proposed a hypothetical model in which GABA is released from astrocytes gradually according to the uptake of glutamate, based on his current experimental work. The release of GABA is Ca^{2+} independent and occurs via transporter reversals of the subtype GAT-2 and GAT-3. In this mechanism Na^+ plays an important role since the GAT-2 and GAT-3 driving forces are believed to depend on the difference of Na^+ between the intracellular and extracellular spaces. Following the generation of APs from the presynaptic neuron, Glu (glutamate) is released and transported along with Na^+ from the extracellular space into the astrocyte's intracellular space by means of the glutamate transporters EAAT1/2. This causes an organic compound called putrescine to synthesize GABA, which is released back into the extracellular space, binding extrasynaptic receptors in the postsynaptic membrane [145]. Another experimental study shows that the anion voltage-dependent channel Best-1 (bestrophin-1) appears to be involved in astrocytic GABA release. Best-1 can be activated by means of elevated intracellular Ca^{2+} in the astrocyte [146].

Studies have also shown that stimulation at one synapse leads to inhibition at a nonoverlapping synapse by the release of ATP from astrocytes [147, 148]. ATP transmitters released from astrocytes through metabotropic P2Y receptors have been found to induce LTD in neighboring hippocampal neurons [147]. Heterosynaptic depression, a form of LTD, where the efficacy of neighboring inactive synapses is decreased by active synapses, can be mediated by the release of ATP or by the release of glutamate from astrocytes. In the former case, ATP is released by astrocytes upon glutamate stimulation from neurons [148]; while in the latter case, GABA released from neurons triggers glutamate release from astrocytes modulating mGluR (a type of glutamate receptor) channels [149]. Heterosynaptic depression is a form of intersynaptic communication in which astrocytes appear to have a significant role. Moreover, about 75% of astrocytes' gap junctions are autologous (intradomain) which means that they can represent the main path for this form of intersynaptic communication [150].

Another form of inhibition by astrocytes is the production of slow outward currents (SOCs) at the extrasynaptic GABA receptors [151]. SOCs have shown to have, like slow inward currents (SICs), slow rise and decay times with a high amplitude. They were shown to inhibit neurons in the olfactory bulb synchronously [152]. They may also be involved in the production of tonic inhibition in the thalamus [151, 153] and thus in the prevention of seizure generation.

1.7.4 Calcium waves: a coding mechanism in astrocytes

The encoding of information in astrocytes occurs via calcium waves that are formed in the cell by the activation of different mechanisms, enabling them to propagate over long distances. Intracellular calcium dynamics is primarily considered to be modulated by an IP3 (inositol trisphosphate)-dependent mechanism. The activation of this mechanism is caused by the stimulation of neurotransmitters released from synapses enwrapped by the astrocyte. These neurotransmitters bind and activate receptors located in the extracellular membrane of the astrocyte. This generates diacylglycerol(DAG) and IP3 [154]. The IP3 production acts on IP3R channels located in the astrocyte's endoplasmic reticulum (ER). Calcium is released from the ER (endoplasmic reticulum) into the astrocyte's *intracellular membrane (cytosol)* in the form of successive puffs through the IP3R channels. The cell is endowed with pumps that take back calcium into the ER. The interplay between these channels causes the calcium wave production and propagation.

IP3 receptors close when the astrocytic extracellular stimulation from the released neurotransmitter decreases and thus the binding of transmitters into the receptors at the astrocytic outer cell membrane is reduced, causing a reduction in the formation of IP3 in the astrocytic *cytosol*. The high concentration of calcium is then reversed by the autocatalytic action of Ca^{2+} release[21] which along with the SERCA-pumps cause the inactivation of IP3R channels in the astrocytes. SERCA-pumps are activated by the increase of calcium in the *cytosol*. Their role is to pump back the excess of intracellular calcium into the endoplasmic reticulum so that calcium in the intracellular space goes back to its natural concentration. The repetition of these events by the constant release of neurotransmitters can lead to calcium oscillations. As the calcium wave propagates, it is self-amplified by the release of calcium from the nearby IP3 receptors located on different sides of the endoplasmic reticulum[22].

It should be highlighted that the transmitter ATP (adenosine triphosphate), which is produced by the mitochondria, is the main source of energy for the astrocyte. Without ATP, SERCA-pumps would not be activated, which could lead to eventual cell death [155, 156]. It is important to mention that the calcium concentration in the endoplasmic reticulum is about 10–15 times higher in calcium than in the intracellular space and proteins are about 1000 times more likely to bind calcium in the intracellular space rather than in the ER [156].

1.7.5 Patterns of astrocytic calcium waves

Experiments have shown that the activation of different types of metabotropic glutamate receptors (mGluR1, mGluR5) induces different patterns of intracellular calcium waves [133]. Biphasic elevations of calcium (initial peak followed by a sustained plateau) are caused by activation of mGluR1 and typically have little influence on the astrocytic release of transmitters. Ca^{2+} oscillations are induced by mGluR5 and can vary in frequency and amplitude over time, triggering the release of transmitters [133]. These are the two most recognized patterns of calcium signaling.

Researchers have shown that biphasic elevations of calcium in astrocytes only evoke a single release of glutamate having little effect on neuronal activity. Calcium

---

[21] Ca^{2+} itself acts as a catalyst to reverse the generation of Ca^{2+}.

[22] The endoplasmic reticulum is a continuous membrane system that forms a series of flattened sacs within the cytoplasm and acts as a transportation mechanism.

oscillations in the astrocyte appear to be more influential by the pulsatile (pulsing) release of glutamate; and have been viewed as a possible representation of synaptic activity by encoding information through frequency variations [133, 157, 158]. In other words, activity induced by astrocytes appears to have different levels. The lowest level induces no release of transmitters from astrocytes due to the lack of or small activity in the neuronal release of glutamate. A medium level is observed with a substantial increase of glutamate, causing the astrocyte to release successive puffs of glutamate. Under excessive stimulation, astrocytes have shown to release only a single event of glutamate. This case is usually seen in pathological diseases, such as epilepsy.

Studies have shown that the amplitude and frequency of calcium waves in astrocytes may be controlled by different biological processes. Nitric oxide (NO), for example, could be implied in the frequency variations of oscillations with little influence on the amplitude and pattern of the calcium wave. Experiments have shown that the increase in the frequency of oscillations is inactivated by inhibition of NO even when mGLUR channels remain active.

1.7.6 Intercellular propagation of calcium waves in astrocytes

Astrocytes have the ability to process a wide range of synaptic information through their *syncytium*, i.e., a network of astrocytes connected by gap junctions. There are suggestions based on a study made in the optic nerve indicating that the strengths of the connections in the syncytium are dynamically regulated by neuronal activity [159]. Astrocytes *in vivo* express *connexin* CX43 localized at gap junctions between processes near the soma, dendritic, and synaptic glomeruli (capillaries that filter waste products) [159]. When astrocytes are working together in a network, they influence each other through intercellular calcium waves or possibly by ATP released into the extracellular space.

Intercellular calcium waves can propagate through nonlinear gap junctions. Gap junctions are the channel by which two non-physically connected cells are able to interchange molecules and proteins. There are two main mechanisms through which the propagation of intercellular calcium waves occur. One is by the diffusion of IP3 molecules from one astrocytic cell to another astrocytic cell through gap junctions [160]. This diffusion causes activation of IP3 channels in the *cytosol* of the cell, thus inducing calcium release through the IP3R channels. A second mechanism found is by the diffusion of ATP in the extracellular space binding plasma receptors and causing the regulation of IP3 production in nearby cells. These two mechanisms are not necessarily mutually exclusive.

It is noteworthy to mention that gap junctions are shared between astrocyte–astrocyte cells as well as astrocyte–oligodendrocyte cells [161]. Oligodendrocyte cells are a subtype of glial cells, known for their role in axon myelination. This represents another complex form of communication by which astrocytes may be able to influence neuronal responses in an indirect manner.

1.7.7 Integration of synaptic information

Glial cells have been proposed as suitable cells for the implementation of information routing mechanisms [162]. The routing of information requires mechanisms that allow astrocytes to modify the strength of a group of synapses which do not necessarily share the same presynaptic and postsynaptic neurons. Some types of interneurons in the cortex [163] only target the axon hillock and are able to deactivate communication between thousands of synapses connected to the neuron by merely inhibiting the neuron through the axon hillock. Some types of neurons in the cortex preferably target the dendritic tree near the soma of their postsynaptic neuron which allows them to modulate a wide number of synapses of the same dendritic tree homogeneously. However, for information routing, selectivity is required. We need to control the synaptic efficacy of a subset of synapses even if they belong to the same dendritic tree. This requires a mechanism which does not modulate synapses in an homogeneous manner. Möller *et al* proposed the astrocyte to play a role in attentional mechanisms, due to the astrocyte's capability to autonomously modulate synapses at different microdomains [162].

Pereira [164] offers theoretical insights for the behavior of a single astrocyte interacting with a group of neurons with aims to explain possible contributions to astrocytes in the conscious binding process. An astrocyte surrounded by a group of neurons is defined as a 'local hub', while an astrocytic network interacting with a group of neurons is described as a 'master hub'.

In a 'master hub', 'local hubs' can interact with each other by means of propagating their calcium waves through gap junctions to combine synaptic information from different 'local hubs'. The 'master hub' can be viewed as a global work space that integrates information from many local neurons to a brain-wide network []. Two mechanisms for the contribution to the formation of the intercellular calcium wave were defined, the 'domino effect' and the 'carousel effect'.

The 'domino effect' is based on previous experimental findings that calcium waves elicit nonlinear saltatory (leaping) behavior; it states that the waves in astrocytes' syncytium may propagate like an effect of domino pieces that fall after another, where in a small group of these dominoes the last piece may fall almost simultaneously with the first piece. For conscious binding, this process is very important, since the binding of information should happen quickly. The 'domino effect' may represent the ATP signaling between astrocyte cells.

The 'carousel effect' is used to describe the possible role of synchronized neurons in the generation of intercellular calcium waves. In this putative (commonly accepted) description, neurons that are synchronized coordinate calcium waves in different microdomains in astrocytic syncytia. Each calcium wave in a different microdomain would be analogous to a horse in the carousel, while the movement of the carousel will be orchestrated by the synchronized neurons. The astrocytes' feedback is to the synchronized neurons, strengthening or weakening the neurons. Pererira *et al* have also defined a theoretical calcium wave model of the perception action cycle [165].

1.7.8 Retrograde signaling

Traditionally, neurotransmission has been thought to be a unidirectional process with information being communicated from the presynaptic neuron to the post-synaptic neuron. However *retrograde* messengers have been found that allow communication in the opposite direction, from postsynaptic to presynaptic neuron [166, 167]. Retrograde messengers are released from postsynaptic neurons and travel in a 'backwards' direction to activate presynaptic receptors, ultimately influencing presynaptic neurotransmitter release. Signaling by retrograde messengers has been implicated in forms of synaptic plasticity and neuroprotection [168]. Neurotransmission effects of retrograde messengers have been found to be related to both neurons and astrocytes [168, 169]. In regard to fault-tolerance, recent computational studies have demonstrated that retrograde signaling could be used to initiate self-repair in neuron-astrocyte networks [170, 171].

In light of these new findings, it would be worthwhile to create neuromorphic systems that include models for astrocytic mechanisms and retrograde signaling. These mechanisms could give neuromorphic circuits extra functionalities that cannot be achieved by networks formed using only neurons.

1.7.9 Homeostatic plasticity

Homeostatic plasticity, or synaptic scaling, refers to plasticity mechanisms that potentiate or depress all of a neuron's synapses in order to maintain stable firing rates. In contrast to Hebbian plasticity, which selectively modulates weights based on the activity of individual synapses, homeostatic plasticity induces global changes over multiple synapses.

In excitatory networks, homeostatic plasticity can be used to prevent runaway excitation caused by Hebbian plasticity by globally depressing synapses once neural activity reaches an activity set point. The effects are illustrated by the cartoon in figure 1.23. Correlated presynaptic and postsynaptic activity potentiates synapses by Hebbian mechanisms. In turn, increased synapse strengths may generate more activity between correlated neurons, creating a positive feedback loop (figure 1.23(a)). Unconstrained potentiation can eventually lead to a loss in synapse specificity of a neuron (figure 1.23(b)). After one synapse experiences LTP, the postsynaptic neuron is driven more strongly, making it easier for the neuron to fire. This could lead to LTP of other synapses that should not be potentiated. Figure 1.23(c) shows what could happen if synaptic scaling is used. The left figure shows the original weight configuration and desired firing rate of the output neuron. In the middle figure, the middle synapse is potentiated by LTP, leading to an increase in output neural activity. In response to increased activity, homeostatic plasticity mechanisms depress all synapses so that a stable firing rate is maintained (right figure). The weight of the middle synapse is still larger than the other synapses, preserving input specificity.

In biology, demonstrations of homeostatic plasticity have been found in the visual and auditory systems [172, 173]. During early stages of postnatal development in the visual cortex, synaptogenesis and the number of synaptic connections is high. It has

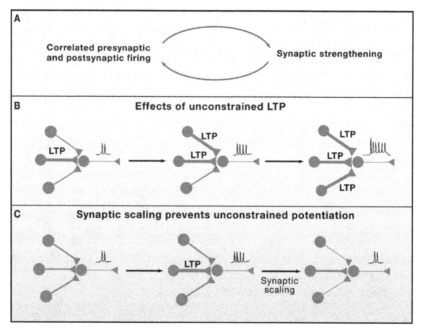

Figure 1.23. Homeostatic plasticity can prevent runaway excitation. Reprinted from [172], copyright (2008), with permission from Elsevier.

been found that there is an inverse relationship between mESPC (miniature excitatory postsynaptic current) frequency and amplitude. Furthermore, this type of relationship does not exist when animals are raised in the dark. These findings suggest that when visual drive and mESPC frequency increase, synaptic strengths are decreased to lower neural firing rates.

Homeostatic plasticity can also be used to increase synaptic strengths when neural activity is too low. It has been found that AMPA-silent synapses are transiently unsilenced following periods of inactivity [174]. After minutes of inactivity, AMPARs move in to the synapse membrane, effectively increasing the synaptic weight. It has also been demonstrated that neurons in the postnatal visual cortex exhibit homeostatic behavior through increased responses following inactivation of the optic nerve over a time period of 2 days [175]. Interestingly, the effects were reversed after vision was restored.

Activity thresholds for homeostatic plasticity have been found to vary over developmental stages. For example, layer 4 cortical neurons respond homeostatically during early development [175]. At later stages of the visual system critical period, homeostatic responses in layer 4 neurons are turned off and moved into layers 2 and 3. In layers 2 and 3, the responses were shown to persist into adulthood [172, 176]. It was hypothesized that homeostatic plasticity in layer 4 neurons were switched off because homeostasis responses to sensory deprivation in adults would amplify noise in layer 4 neurons, an undesirable effect. Layer 2 and 3 neurons, on the other hand, receive many lateral and feedback connections from other areas in the cortex. Switching on homeostatic plasticity in these neurons during adulthood could encourage remapping of cortical areas deprived of sensory drive. Areas that receive low levels of sensory input activity could be taken over by areas with intact sensory drive, increasing the signal processing efficiency of intact regions.

1.8 The retina

The retina pre-processes visual information with millions of neurons and glial cells, and with billions of synapses[23,24]. Motion sensing in particular is found in some vertebrate retinas. There are at least 50 distinct cell types that have been found. The retinal neurons are arranged in three cellular layers (i.e. outer nuclear layer, inner nuclear layer, and retinal ganglion cell layer) and are interconnected in the intervening two synaptic layers (i.e. outer plexiform layer and inner plexiform layer). The outer plexiform layer is a layer of neuronal synapses that consists of a dense network of synapses between dendrites of horizontal cells, bipolar cells (from the inner nuclear layer), and photoreceptor cell inner segments (from the outer nuclear layer). The inner plexiform layer is a layer of neural synapses consisting of a dense reticulum of fibrils formed by interlaced dendrites of retinal ganglion cells, bipolar cells, and amacrine cells.

Lateral communications formed by the amacrine cells and horizontal cells are noteworthy because they increase connectivity significantly. The feedback and lateral communications found in these two layers are believed to be important to modulate the responses of the retinal network in order to perform some essential functions. For instance, the existence of lateral connections helps to employ center-surround antagonism in the ganglion cell's receptive field that may sharpen the image in time and space. Neuroscientists have found another example in which starburst amacrine cells (SACs) in the vertebrate retina (such as the rabbit's retina) perform the neural computations that induce directional selectivity in the ganglion cell. Other functions such as differential motion detection have also been observed in the vertebrate retina [178]. To perform these functions, the feedback and lateral signaling pathways play important roles.

The retina is a complex multi-layered neural tissue consisting of many neurons interconnected by synapses and located in the back of the eye. In mammalian retinas, the output is conveyed to the brain by about 15 different retinal ganglion cell (RGC) types.

Light is first absorbed by photoreceptors and then converted into electrical signals, namely graded potentials. There are two main types of photoreceptors in the retina: rods and cones. Compared to the rod cells, the cone cells are less sensitive to light, but allow the perception of color. Furthermore, the cone cells become sparser towards the periphery of the retina while the rod cells become denser towards the periphery of the retina. Horizontal cells that synapse with the photoreceptor cells can facilitate the communication between photoreceptors. Horizontal cells are

---

[23] This section supports the material found in chapter 12, and should be read prior to reading that chapter.
[24] This information comes from Tseng's thesis [171].

believed to play a key role in forming center-surround antagonism, which enables edge detection and contrast enhancement. The signals from photoreceptor cells and horizontal cells are relayed by bipolar cells through which they reach amacrine cells and ganglion cells. There are about 40 different types of amacrine cells in the retina. They work laterally affecting other amacrine cells, bipolar cells, and ganglion cells. It is widely accepted that amacrine cells perform more specialized tasks than horizontal cells. The retinal signals from bipolar cells and amacrine cells reach ganglion cells which convert graded potentials into APs, namely spikes. Some neuroscientists believe that each ganglion cell type computes rather differently, based on the contents of the visual scene [178]. Lastly, the spikes from retinal ganglion axons forming the optic nerve are delivered to the visual cortex. Besides these retinal cells, retinal glial cells spanning the entire thickness of the retinal layers may modulate the electrical activity of neurons within the retina [179, 180]. There are three basic types of glial cells found in the human retina: Müller, astroglia, and microglia cells [181]. Conventionally, Müller cells are the principal glial cell of the retina and are believed to be vital to the health of the retinal neurons [181, 182]. A two-way communication between retinal neurons and glial cells may exist and suggest that the glia contributes to information processing in the retina [183]. For the basic structure of a retina, please refer to figure 1.24 that shows the organization of the principal retinal cells.

Figure 1.25 illustrates the major pathways of principle retinal cells. As described previously, photoreceptors and horizontal cells form reciprocal synapses that help to increase the dynamic range of photoreceptors and to perform many functions such as contrast enhancement and center-surround antagonism. The channels between horizontal cells are confirmed to be gap junctions that facilitate the communication across different horizontal cells. The pathway from horizontal cell to bipolar cell may be weak [185]. Bipolar cells relay the signal from photoreceptors to amacrine cells, as well as to retinal ganglion cells. They may also receive feedback from amacrine cells. Similar to horizontal cells, reciprocal synapses between amacrine cells are also identified. They may be electrical synapses or chemical synapses. Ganglion cells may synapse with amacrine cells as well as bipolar cells, and then convert the graded potentials into APs, namely spikes. Müller cells can influence the response of retinal cells [186]. Note that figure 1.25 only illustrates the principal neurons of the retina that we will discuss in the following sections.

1.8.1 The outer retina

In the outer retina, the photoreceptors absorb photons and convert them into electrical signals that modulate the release of glutamate from photoreceptor ribbon synapses. The horizontal cells (HCs) receive the glutamate released from photo-receptors and provide feedback to the photoreceptors. The feedback from the horizontal cells to the photoreceptor cells helps to ensure the transmission of sensory patterns with proper contrast, modulates the dynamic range of retinal cells' responses, and enhances spatial contrast in the retina [187]. Three synaptic mechanisms have been proposed to explain the underlying mechanisms for the

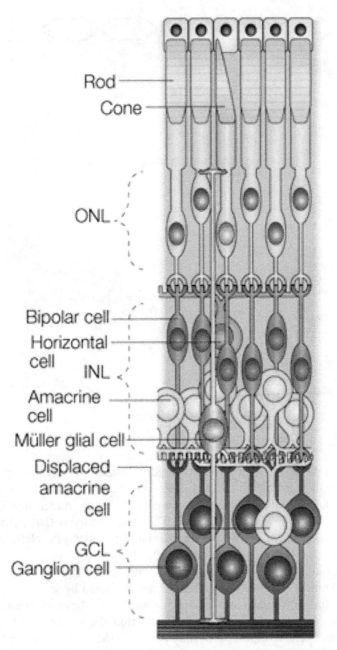

Rod

Cone

ONL

Bipolar cell

Horizontal cell

INL

Amacrine cell

Müller glial cell

Displaced amacrine cell

GCL

Ganglion cell

Figure 1.24. A cross-sectional view of a biological retina. Reprinted from [184], with permission of Springer Nature.

feedback [188]. The first mechanism is that HCs release the inhibitory GABA neurotransmitter in darkness, which opens chloride channels in cones. When a light stimulus hyperpolarizes the HCs, HCs release less GABA neurotransmitter, which suppresses feedback transmitter release and depolarizes the cones [189, 190]. The

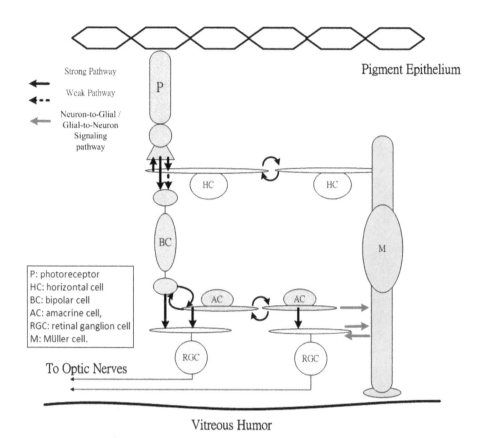

Figure 1.25. Retinal circuitry showing major pathways [177].

second theory is that a light stimulus hyperpolarizes HCs, resulting in an inward current through hemichannels in their dendrites near the cones, charging the cone membrane and modulating calcium currents in cones, increasing their calcium-dependent glutamate release [191, 192]. The third theory is that light-induced HC hyperpolarization elevates the pH in the HC-cone synaptic cleft, leading to an increase in calcium current in the cones [193, 194].

The horizontal cells may communicate with their neighboring horizontal cells through gap junctions whose permabilities are mediated by some neurotransmitters [195]. Both the photoreceptors and horizontal cells have connections with the bipolar cells. However, neuroscientists found that the strength of the connections from horizontal cells to bipolar cells may be weak [185]. Thus, the feedback from the horizontal cells to the photoreceptors that regulates the responses of photoreceptors is believed to play the more important role in producing some important computations observed in bipolar cells. Due to the lateral communications between the horizontal cells and the feedback from the horizontal cells to photoreceptor cells, the outer retina is, therefore, considered the start of the center-surround mechanism in the whole visual system. Eventually, the visual information is relayed by the bipolar cells and sent to the inner retina.

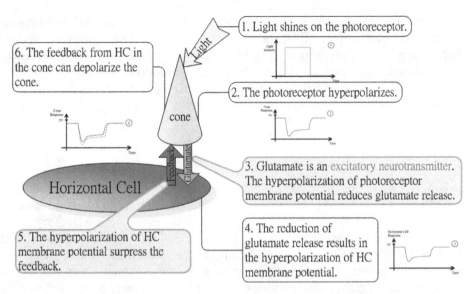

Figure 1.26. Functional diagram of the interaction between cone and horizontal cell [177].

We show the interaction between the photoreceptors and horizontal cells in figure 1.26. In a biological retina, one horizontal cell can synapse with multiple photoreceptors in the retina. But, we only show one photoreceptor, which is a cone, in figure 1.26. When the photon enters the retina, it is first absorbed by the photoreceptor. The photoreceptor converts the light into electrical signals, i.e. the photo transduction process. During the resting state, the photoreceptor releases glutamate tonically. Hyperpolarization of the photoreceptor will reduce the release of glutamate, which is an excitatory neurotransmitter. Since the horizontal cell receives less excitation from the photoreceptors through ribbon synapses, the horizontal cell, therefore, hyperpolarizes as well. Hyperpolarization of the horizontal cell provides an inhibition to the photoreceptor as a net effect. The overall interaction is analogous to providing negative feedback from the horizontal cell to the photoreceptors.

A positive feedback synapse from horizontal cells to cone photoreceptors has recently been found in the outer retina [196]. Unlike the negative feedback that spreads throughout a horizontal cell to affect many surrounding photoreceptors, the positive feedback signal is constrained to individual horizontal cell-photoreceptor connections. The positive feedback locally offsets the effects of negative feedback and amplifies photoreceptor synaptic release without sacrificing HC-mediated contrast enhancement.

1.8.2 The inner retina

The inner retina is believed to be the place where retinal motion detection originates. The bipolar cell relays the visual information from the outer retina and sends it to the amacrine cells and ganglion cells. In the inner retina, multiple feedback pathways have been identified recently between amacrine cells [197] and between amacrine cells and bipolar cells [198, 199]. With these feedback pathways and the collaboration of diverse retinal cell types, the inner retina may perform various retinal computations such as differential motion detection [200, 201], directional selectivity [202, 203], approaching motion detection [204], and others. In addition to the feedback, lateral communication also contributes to regulating the responses of other retinal cells [205]. We will describe two functions in this section: directional selectivity and differential motion detection.

1.8.2.1 Directional selectivity

The SAC, found in the mammalian retina, with a characteristic radially symmetric morphology, is thought to provide directional inhibitory input to direction-selective ganglion cells (DSGCs) [206–208]. The computation of directional selectivity occurs at individual dendritic branches of each SAC and each dendritic branch acts as an independent computation module [209]. Both the dendritic calcium signal and membrane voltage in the dendritic tip may generate a stronger response by the stimuli moving from the soma towards the dendritic tip (namely centrifugal motion) than moving the opposite direction (namely centripetal motion) [209]. To explain the directional selectivity observed in the SACs, neuroscientists have proposed at least two fundamentally different mechanisms [210]: dendrite-intrinsic electrotonics [211, 212] and lateral inhibition [202, 213]. Euler *et al* demonstrated that the intrinsic electrical mechanisms of SACs may produce directional selectivity without inhibitory network interactions [210]. Further, the lateral inhibition between two SACs may enhance the difference in response and generate a robust directional selectivity [202]. SACs may receive glutamate release from bipolar cells (BCs). Furthermore, the dendritic tip may release and receive GABA neurotransmitter. Euler *et al* observed a weak directional selectivity at the soma but a strong directional selectivity in the dendritic tips [209]. They also found that SACs may have directional responses even if GABA inhibitory interactions between the SACs are blocked pharmacologically [209]. Their results suggest directional selectivity in the starburst cell arises intrinsically from its distinctive morphology. A centrifugal motion generates an in-phase response which can be summed effectively with the response in the distal compartment. However, centripetal motion generates an out-of-phase response that cannot be summed effectively with the response in the distal compartment. Hence, a SAC produces a stronger response in the distal tip with respect to centrifugal motion. The lateral inhibition between two overlapping SACs may make the directional selectivity response more robust [202]. The distal dendrite of SACs may release GABA neurotransmitters and GABA receptors are also found in the SAC dendrites. Therefore, as long as the processes of two neighboring starburst cells overlap, they are likely to form reciprocal connections. The reciprocal synapse that forms a positive feedback loop can enhance the difference in response between the two SACs. The interactions between SACs are illustrated in figure 1.27. When the light moves to BC2, the distal dendrite of SAC1 produces a voltage response and releases more GABA, which inhibits the response of distal dendrites in

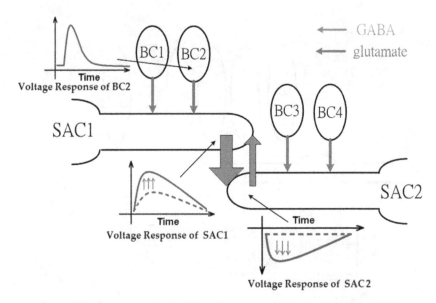

Figure 1.27. The reciprocal interactions between two branches of the SACs [177].

SAC2. SAC2 in turn produces less GABA release, which enhances the response of the distal dendrite in SAC1.

Although SACs play an important role in producing directional selectivity, the actual directional selectivity output in the retina is at directional selectivity GCs. Signaling between the bipolar cell, SAC, and directional selectivity GC constitutes a neural network that generates the directional selectivity light responses of the directional selectivity GC [214], as shown in figure 1.28. The glutamate released from the BC is an excitatory neurotransmitter to the directional selectivity GC while the GABA released from SAC is an inhibitory neurotransmitter to the directional selectivity GC. Due to a strong response of SAC1 that induces more GABA release, the directional selectivity GC is being more strongly inhibited from firing. In the example shown in figure 1.28, the directional selectivity GC synapses with BC2 and SAC1. The light stimulus moving from BC1 to BC2 evokes a larger response at the distal tip of SAC1 that cancels out the excitatory input from BC2 and inhibits the directional selectivity GC from firing. If the light stimulus moves from BC2 to BC1, SAC1 does not provide enough inhibitory input to directional selectivity GC. Hence, the directional selectivity GC fires.

1.8.2.2 Saccadic suppression/object motion detection
Large retinal shifts such as saccadic eye movements of humans and other animals may cause great excitation across the entire retina. These eye movements can be surprisingly large, up to 0.5° in amplitude (the width of the full moon) and up to 1° per second. However, humans do not perceptually report this effect. Although the brain-motor command may suppress the perception of saccadic eye movements, research results suggest that retinal motion alone is sufficient to produce this perceptual suppression [215]. Certain retinal ganglion cells are strongly inhibited

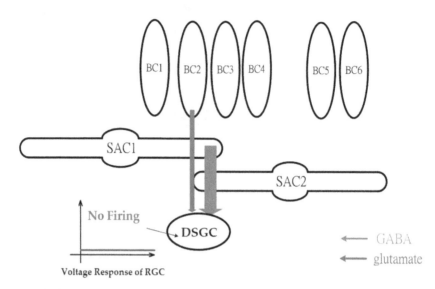

Figure 1.28. The interaction of a direction-selective ganglion cell (DSGC) with bipolar cells and SACs [177].

with brief, well-timed inhibition during saccades [216]. The mechanisms that suppress the visual effects of eye movements are found in the inner retina.

An object-motion-sensitivity ganglion cell remains silent under global motion of the entire image but fires when the image patch in its receptive field moves differently from the background [200, 201]. Object-motion-sensitivity ganglion cells meet two seemingly conflicting requirements: they are highly tuned to a condition of differential motion between the receptive field center and the surround, but at the same time remarkably insensitive to the actual visual pattern in the center or the surround. The polyaxonal amacrine cell appears to be a plausible candidate to transmit inhibition from the background region [200]. The inhibition signal may derive from amacrine cells that inhibit the bipolar cell synaptic terminal, close to the site of transmission but at some electrotonic distance from the soma. Only the polyaxonal amacrine cells have the response properties required to implement inhibition from global motion. The underlying retinal circuitry for performing differential motion detection is shown in figure 1.29. The visual inputs from the peripheral and central receptive fields are relayed by the bipolar cells (BC). The amacrine cell (AC) delivers timed inhibition from the peripheral receptive field to suppress the responses of central bipolar cell terminals. The object-motion-sensitivity ganglion cell (OMS) synapses with the bipolar cells of the central receptive field. An object-motion-sensitivity (OMS) ganglion cell remains silent under global motion of the entire receptive field but fires when the image patch in the peripheral receptive field moves differently from the central receptive field. Moreover, the underlying retinal circuitry compares only the speed of motion of the object and the background, not the direction. Both object motion sensitivity and saccadic suppression involving timed inhibition from globally correlated shifting stimuli may share common circuitry.

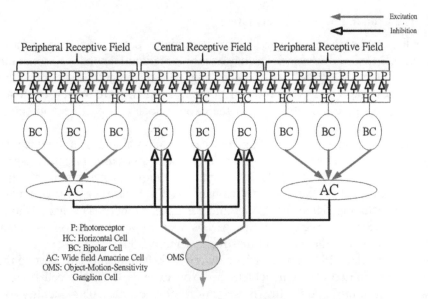

Figure 1.29. The underlying retinal circuitry for performing differential motion detection and saccadic suppression [177].

A dissertation covering many neuromorphic retinal circuits was written by Tseng, based on retinal designs he produced, and is summarized and referenced later in chapter 12.

1.9 The neural code

This section supports the material found in chapter 5, and should be read prior to reading that chapter.

Most biological neurons fire by emitting several closely-spaced spikes or a burst of spikes when input stimulation is sufficient to cause spiking. The biological mechanism behind a neural spike is well understood [217]. Bursts of spikes or higher-frequency spike trains are more likely to result in relaying sensory inputs to the cortex than lower-frequency trains [218]. For example, neurons in the visual cortex respond with varying frequency when there is a detection of an edge at a particular orientation [219], depending on the contrast of the edge.

Spiking neurons can be classified into many types [220]. Neurons can emit single spikes, spike trains or bursts of spikes. Many neurons are either all-or-nothing spiking neurons or exhibit spiking frequency increase as the somatic membrane potential increases. A recent publication [221] describes neurons in the somatosensory cortex that are classified as either regular spiking (RS) pyramidal or fast spiking (FS) interneurons. RS neurons have a higher spiking rate from the onset of spiking and settle down to a base frequency, whereas FS cells have a high frequency from onset itself, and cease spiking completely when the cell membrane potential drops below a critical threshold.

More on spiking neuron types can be found later in this section, in chapters 4 and 13 and in other BioRC dissertations, including [2, 104, 222].

1.9.1 The axon initial segment definition

As we discussed earlier, biological neurons are highly polarized cells in terms of the direction of signal flow, by which they ensure directional signaling throughout the mammalian CNS. They do that by converting the received graded synaptic inputs at the dendrites and soma (somatodendritic compartment) into APs. The generated APs then propagate reliably through the axon hillock compartment to signal the targeted postsynaptic neurons [223].

Superior to the classical view that describes the axon hillock as a reliable medium for the initiation and propagation of the AP to the postsynaptic targets, the physical and geometrical properties of the axon, and the unique properties of the reported ions channels at the axon initial segment (AIS), determines various complex behaviors, including signal processing and timing of numerous events in the brain. The highly excitable region of the AIS is located at the region between the somatodendritic and the axon compartments (figure 1.30).

On average, the AIS location varies between 20–60 μm distance relative to the cell body for myelinated axons in which the axon extends from the cell body. This physical separation allows the preservation of the molecular identity of the somatodendritic and axon compartments. **Therefore, knowing where the spikes are initiated is crucial to understand how different graded synaptic inputs are converted to different action potential patterns.**

In cortical neurons, the initiation (sudden rise) of AP occurs at the AIS because the AP generation threshold is lowest in this region compared to the somatodendritic and axon compartments [44, 225, 226]. Several reasons explain why the threshold required for the AP initiation at the AIS is lowest. First, the AIS diameter is an order of magnitude smaller than the soma, which implies a smaller characteristic capacitance; thus, a less inward current is required to provoke APs [224]. Second, there is a higher density of voltage-gated ion channels per unit area than at the soma, specifically, the low threshold voltage-gated ion channels [225]. The voltage-gated ion channels reported at the AIS site include **voltage-gated sodium channels** (Na_V) and **voltage-gated potassium channels** (K_V).

1.9.2 Voltage gated ion channels at the AIS

Voltage-gated ion channels are distributed into specific neuron locations to perform specific functions. Hence, inaccurate distribution of the voltage-gated ion channels can cause a deficiency in the neural network. Therefore, investigating each type of voltage-gated ion channel and its role in neural signaling is crucial in understanding how neurons encode and transfer information [227].

The Na_V channels are the main ion channels responsible for generating the inward current. There are four subtypes of the Na_V channels found throughout the CNS ($Na_V1.1$, $Na_V1.2$, $Na_V1.3$, $Na_V1.6$), however, the main Na_V subtype that can be found at the AIS region is the $Na_V1.6$ at a distal location from the soma [228, 229]. On the other hand, the $Na_V1.1$ and $Na_V1.2$ target in mainly a cell-type-specific manner and can be clustered at a proximal distance from the soma [230, 231]. The Na_V channels found at the AIS are specialized and have different properties compared to those found

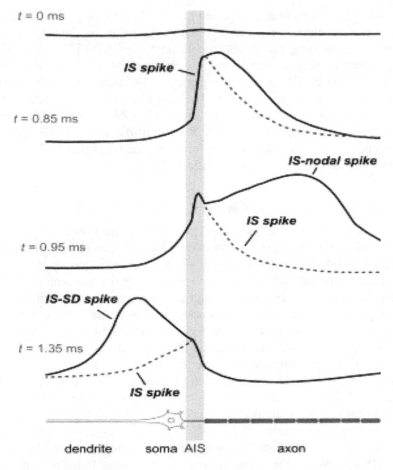

Figure 1.30. A graphical representation of the voltage-space distribution for a generated AP in pyramidal neurons (adopted from [224], copyright (2012), with permission from Elsevier). SD and IS represent the somatodendritic and the axon initial segment regions, respectively. The dotted line shows the voltage-space distribution without the Na^+ ion channels in the nodal region ($t = 0.85$ ms and $t = 0.95$ ms) and the somatodendritic region ($t = 1.35$ ms).

in the somatodendritic compartment in which they control the neuronal firing properties. For example, the Na_V channels expressed at the AIS region have an activation/deactivation threshold voltage of 0 mV lower than those at the somatodendritic compartment [230, 232]. Interestingly, the Na_V located at the AIS of the Granule cells (found in the granular layer of the cerebellum) can be activated/deactivated by a factor of two times the speed of those located at the soma [233]. Moreover, in some cases, researchers studying the Na_V at the AIS region have reported some capabilities of not undergoing a complete deactivation phase, leading to the generation of the persistent Na current. Such current contributes to the generation of higher frequency APs (burst generation); therefore, the Na_V channels found at the AIS contribute mainly to lowering the neural threshold, and consequently, increase excitability.

Another type of ion channel reported at the AIS is the K_V ion channel. The K_V channels play a significant role in shaping APs due to their lower threshold activation and shunting properties (repolarization of APs) [234, 235]. Moreover, the K_V channels play a significant role in modulating the neural thresholds, interspike time intervals, and the frequency of the generated APs patterns. The main type of K_V channels is the K_V1. The K_V1 channels, in particular, have a fast activation time, yet slower deactivation time [235, 236]. Such properties lead to the conclusion that the K_V1 at the AIS is responsible for the AP repolarization independently of the somatic AP waveform and the transmitter release regulation at the synaptic terminals of the axon hillock [235].

1.9.3 Dynamical neural modulation and signal processing at the AIS

With the advances in the electrical and optical recording methods used in experimental neuroscience, recent discoveries have suggested that the AIS's role is more complicated than being a trigger site for AP initiation. It is also a site of complex neural modulation and adaptive neural signal processing [225, 237, 238]. Such capabilities can be realized through the AIS's *structural plasticity*. The term *structural plasticity* describes the continuous physical changes of the AIS length and location relative to the soma in an activity-dependent manner. Therefore, the AIS is the site of neural structural plasticity, and neuronal activity regulation [239, 240] by which the AIS governs the dynamical neural signal processing.

Structurally, the AIS length and location relative to the soma vary with neural activities [241]. This structural plasticity of the AIS is capable of altering neuronal excitability through slow adaptation processes. With such variations, for example, neurons in the avian nucleus laminaris (NL) pathway can adapt to particular frequencies during sound localization processes because the length and the location of the AIS relative to the soma vary with the tuning frequency (characteristic frequency (CF)) of the neuron. In other words, the shorter the AIS and more distal from the soma in a neuron, the higher the tuning frequency of that neuron because at a distal location, the AIS has a smaller shunting conductance of the K_V ion channels, and the loading effect of the somatodendritic compartment is reduced at further distances from the soma [242, 243]. In contrast, the neuron's excitability is reduced and the odds of spiking reduced when the AIS is located distally from the soma because of the increase in charge dissipation along the AIS region. Thus, the AP's depolarization becomes more difficult, especially in the presence of the shunting conductance of the K_V ion channels.

Therefore, the negative correlation between length and the location of the AIS can maximize excitability. Also, the unique structural property of the AIS allows the nucleus laminaris neurons to interpret and respond accurately to their synaptic inputs at the desired characteristic frequency; hence, ensuring a precise calculation of the inter-aural time difference (ITD) between the two ears in the mammalian against a wide range of sound frequencies [244]. For example, in figure 1.31(A), the AIS's elongation and the replacement of K_V1 with K_V7 cause an increase in the neuron's excitability. Such structural elongation requires 3–7 days to take place. Another

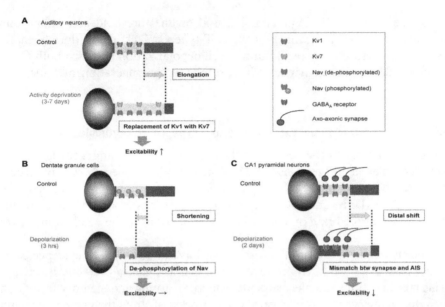

Figure 1.31. Structural and biophysical interaction during axon initial segment (AIS) plasticity (adopted from [245] CC BY 4.0). (A) shows the effect of the AIS elongation in NL neurons. (B) represents the effect on depolarizing the hippocampal dentate granule cells for 3 hours, that shortens the AIS. (C) shows a depolarization effect for two days on the pyramidal neurons that causes the AIS to move distally, yet the axo-axonic synapses remain at the original location, boosting the suppressive effects of distal movement on excitability.

example of the AIS structural plasticity can be shown in figure 1.31(C), where the further the AIS location is relative to the soma, the less excitable the neuron is. Such change in location can take place within two days period.

Moreover, in cortical and hippocampal regions, the AIS is the only targeted site for the Chandelier cells (a specialized type of GABAergic interneurons known for their remarkable precision in targeting only the AIS of pyramidal neurons) [246]. Interestingly, they have peculiar morphological characteristics by which they form their synaptic connections with the AIS of pyramidal neurons symmetrically; hence, they are referred to as axo-axonic cells.

Therefore, the Chandelier cells can directly modulate the AP's generation of the excitatory neurons through the axo-axenic synapses located at the AIS region of the targeted neurons [247, 248], and synchronize neural activities [249] (figure 1.31).

1.9.4 Bursting through calcium ion channels

In addition, the intracellular Ca^{2+} mechanism plays a significant role in neural signaling, where this mechanism increases the neural firing rate (burst generation) [250]. Bursting APs can be generated externally throughout a network of neurons to generate rhythmic motor patterns [251], such as the neurons found in the central pattern generator (CPG) [252], or intrinsically using voltage-gated calcium channels (Ca_V). In general, Ca_V channels can be categorized into high-voltage (HVA) and low-voltage activated (LVA) channels based on the threshold activation voltage. The activation of HVA channels, such as T-type Ca^{2+} channels, during small cell depolarization causes a more substantial cell depolarization at which both Ca_V and Na_V channels become activated, which results in the generation of bursting APs [253].

1.9.5 Astrocytes roles in neural signaling and synaptic strengthening

Glial cells, such as astrocytes, are critical to neural signaling and contribute to various complex neural responses [254]. Astrocytes have been shown to participate in neural activity modulation for a specific neural network within a specific region in the brain [255]. Thus, understanding astrocyte's roles is crucial when simulating a specific region of the brain or simulating the oscillations of the whole-brain rhythms [256].

In recent years, laboratory neuroscientists have revealed much evidence suggesting that astrocytes are far more involved in **neural signal processing, learning, and storing memory**. For example, astrocytes support learning and memory formation by which they influence synaptic plasticity, the process of strengthening or weakening a synaptic connection between two neurons [256, 257]. Besides, astrocytes improve the synchronization of neural activity at hippocampal CA1 neurons [129]. Moreover, several proposed hypotheses suggest that astrocytes store memory by the organization of their ion channels [258], promote motor skills learning [259], and can modulate other cognitive processes [260].

Long-term synaptic plasticity is a widely accepted concept in neuroscience that correlates cellular changes with learning and memory [261]. In general, there are two types of long-term plasticity. First, LTP, the process by which the synaptic connection between a presynaptic neuron to a postsynaptic neuron is strengthened, resulting in a larger induced EPSP at the latter's dendrite. Second, LTD, is the process by which the synaptic connection between a presynaptic neuron to a postsynaptic neuron is weakened, resulting in a decreased induced EPSP at the latter's dendrite [262, 263]. Several protocols are associated with the formation of LTP and LTD, including: (1) repeated presynaptic stimulus-based plasticity where individual synapse strengthening depends on the rate of the presynaptic AP from the presynaptic neuron; and (2) precise spikes timing of presynaptic and postsynaptic-based plasticity, also known as STDP [12, 264].

The astrocyte plays a role in synaptic plasticity. When an intrinsic AP reaches the presynaptic terminal, the voltage-gated Ca^{2+} channels open to allow the influx of Ca^{2+}. The influx of Ca^{2+} causes the synaptic vesicles to fuse with the presynaptic neuron's membrane (exocytosis) to release neurotransmitters (NTs) into the synaptic cleft. Consequently, the released NTs diffuse to the postsynaptic terminal. At the same time, the astrocyte senses the released NT at the synaptic cleft using particular NT receptor types, resulting in intrinsic astrocytic Ca^{2+} oscillations within the astrocyte. The intrinsic astrocytic Ca^{2+} oscillations then cause chemical substances to be released back to the presynaptic terminal, thus, creating a *controlled positive feedback* signaling between the presynaptic neuron and the astrocyte. In particular, this communication protocol is governed by the release of glutamate NT from the astrocyte to the presynaptic terminal, that eventually increases the Ca^{2+} influx of the presynaptic neuron by which synaptic connection is strengthened.

1.10 Chapter conclusions and future thoughts

This chapter introduced the concept of neuromorphic circuits, and gave an overview of a neuron and basic neuroscience helpful to understanding these circuits. While the neuron depicted here is very simple, human neurons are orders of magnitude more complex, with new research findings emerging daily. There is significant variability from neuron to neuron, and from species to species but what is stated here is predominantly the case in research findings in human neuroscience. New research results usually explain and amplify well-understood mechanisms, but can uncover more revolutionary information, like DNA–RNA–protein expression [265], that has impact on memory in biological neurons [217][25]. Furthermore, neurons are not only complex, but contributing to the complexity is that each is different. One of the most striking differences is that virtually every neuron performs gene expression slightly differently [266]. The way that DNA uses messenger RNA to synthesize proteins varies from cell to cell. One neuron might wake up *silent synapses* (dormant synapses that do not respond to stimulation) differently than another, for example. Further, during development, gene expression can cause a variety of neurons to be specialized, with different cell fates depending on the location of the neurons and other circumstances. If engineers are to build neural electronics that models the cortex, with its intelligence, memory, reasoning and problem-solving ability, mastering at least some of this complexity seems to be required, and adapting and evolving the electronics is required as research is published that clarifies, modifies and changes biological understanding. Given this complicated, active, interdisciplinary problem domain, how can an engineer construct neural circuits that model the human cortex (and other parts of the brain) for autonomous robotics, brain prosthetics and medical research? The circuits should themselves be amenable to evolution and change, as well as to extensions and modifications to add additional neural features that contribute to intelligence, reasoning and memory. A recent article discusses how motor neurons differentiate due to gene expression [267]. The text provides some hints in later chapters to illustrate how change is accomplished without altering basic structures of each circuit.

Another challenge in this research is that there remains much unknown about how the brain responds in a certain way, hence it is difficult to prove directly that a particular mechanism is both necessary and sufficient to the computational behavior in a biological neural network. In addition to the aforementioned neural complexity challenges, an engineering challenge arises: how to implement artificial dendrites

---

[25] This particular revolutionary research shows that RNA modulates gene expression performed by cellular DNA, acting more like a change agent than a simple messenger. This research is included here to give the reader a sense for how the understanding of a 'well-understood' biological mechanism can change drastically as new research results are obtained. The protein expression Kandel researched in his Nobel-prize winning research on neural synaptic strength involves this DNA–RNA–protein mechanism.

with similar complexity to the biological ones with little hardware requirement, a trade-off between biomimetic accuracy and efficiency.

Before the book introduces modern neuromorphic circuits, the next chapter gives a brief history of neuromorphic circuits, and presents challenges facing designers of neuromorphic circuits.

1.11 Exercises

1. Biological neurons signal between each other with (mark all correct answers):
   (a) Chemicals called neurotransmitters that flow in the synapses between neurons;
   (b) Electrical signals (flow of ions between neurons);
   (c) Retrograde messengers that signal from the postsynaptic neuron to the presynaptic neuron;
   (d) Graded potentials—resembling membrane potentials.
2. Dendritic spikes (mark all correct answers):
   (a) Are nonlinear responses to presynaptic spikes;
   (b) Can be caused by potassium and chloride ions;
   (c) Can be caused by NMDA channels;
   (d) Can be less likely to occur right after they have occurred.
3. Several synapses on the same dendritic branch that are excited at about the same time can cause a neuron with thousands of synapses to fire. Why?
4. An inhibitory synapse on one dendritic branch can keep any of the excitatory synapses from having an effect on the neuron. Draw a picture of the branch and a small part of the dendritic trunk, with labels to show the location of the inhibitory synapse.
5. Oligodendrocytes (mark all correct answers):
   (a) cause the spike traveling down the axon to be regenerated;
   (b) insulate the axon, speeding up the signal;
   (c) contain the nodes of Ranvier;
   (d) are glial cells.

References

[1] Spruston N 2008 Pyramidal neurons: dendritic structure and synaptic integration *Nat. Rev. Neurosci.* **9** 206–21
[2] Hsu C-C 2014 Dendritic computation and plasticity in neuromorphic circuits *PhD Thesis* University of Southern California
[3] Shepherd G M (ed) 2004 Introduction to synaptic circuits *Synaptic Organization of the Brain* vol 5 (Oxford: Oxford University Press)
[4] Blausen.com Staff 2014 *Medical gallery of Blausen Medical 2014* https://en.wikiversity.org/wiki/WikiJournal_of_Medicine/Medical_gallery_of_Blausen_Medical_2014
[5] Hensch T K 2005 Critical period plasticity in local cortical circuits *Nat. Rev. Neurosci.* **6** 877–88
[6] SynapseIllustration2 2006 URL: https://commons.wikimedia.org/wiki/File:SynapseIllustration2.png

[7] 2001 Synapses. illustrated edition *Synapses* ed W M Cowan, T C Sudhof and C F Stevens (Baltimore, MD: Johns Hopkins University Press)

[8] Sandoiu A 2020 What happens in the brain when we sleep? (MedicalNewsToday) https://www.medicalnewstoday.com/articles/what-happens-in-the-brain-when-you-sleep

[9] Neuroscience of sleep URL: https://en.wikipedia.org/wiki/Neuroscience_of_sleep

[10] Dan Y and Poo M M 2004 Spike timing-dependent plasticity of neural circuits *Neuron* **44** 23–30

[11] Kampa B M *et al* 2004 Kinetics of Mg^{2+} unblock of NMDA receptors: implications for spike-timing dependent synaptic plasticity *J. Physiol.* **556** 337–45

[12] Markram H *et al* 1997 Regulation of synaptic efficacy by coincidence of postsynaptic APs and EPSPs *Science* **275** 213–5

[13] Tsodyks M V and Markram H 1997 The neural code between neocortical pyramidal neurons depends on neurotransmitter release probability *Proc. Natl Acad. Sci.* **94** 719–23

[14] Kandel E R 2001 The molecular biology of memory storage: a dialogue between genes and synapses *Science* **294** 1030–8

[15] Connors B W and Long M A 2004 Electrical synapses in the mammalian brain *Annu. Rev. Neurosci.* **27** 393–418

[16] Behabadi B F *et al* 2012 Location-dependent excitatory synaptic interactions in pyramidal neuron dendrites *PLoS computational biology* **8** e1002599

[17] Katz Y *et al* 2009 Synapse distribution suggests a two-stage model of dendritic integration in CA1 pyramidal neurons *Neuron* **63** P171–7

[18] Nevian T *et al* 2007 Properties of basal dendrites of layer 5 pyramidal neurons: a direct patch-clamp recording study *Nat. Neurosci.* **10** 206–14

[19] Jesper P, Sjöström J and Häusser M 2006 A cooperative switch determines the sign of synaptic plasticity in distal dendrites of neocortical pyramidal neurons *Neuron* **51** 227–38

[20] Polsky A, Mel B W and Schiller J 2004 Computational subunits in thin dendrites of pyramidal cells *Nat. Neurosci.* **7** 621–7

[21] Brannon T, Poirazi P and Mel B W 2003 Pyramidal neuron as two-layer neural network *Neuron* **37** 989–99

[22] Mel B W and Schiller J 2004 On the fight between excitation and inhibition: location is everything *Sci. STKE* **250** e44

[23] Larkum M E and Nevian T 2008 Synaptic clustering by dendritic signalling mechanisms *Curr. Opin. Neurobiol.* **18** 321–31

[24] Ariav G, Polsky A and Schiller J 2003 Submillisecond precision of the input-output transformation function mediated by fast sodium dendritic spikes in basal dendrites of CA1 pyramidal neurons *J. Neurosci.* **23** 7750–8

[25] Losonczy A, Makara J K and Magee J C 2008 Compartmentalized dendritic plasticity and input feature storage in neurons *Nature* **452** 436–41

[26] Hardie J and Spruston N 2009 Synaptic depolarization is more effective than back-propagating action potentials during induction of associative long-term potentiation in hippocampal pyramidal neurons *J. Neurosci.* **29** 3233–41

[27] Holthoff K *et al* 2004 Single-shock LTD by local dendritic spikes in pyramidal neurons of mouse visual *Physiol. J.* **560** 27–36

[28] Kampa B M, Letzkus J J and Stuart G J 2007 Dendritic mechanisms controlling spike-timing-dependent synaptic plasticity *Trends Neurosci.* **30** 456–63

[29] Letzkus J J, Kampa B M and Stuart G J 2006 Learning rules for spike timing-dependent plasticity depend on dendritic synapse location *J. Neurosci.* **26** 10420–9

[30] Williams S and Atkinson S 2008 Dendritic synaptic integration in central neurons *Curr. Biol.* **18** R1045–7

[31] Stuart G, Schiller J, Schiller Y and Sakmann B 1997 Calcium action potentials restricted to distal apical dendrites of rat neocortical pyramidal neurons *J. Physiol.* **505** 605–16

[32] Larkum M E, Julius Zhu J and Sakmann B 1999 A new cellular mechanism for coupling inputs arriving at different cortical layers *Nature* **398** 338–41

[33] Kampa B M and Stuart G J 2006 Calcium spikes in basal dendrites of layer 5 pyramidal neurons during action potential bursts *J. Neurosci.* **26** 7424–32

[34] Larkum M E and Zhu J J 2002 Signaling of layer 1 and whisker-evoked Ca^{2+} and Na^{+} action potentials in distal and terminal dendrites of rat neocortical pyramidal neurons *in vitro* and *in vivo J. Neurosci.* **22** 6991–7005

[35] Schaefer A T *et al* 2003 Coincidence detection in pyramidal neurons is tuned by their dendritic branching pattern *J. Neurophysiol.* **89** 3143–54

[36] Gasparini S and Magee J C 2006 State-dependent dendritic computation in hippocampal CA1 pyramidal neurons *J. Neurosci.* **26** 2088–100

[37] Remy S, Csicsvari J and Beck H 2009 Activity-dependent control of neuronal output by local and global dendritic spike attenuation *Neuron* **61** 906–16

[38] Larkum M E *et al* 2009 Synaptic integration in tuft dendrites of layer 5 pyramidal neurons: a new unifying principle *Science (New York)* **325** 756–60

[39] Schiller J *et al* 2000 NMDA spikes in basal dendrites of cortical pyramidal neurons *Nature* **404** 285–9

[40] Polsky A, Mel B and Schiller J 2009 Encoding and decoding bursts by NMDA spikes in basal dendrites of layer 5 pyramidal neurons *The J. Neurosci.* **29** 11891–903

[41] Williams S R, Wozny C and Mitchell S J 2007 The back and forth of dendritic plasticity *Neuron* **56** P947–53

[42] Legenstein R and Maass W 2011 Branch-specific plasticity enables self-organization of nonlinear computation in single neurons *J. Neurosci.* **31** 10787–802

[43] Longtin A 1993 Stochastic resonance in neuron models *J. Stat. Phys.* **70** 309–27

[44] Mainen Z F and Sejnowski T J 1995 Reliability of spike timing in neocortical neurons *Science* **268** 1503–6

[45] Mahvash Mohammadi M 2012 Emulating variability in the behavior of artificial central neurons *PhD Thesis* University of Southern California

[46] Maye A *et al* 2007 Order in spontaneous behavior *PLoS One* **2** e443

[47] Faisal A A, Selen L P J and Wolpert D M 2008 Noise in the nervous system *Nat. Rev. Neurosci.* **9** 292–303

[48] Stein R B, Gossen E R and Jones K E 2005 Neuronal variability: noise or part of the signal? *Nat. Rev. Neurosci.* **6** 389–97

[49] King C C 1991 Fractal and chaotic dynamics in nervous systems *Prog. Neurobiol.* **36** 279–308

[50] Faure P, Kaplan D and Korn H 2000 Synaptic efficacy and the transmission of complex firing patterns between neurons *J. Neurophysiol.* **84** 3010–25

[51] Kleppe I C and Robinson H P C 2006 Correlation entropy of synaptic input-output dynamics *Phys. Rev. E Stat. Nonlin. Soft Matter Phys.* **74** 041909

[52] Calvin W H and Stevens C F 1968 Synaptic noise and other sources of randomness in motoneuron interspike intervals *J. Neurophysiol* **31** 574–87

[53] Calvin W H and Stevens C F 1967 Synaptic noise as a source of variability in the interval between action potentials *Science* **155** 842–4

[54] Diba K, Lester H A and Koch C 2004 Intrinsic noise in cultured hippocampal neurons: experiment and modeling *J. Neurosci.* **24** 9723–33

[55] Carelli P V *et al* 2005 Whole cell stochastic model reproduces the irregularities found in the membrane potential of bursting neurons *J. Neurophysiol.* **94** 1169–79

[56] Pecher C 1939 La fluctuation diexcitabilite de la fibre nerveuse *Arch Intern Physiol* **49** 129

[57] Fatt P and Katz B 1950 Some observations on biological noise *Nature* **166** 597

[58] Fatt P and Katz B 1952 Spontaneous subthreshold activity at motor nerve endings *J. Physiol. (Lond)* **117** 109

[59] Bezrukov S M and Vodyanoy I 1995 Noise-induced enhancement of signal transduction across voltage-dependent ion channels *Nature* **378** 362–4

[60] Collins J J, Imhoff T T and Grigg P 1996 Noise-enhanced information transmission in rat SA1 cutaneous mechanoreceptors via aperiodic stochastic resonance *J. Neurophysiol.* **76** 642–5

[61] Douglass J K *et al* 1993 Noise enhancement of information transfer in crayfish mechanoreceptors by stochastic resonance *Nature* **365** 6444

[62] Levin J E and Miller J P 1996 Broadband neural encoding in the cricket cercal sensory system enhanced by stochastic resonance *Nature* **380** 165–8

[63] Knight B W 1972 Dynamics of encoding in a population of neurons *J. Gen.* **59** 734–66

[64] Gerstner W 2000 Population dynamics of spiking neurons: fast transients, asynchronous states, and locking *Neural Comput.* **12** 43–89

[65] Fourcaud N and Brunel N 2002 Dynamics of the firing probability of noisy integrate-and-fire neurons *Neural Comput.* **14** 2057–110

[66] Kara P, Reinagel P and Reid R C 2000 Low response variability in simultaneously recorded retinal, thalamic, and cortical neurons *Neuron* **27** P635–46

[67] Cecchi G A *et al* 2000 Noise in neurons is message dependent *Proc. Natl Acad. Sci.* **97** 5557–61

[68] Butts D A *et al* 2007 Temporal precision in the neural code and the timescales of natural vision *Nature* **449** 92–5

[69] Ermentrout G B, Gal n R F and Urban N N 2008 Reliability, synchrony and noise *Trends Neurosci.* **31** 428–34

[70] Galan R F, Ermentrout G B and Urban N N 2008 Optimal time scale for spike-time reliability: theory, simulations and experiments *J. Neurophysiol.* **99** 277–83

[71] Manwani A 2001 Detecting and estimating signals over noisy and unreliable synapses: information-theoretic analysis *Neural Comp.* **13** 1–33

[72] Jaramillo F and Wiesenfeld K 1998 Mechanoelectrical transduction assisted by Brownian motion: a role for noise in the auditory system *Nat. Neurosci.* **1** 384–8

[73] Bialek P W 1987 Limits to sensation and perception *Annu. Rev. Biophys. Biophys. Chem.* **16** 455–78

[74] Berg H C and Purcell E M 1977 Physics of chemoreception *Biophys. J* **20** 193–219

[75] Bialek W and Setayeshgar S 2005 Physical limits to biochemical signaling *Proc. Natl Acad. Sci. USA* **102** 10040–5

[76] Barlow H B, Levick W R and Yoon R M 1971 to single quanta of light in retinal ganglion cells of the cat *Vision Res.* **11** 87–101

[77] Laughlin S B, Anderson J C, O'Carroll D and De Ruyter Van Steveninck R *et al* 2000 Coding efficiency and the metabolic cost of sensory and neural information *Information Theory and the Brain* ed R Baddeley, P Hancock and P Foldiak (Cambridge: Cambridge University Press)

[78] van Beers R J 2007 The sources of variability in saccadic eye movements *J. Neurosci.* **27** 8757–70

[79] ven Beers R J, Haggard P and Wolpert D M 2004 The role of execution noise in movement variability *J. Neurophysiol.* **91** 1050–63

[80] Conti R, Tan Y and Llano I 2004 Action potential-evoked and ryanodine-sensitive spontaneous Ca^{2+} transients at the presynaptic terminal of a developing CNS inhibitory synapse *J. Neurosci.* **24** 6946–57

[81] Destexhe A *et al* 2001 Fluctuating synaptic conductances recreate *in vivo*-like activity in neocortical neurons *Neuroscience* **107** P13–24

[82] Fellous J M *et al* 2003 Synaptic background noise controls the input–output characteristics of single cells in an *in vitro* model of *in vivo* activity *Neuroscience* **122** P811–29

[83] Lou X, Scheuss V and Schneggenburger R 2005 Allosteric modulation of the presynaptic Ca^{2+} sensor for vesicle fusion *Nature* **435** 497–502

[84] Wang S Q *et al* 2001 Ca^{2+} signalling between single L.type Ca^{2+} channels and ryanodine receptors in heart cells *Nature* **410** 592–6

[85] Koch C 1999 *Biophysics of Computation* (New York: Oxford University Press)

[86] Sulzer D and Edwards R 2000 Vesicles: equal in neurotransmitter concentration but not in volume *Neuron* **28** 5–7

[87] Wu X-S *et al* 2007 The origin of quantal size variation: vesicular glutamate concentration plays a significant role *J. Neurosci.* **27** 3046–56

[88] Bair W 1999 Spike timing in the mammalian visual system *Curr. Opin. Neurobiol.* **9** 447

[89] Stuart G J and Hausser M 2011 Dendritic coincidence detection of epsps and action potentials *Nat. Neurosci.* **4** 63

[90] Rubinstein J T 1995 Threshold fluctuations in an N sodium channel model of the node of Ranvier *Biophys. J.* **68** 779–85

[91] Faisal A A and Laughlin S B 2007 Stochastic simulations on the reliability of action potential propagation in thin axons *PLoS Comput. Biol.* **3** 783–95

[92] Faisal A A, White J A and Laughlin S B 2005 Ion-channel noise places limits on the miniaturization of the brain's wiring *Curr. Biol.* **5** 1143–9

[93] Chow C C and White J A 1996 Spontaneous action potentials due to channel fluctuations *Biophys. J.* **71** 3012–21

[94] Chklovskii D B, Mel B W and Svoboda K 2004 Cortical rewiring and information storage *Nature* **431** 782–8

[95] Verderio C *et al* 1999 Synaptogenesis in hippocampal cultures *Cell. Mol. Life Sci.* **55** 1448–62

[96] Ziv N E 2001 Recruitment of synaptic molecules during synaptogenesis *Neuroscientist* **7** 365–70

[97] Kapitsky S *et al* 2005 Recruitment of synapses in the neurosecretory process during long-term facilitation at the lobster neuromuscular junction *Neuroscience* **134** 1261–72

[98] Fiala J C *et al* 1998 Synaptogenesis via dendritic filopodia in developing hippocampal area CA1 *J. Neurosci.* **18** 8900–11

[99] Trachtenberg J T *et al* 2002 Long-term *in vivo* imaging of experience-dependent synaptic plasticity in adult cortex *Nature* **420** 788–94

[100] Cline H and Haas K 2008 The regulation of dendritic arbor development and plasticity by glutamatergic synaptic input: a review of the synaptotrophic hypothesis *Physiol. J* **586** 1509–17

[101] Engert F and Bonhoeffer T 1999 Dendritic spine changes associated with hippocampal long-term synaptic plasticity *Nature* **399** 66–70

[102] Knott G W *et al* 2006 Spine growth precedes synapse formation in the adult neocortex *in vivo Nat. Neurosci.* **9** 1117–24

[103] De Paola V *et al* 2006 Cell type-specific structural plasticity of axonal branches and boutons in the adult neocortex *Neuron* **49** P861–75

[104] Joshi J 2013 Plasticity in CMOS neuromorphic circuits *PhD Thesis* University of Southern California

[105] Antanitus D S 1998 A theory of cortical neuron-astrocyte interaction *Neuroscientist* **4** 154–9

[106] Douglas Fields R 2009 *The Other Brain: From Dementia to Schizophrenia, How New Discoveries about the Brain Are Revolutionizing Medicine and Science* (New York: Simon & Schuster) 1st edn

[107] Verkhratsky A and Butt A 2007 *Glial Neurobiology* (New York: Wiley) 1st edn

[108] Haydon P G and Carmignoto G 2006 Astrocyte control of synaptic transmission and neurovascular coupling *Physiol. Rev.* **86** 1009–31

[109] Theodosis D T, Poulain D A and Oliet S H R 2008 Activity-dependent structural and functional plasticity of astrocyte–neuron interactions *Physiol. Rev.* **88** 983–1008

[110] Volterra A and Meldolesi J 2005 Astrocytes, from brain glue to communication elements: the revolution continues *Nat. Rev. Neurosci.* **6** 626–40

[111] Fellin T 2009 Communication between neurons and astrocytes: relevance to the modulation of synaptic and network activity *J. Neurochem.* **108** 533–44

[112] Perea G, Navarrete M and Araque A 2009 Tripartite synapses: astrocytes process and control synaptic information *Trends Neurosci.* **32** 421–31

[113] Barker A J and Ullian E M 2010 Astrocytes and synaptic plasticity *Neuroscientist* **16** 40–50

[114] Kofuji P *et al* 2002 Kir potassium channel subunit expression in retinal glial cells: implications for spatial potassium buffering *Glia* **39** 292–303

[115] Parpura V and Verkhratsky A 2012 Homeostatic function of astrocytes: Ca^{2+} and Na^+ signalling *Transl. Neurosci.* **3** 334–44

[116] Joshi J, Parker A C and Tseng K-C 2011 An synchronization glial microdomain to invoke excitability in cortical neural networks *2011 Int. Symp. of Circuits and Systems (ISCAS)* (Piscataway, NJ: IEEE) 681–4

[117] Izhikevich E M 2009 Polychronization: computation with spikes *Neural Comput.* **18** 245–82

[118] Treisman A 1999 Solutions to the binding problem: progress through controversy and convergence *Neuron* **24** 105–25

[119] Araque A 2008 Astrocytes process synaptic information *Neuron Glia Biology* **4** 3–10

[120] Berridge M J 2014 *Cell Signalling Biology* (London: Portland Press)

[121] Agulhon C *et al* 2008 What is the role of astrocyte calcium in neurophysiology? *Neuron* **59** 932–46

[122] Huang Y H *et al* 2004 Astrocyte glutamate transporters regulate metabotropic glutamate receptor-mediated excitation of hippocampal interneurons *J. Neurosci.* **24** 4551–9

[123] Bergles D E and Jahr C E 1997 Synaptic activation of glutamate transporters in hippocampal astrocytes *Neuron* **19** 1297–308

[124] Huang Y H and Bergles D E 2004 Glutamate transporters bring competition to the synapse *Curr. Opin. Neurobiol.* **14** 346–52

[125] Danbolt N C 2001 Glutamate uptake *Prog. Neurobiol.* **65** 1–105

[126] Gillingwater T H and Ribchester R R 2001 Compartmental neurodegeneration and synaptic plasticity in the Wld^s mutant mouse *J. Physiol.* **534** 627–39

[127] Irizarry-Valle Y 2016 Modeling astrocyte-neural interactions in CMOS neuromorphic circuits *PhD Thesis* University of Southern California

[128] Diamond J S 2001 Neuronal glutamate transporters limit activation of NMDA receptors by neurotransmitter spillover on CA1 pyramidal cells *J. Neurosci.* **21** 8328–38

[129] Fellin T *et al* 2004 Neuronal synchrony mediated by astrocytic glutamate through activation of extrasynaptic NMDA receptors *Neuron* **43** 729–43

[130] Pereira A Jr and Furlan F A 2010 Astrocytes and human cognition: modeling information integration and modulation of neuronal activity *Prog. Neurobiol.* **92** 405–20

[131] Koizumi S 2010 Synchronization of Ca^{2+} oscillations: involvement of ATP release in astrocytes *The FEBS Journal* **277** 286–92

[132] Oberheim N A *et al* 2009 Uniquely hominid features of adult human astrocytes *J. Neurosci.* **29** 3276–87

[133] Carmignoto G 2000 Reciprocal communication systems between astrocytes and neurones *Prog. Neurobiol.* **62** 561–81

[134] Izhikevich E M 2006 Polychronization: computation with spikes *Neural Comput.* **18** 245–82

[135] Treisman A 1999 Solutions to the binding problem: progress through controversy and convergence *Neuron* **24** 105–25

[136] Robertson J M 2002 The astrocentric hypothesis: proposed role of astrocytes in consciousness and memory formation *J. Physiol. Paris* **96** 251–5

[137] Pereira A and Augusto Furlan F 2009 On the role of synchrony for neuron-astrocyte interactions and perceptual conscious processing *J. Biol. Phys.* **35** 465–80

[138] Perea G and Araque A 2009 Synaptic information processing by astrocytes *J. Physiol. Paris.* **99** 287–300

[139] Perea G, Navarrete M and Araque A 2009 Tripartite synapses: astrocytes process and control synaptic information *Trends Neurosci.* **32** 421–31

[140] Araque A *et al* 2002 Synaptically released acetylcholine evokes Ca^{2+} elevations in astrocytes in hippocampal slices *J. Neurosci.* **22** 2443–50

[141] Perea G and Araque A 2005 Properties of synaptically evoked astrocyte calcium signal reveal synaptic information processing by astrocytes *J. Neurosci.* **25** 2192–203

[142] Benedetti B, Matyash V and Kettenmann H 2011 Astrocytes control GABAergic inhibition of neurons in the mouse barrel cortex *Physiol. J* **589** 1159–72

[143] Héja L *et al* 2012 Astrocytes convert network excitation to tonic inhibition of neurons *BMC biology* **10** 1–21

[144] Beenhakker M P and Huguenard J R 2010 Astrocytes as gatekeepers of GABAB receptor function *J. Neurosci.* **30** 15262–76

[145] Heja L, Nyitrai G, Kekesi O, Dobolyi A, Szabo P, Fiath R, Ulbert I, Pal-Szenthe B, Palkovits M and Kardos J 2012 Astrocytes convert network excitation to tonic inhibition of neurons *BMC Biol.* **10** 26

[146] Lee S *et al* 2010 Channel-mediated tonic GABA release from glia *Science* **330** 790–6

[147] Chen J *et al* 2013 Heterosynaptic long-term depression mediated by ATP released from astrocytes *Glia* **61** 178–91

[148] Zhang J-M *et al* 2003 ATP released by astrocytes mediates glutamatergic activity-dependent heterosynaptic suppression *Neuron* **40** 971–82

[149] Andersson M, Blomstrand F and Hanse E 2007 Astrocytes play a critical role in transient heterosynaptic depresion in the hippocampal CA1 region *J. Physiol.* **585** 843–52

[150] Andersson M, Blomstrand F and Hanse E 2007 Astrocytes play a critical role in transient heterosynaptic depression in the rat hippocampal CA1 region *J. Physiol.* **585** 843–52

[151] Kozlov A S *et al* 2006 Target cell-specific modulation of neuronal activity by astrocytes *Proc. Natl Acad. Sci.* **103** 10058–63

[152] Kozlov A S, Angulo M C, Audinat E and Charpak S 2006 Target cell-specific modulation of neuronal activity by astrocytes *Proc. Natl Acad. Sci USA* **103** 10058–63

[153] Jiménez-González C *et al* 2011 Non-neuronal, slow GABA signalling in the ventrobasal thalamus targets δ-subunit-containing GABAA receptors *European J. Neurosci.* **33** 1471–82

[154] Agulhon C *et al* 2012 Calcium signaling and gliotransmission in normal versus reactive astrocytes *Front. Med.* **3** 139

[155] De Pittà M *et al* 2009 Glutamate regulation of calcium and IP3 oscillating and pulsating dynamics in astrocytes *J. Biol. Phys.* **35** 383–411

[156] Koob A 2009 *The Root of Thought: Unlocking Glia–The Brain Cell That Will Help Us Sharpen Our Wits, Heal Injury, and Treat Brain Disease* (Upper Saddle River, NJ: FT Press)

[157] Pasti L *et al* 1997 Intracellular calcium oscillations in astrocytes: a highly plastic, bidirectional form of communication between neurons and astrocytes *J. Neurosci.* **17** 7817–30

[158] Zonta M and Carmignoto G 2002 Calcium oscillations encoding neuron-to-astrocyte communication *J. Physiol. Paris* **96** 193–8

[159] Nagy J I and Rash J E 2000 Connexins and gap junctions of astrocytes and oligodendrocytes in the CNS *Brain Res. Rev.* **32** 29–44

[160] Goldberg M *et al* 2010 Nonlinear gap junctions enable long-distance propagation of pulsating calcium waves in astrocyte networks *PLoS Comput. Biol.* **6** e1000909

[161] Nagy J I and Rash J E 2003 Astrocyte and oligodendrocyte connexins of the glial syncytium in relation to astrocyte anatomical domains and spatial buffering *Cell Commun. Adhes* **10** 401–6

[162] Möller C *et al* 2007 Glial cells for information routing? *Cogn. Syst. Res.* **8** 28–35

[163] Silberberg G *et al* 2005 Synaptic pathways in neural microcircuits *Trends Neurosci.* **28** 541–51

[164] Pereira A Jr 2010 Astrocytes and human cognition: modeling information integration and modulation of neuronal activity *Prog. Neurobiol.* **92** 405–20

[165] Pereira A Jr, Santos R P and Barrros R F 2013 The calcium wave model of the perception-action cycle: evidence from semantic relevance in memory experiments *Front. Psychol.* **4** 252

[166] Alger B 2002 Retrograde signaling in the regulation of synaptic transmission: Focus on endocannabinoids *Prog. Neurobiol.* **68** 247–86

[167] Reghr W, Carey M and Best A 2009 Activity-dependent regulation of synapses by retrograde messengers *Neuron* **63** 154–70

[168] Navarrete M and Araque A 2010 Endocannabinoids potentiate synaptic transmission through stimulation of astrocytes *Neuron* **68** 113–26

[169] Min R and Nevian T 2012 Astrocyte signaling controls spike timing dependent depression at neocortical synapses *Nat. Neurosci.* **15** 746–53

[170] Naeem M *et al* 2015 On the role of astroglial synctia in self-repairing spiking neural networks *IEEE Trans. Neural Netw. Learn. Syst.* **26** 2370–80

[171] Wade J *et al* 2012 Self-repair in a bidirectionally coupled astrocyte-neuron (an) system based on retrograde signaling *Front. Comput. Neurosci.* **6** 76

[172] Turrigiano G G 2008 The self-tuning neuron: synaptic scaling of excitatory synapses *Cell* **135** 422–35

[173] Teichert M *et al* 2017 Homeostatic plasticity and synaptic scaling in the adult mouse auditory cortex *Sci. Rep.* **7** 17423

[174] Hanse E, Seth H and Riebe I 2013 AMPA-silent synapses in brain development and pathology *Nat. Rev.* **14** 839–50

[175] Maffei A, Nelson S B and Turrigiano G G 2004 Selective reconfiguration of layer 4 visual cortical circuitry by visual deprivation *Nat. Neurosci.* **7** 1353–9

[176] Maffei A and Turrigiano G G 2008 Multiple modes of network homeostasis in visual cortical layer 2/3 *The J. Neurosci.* **28** 4377–84

[177] Tseng K-C 2012 Neuromorphic motion sensing circuits in a silicon retina *PhD Thesis* (ProQuest Dissertations Publishing)

[178] Gollisch T and Meister M 2010 Eye smarter than scientists believed: neural computations in circuits of the retina *Neuron* **65** 150–64

[179] Squire L R 2008 *Encyclopedia of Neuroscience* (Oxford: Academic) 10 pp 225–32

[180] Higgs M H and Lukasiewicz P D 1999 Glutamate uptake limits synaptic excitation of retinal ganglion cells *J. Neurosci.* **19** 3691–700

[181] Kolb H 2007 *Glial Cells of the Retina* (Salt Lake City, UT: University of Utah Health Sciences Center)

[182] Bringmann A *et al* 2006 Müller cells in the healthy and diseased retina *Prog. Retin. Eye Res.* **25** 397–424

[183] Newman E A 2005 Calcium increases in retinal glial cells evoked by light-induced neuronal activity *J. Neurosci.* **25** 5502–10

[184] Dyer M A and Cepko C L 2001 Regulating proliferation during retinal development *Nat. Rev. Neurosci.* **2** 333–42

[185] Zhang A-J and Wu S M 2009 Receptive fields of retinal bipolar cells are mediated by heterogeneous synaptic circuitry *J. Neurosci.* **29** 789–97

[186] Newman E A and Zahs K R 1998 Modulation of neuronal activity by glial cells in the retina *J. Neurosci.* **18** 4022–8

[187] Wu S M 1992 Feedback connections and operation of the outer plexiform layer of the retina *Curr. Opin. Neurobiol.* **2** 462–8

[188] Wu S M 2010 Synaptic organization of the vertebrate retina: general principles and species-specific variations *Investig. Ophthalmol. Vis. Sci.* **51** 1264–74

[189] Murakami M *et al* 1982 GABA-mediated negative feedback from horizontal cells to cones in carp retina *Jpn. J. Physiol.* **32** 911–26

[190] Wu S M 1991 Input-output relations of the feedback synapse between horizontal cells and cones in the tiger salamander retina *J. Neurophysiol.* **65** 1197–206

[191] Kamermans M and Fahrenfort I 2004 Ephaptic interactions within a chemical synapse: hemichannel-mediated ephaptic inhibition in the retina *Curr. Opin. Neurobiol.* **14** 531–41

[192] Kamermans M *et al* 2001 Hemichannel-mediated inhibition in the outer retina *Science* **292** 1178–80

[193] Hirasawa H and Kaneko A 2003 pH changes in the invaginating synaptic cleft mediate feedback from horizontal cells to cone photoreceptors by modulating Ca^{2+} channels *J. Gen. Physiol.* **122** 657–71

[194] Vessey J P *et al* 2005 Proton-Mediated Feedback Inhibition of Presynaptic Calcium Channels at the Cone Photoreceptor Synapse *The J. Neurosci.* **25** 4108–17

[195] Xin D and Bloomfield S A 1999 Dark- and light-induced changes in coupling between horizontal cells in mammalian retina *J. Comp. Neurol.* **405** 75–87

[196] Jackman S L *et al* 2011 A Positive Feedback Synapse from Retinal Horizontal Cells to Cone Photoreceptors *PLoS Biol.* **9** e1001057+

[197] Hsueh H-A, Molnar A and Werblin F S 2008 Amacrine-to-amacrine cell inhibition in the rabbit retina *J. Neurophysiol.* **100** 2077–88

[198] Eggers E D and Lukasiewicz P D 2006 GABAA, GABAC and glycine receptor-mediated inhibition differentially affects light-evoked signalling from mouse retinal rod bipolar cells *Physiol. J.* **572** 215–25

[199] Molnar A and Werblin F 2007 Inhibitory feedback shapes bipolar cell responses in the rabbit retina *J. Neurophysiol.* **98** 3423–35

[200] Baccus S A *et al* 2008 A retinal circuit that computes object motion *J. Neurosci.* **28** 6807–17

[201] Olveczky B P, Baccus S A and Meister M 2003 Segregation of object and background motion in the retina *Nature* **423** 401–8

[202] Lee Sand Jimmy Zhou Z 2006 The synaptic mechanism of direction selectivity in distal processes of starburst amacrine cells *Neuron* **51** 787–99

[203] Münch T A and Werblin F S 2004 Symmetric interactions within a homogenous starburst cell network can lead to robust asymmetries in starburst dendrites *Invest. Ophthalmol. Vis. Sci.* **45** 4274

[204] Munch T A *et al* 2009 Approach sensitivity in the retina processed by a multifunctional neural circuit *Nat. Neurosci.* **12** 1308–16

[205] Cook P B and McReynolds J S 1998 Lateral inhibition in the inner retina is important for spatial tuningof ganglion cells *Nat. Neurosci.* **1** 714–9

[206] Amthor F R, Keyser K T and Dmitrieva N A 2002 Effects of the destruction of starburst-cholinergic amacrine cells by the toxin AF64A on rabbit retinal directional selectivity *Vis. Neurosci.* **19** 495–509

[207] Fried S I, Münch T A and Werblin F S 2002 Mechanisms and circuitry underlying directional selectivity in the retina *Nature* **420** 411–4

[208] Yoshida K *et al* 2001 A key role of starburst amacrine cells in originating retinal directional selectivity and optokinetic eye movement *Neuron* **30** 771–80

[209] Euler T, Detwiler P B and Denk W 2002 Directionally selective calcium signals in dendrites of starburst amacrine cells *Nature* **418** 845–52

[210] Hausselt S E *et al* 2007 A dendrite-autonomous mechanism for direction selectivity in retinal starburst amacrine cells *PLoS Biol.* **5** e185

[211] Poznanski R R 1992 Modelling the electrotonic structure of starburst amacrine cells in the rabbit retina: a functional interpretation of dendritic morphology *Bull. Math. Biol.* **54** 905–28

[212] Tukker J J, Rowland Taylor W and Smith R G 2004 Direction selectivity in a model of the starburst amacrine cell *Vis. Neurosci.* **21** 611–25

[213] Borg Graham L J and Grzywacz N M 1992 *A Model of the Directional Selectivity Circuit in Retina: Transformations by Neurons Singly and in Concert* (San Diego, CA: Academic) pp 347–75

[214] Enciso G A *et al* 2010 A model of direction selectivity in the starburst amacrine cell network *J. Comput. Neurosci.* **28** 567–78

[215] MacKay D M 1970 Elevation of visual threshold by displacement of retinal image *Nature* **225** 90–2

[216] Roska B and Werblin F 2003 Rapid global shifts in natural scenes block spiking in specific ganglion cell types *Nat. Neurosci.* **6** 600–8

[217] Kandel E, Schwartz J and Jessel T 2004 *Principles of Neural Science* (New York: McGraw-Hill) vol 4

[218] Beierlein M *et al* 2002 Thalamocortical bursts trigger recurrent activity in neocortical networks: layer 4 as a frequency-dependent gate *J. Neurosci.* **22** 9885–94

[219] von der Heydt R, Zhou H and Friedman H S 2000 Representation of stereoscopic edges in monkey visual cortex *Vis. Res.* **40** 1955–67

[220] Izhikevich E M 2003 Simple model of spiking neurons *IEEE Trans. Neural Netw.* **14** 1569–72

[221] Tateno A, Harsch T and Robinson H P C 2004 Threshold firing frequency-current relationship on neurons in rat somatosensory cortex: type 1 and type 2 dynamics *J. Neurophysiol.* **92** 2283–94

[222] Alzahrani R 2022 Dynamic neuronal encoding in neuromorphic circuits *PhD Thesis* University of Southern California

[223] Shu Y *et al* 2007 Properties of action-potential initiation in neocortical pyramidal cells: evidence from whole cell axon recordings *J. Neurophysiol.* **97** 746–60

[224] Kole M H P and Stuart G J 2012 Signal processing in the axon initial segment *Neuron* **73** 235–47

[225] Debanne D *et al* 2011 Axon physiology *Physiol. Rev.* **91** 555–602

[226] Palmer L M and Stuart G J 2006 Site of action potential initiation in layer 5 pyramidal neurons *J. Neurosci.* **26** 1854–63

[227] Lai H C and Jan L Y 2006 The distribution and targeting of neuronal voltage-gated ion channels *Nat. Rev. Neurosci.* **7** 548–62

[228] Boiko T *et al* 2003 Functional specialization of the axon initial segment by isoform-specific sodium channel targeting *J. Neurosci.* **23** 2306–13

[229] Van Wart A, Trimmer J S and Matthews G 2007 Polarized distribution of ion channels within microdomains of the axon initial segment *J. Comp. Neurol.* **500** 339–52

[230] Hu W *et al* 2009 Distinct contributions of Na_v 1.6 and Na_v 1.2 in action potential initiation and backpropagation *Nat. Neurosci.* **12** 996–1002

[231] Lorincz A and Nusser Z 2008 Cell-type-dependent molecular composition of the axon initial segment *J. Neurosci.* **28** 14329–40

[232] Rush A M, Dib-Hajj S D and Waxman S G 2005 Electrophysiological properties of two axonal sodium channels, $Na_v1.2$ and $Na_v1.6$, expressed in mouse spinal sensory neurones *Physiol. J.* **564** 803–15

[233] Schmidt-Hieber C and Bischofberger J 2010 Fast sodium channel gating supports localized and efficient axonal action potential initiation *J. Neurosci.* **30** 10233–42

[234] Johnston J, Forsythe I D and Kopp-Scheinpflug C 2010 SYMPOSIUM REVIEW: going native: voltage-gated potassium channels controlling neuronal excitability *J. Physiol.* **588** 3187–200

[235] Kole M H P, Letzkus J J and Stuart G J 2007 Axon initial segment Kv1 channels control axonal action potential waveform and synaptic efficacy *Neuron* **55** 633–47

[236] Shu Y *et al* 2007 Selective control of cortical axonal spikes by a slowly inactivating K+ current *Proc. Natl Acad. sci.* **104** 11453–8

[237] Chang K-J and Rasband M N 2013 Excitable domains of myelinated nerves: axon initial segments and nodes of Ranvier *Current Topics in Membranes* (Amsterdam: Elsevier) vol 72 pp 159–92

[238] Leterrier C and Dargent B 2014 No Pasaran! Role of the axon initial segment in the regulation of protein transport and the maintenance of axonal identity *Seminars in Cell & Developmental Biology* (Amsterdam: Elsevier) 27 pp 44–51

[239] Grubb M S *et al* 2011 Short-and long-term plasticity at the axon initial segment *J. Neurosci.* **31** 16049–55

[240] Kuba H *et al* 2015 Redistribution of Kv1 and Kv7 enhances neuronal excitability during structural axon initial segment plasticity *Nat. Commun.* **6** 1–12

[241] Grubb M S and Burrone J 2010 Activity-dependent relocation of the axon initial segment fine-tunes neuronal excitability *Nature* **465** 1070–4

[242] Gulledge A T and Bravo J J 2016 Neuron morphology influences axon initial segment plasticity *Eneuro* **3** e0085-15

[243] Kuba H, Ishii T M and Ohmori H 2006 Axonal site of spike initiation enhances auditory coincidence detection *Nature* **444** 1069–72

[244] Kuba H, Adachi R and Ohmori H 2014 Activity-dependent and activity-independent development of the axon initial segment *J. Neurosci.* **34** 3443–53

[245] Yamada R and Kuba H 2016 Structural and functional plasticity at the axon initial segment *Front. Cell. Neurosci.* **10** 250

[246] Clark B D, Goldberg E M and Rudy B 2009 Electrogenic tuning of the axon initial segment *Neuroscientist* **15** 651–68

[247] Howard A, Tamas G and Soltesz I 2005 Lighting the chandelier: new vistas for axo-axonic cells *Trends Neurosci.* **28** 310–6

[248] Woodruff A R *et al* 2011 State-dependent function of neocortical chandelier cells *J. Neurosci.* **31** 17872–86

[249] Cobb S R *et al* 1995 Synchronization of neuronal activity in hippocampus by individual GABAergic interneurons *Nature* **378** 75–8

[250] Shai A S *et al* 2015 Physiology of layer 5 pyramidal neurons in mouse primary visual cortex: coincidence detection through bursting *PLoS Comput. Biol.* **11** e1004090

[251] Elices I and Varona P 2017 Asymmetry factors shaping regular and irregular bursting rhythms in central pattern generators *Front. Comput. Neurosci.* **11** 9

[252] Marder E and Bucher D 2001 Central pattern generators and the control of rhythmic movements *Curr. Biol.* **11** R986–96

[253] Cooper D C 2002 The significance of action potential bursting in the brain reward circuit *Neurochem. Int.* **41** 333–40

[254] Halassa M M and Haydon P G 2010 Integrated brain circuits: astrocytic networks modulate neuronal activity and behavior *Annu. Rev. Physiol.* **72** 335–55

[255] Perea G, Sur M and Araque A 2014 Neuron-glia networks: integral gear of brain function *Front. Cell. Neurosci.* **8** 378

[256] Santello M, Toni N and Volterra A 2019 Astrocyte function from information processing to cognition and cognitive impairment *Nat. Neurosci.* **22** 154–66

[257] De Pittà M, Brunel N and Volterra A 2016 Astrocytes: orchestrating synaptic plasticity? *Neuroscience* **323** 43–61

[258] Caudle R M 2006 Memory in astrocytes: a hypothesis *Theor. Biol. Med. Model.* **3** 1–10

[259] Padmashri R *et al* 2015 Motor-skill learning is dependent on astrocytic activity *Neural Plast.* **2015** 938023

[260] Halassa M M *et al* 2009 Astrocytic modulation of sleep homeostasis and cognitive consequences of sleep loss *Neuron* **61** 213–9

[261] Bliss T V P and Lømo T 1973 Long-lasting potentiation of synaptic transmission in the dentate area of the anaesthetized rabbit following stimulation of the perforant path *J. Physiol.* **232** 331–56

[262] Henneberger C *et al* 2010 Long-term potentiation depends on release of D-serine from astrocytes *Nature* **463** 232–6

[263] Lüscher C and Malenka R C 2012 NMDA receptor-dependent long-term potentiation and long-term depression (LTP/LTD) *Cold Spring Harb. Perspect. Biol.* **4** a005710

[264] Turrigiano G G and Nelson S B 2004 Homeostatic plasticity in the developing nervous system *Nat. Rev. Neurosci.* **5** 97–107

[265] Liu J *et al* 2020 N6-methyladenosine of chromosome-associated regulatory RNA regulates chromatin state and transcription *Science* **367** 580–6

[266] Allen P 2020 Allen Brain Map https://portal.brain-map.org/

[267] Zhang H *et al* 2022 The histone demethylase Kdm6b regulates the maturation and cytotoxicity of TCR$\alpha\beta^+$ CD8$\alpha\alpha^+$ intestinal intraepithelial lymphocytes *Cell Death Differ.* **29** 1349–63

Chapter 2

Introduction to neuromorphic circuits

Alice C Parker and Rick Cattell

This chapter covers a short summary of the early history of neuromorphic circuits, followed by a discussion of the complexities of building neuromorphic circuits that occupies most of the chapter. Most of these complexities lay the groundwork for neuromorphic solutions in later chapters. References to other surveys concerning neuromorphic circuits are given at the end of the chapter.

2.1 The history of neuromorphic circuits

Beginning with the early days of vacuum tube and relay electronics, researchers have developed electronic models of neurons designed to emulate neural behavior with electrical signals that mimic the measured potentials of biological neurons in some simplified ways. However, in the past, the size and cost of available electronics made construction of complex brain-like structures impractical. As technologies have become increasingly smaller (nanoscale) and much less expensive, there is a possibility of constructing neural structures on the scale of a human brain in the foreseeable future. Alice Parker's BioRC group[1] has spent the last decade examining the feasibility of building extremely large-scale neural systems with realistic behavior, and nanotechnologies have been investigated, as described in chapter 15.

In 1943, McCulloch and Pitts published a noteworthy paper on a logical calculus for describing neural circuits mathematically [48]. This led to construction of a Mark 1 Perceptron machine with multiple neurons modeled as perceptrons. The perceptrons added the weighted inputs and then output a 1 if the value was high enough and a zero if it was not (sometimes modeled as a simple step function). A sketch of the perceptron is shown in figure 2.1. This oversimplified model has persisted today as the discipline known as neural networks evolved from this model. However, many modern neural networks incorporate significantly more biological features, including spiking outputs, and there remain fewer (but perhaps important) differences

---

[1] BIOmimetic Real-time Cortex.

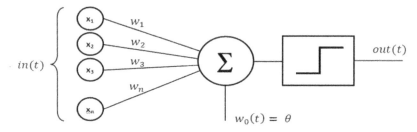

Figure 2.1. Sketch of a perceptron modeling a simplified neuron. This File:Perceptron moj.png image has been obtained by the authors from the Wikimedia website https://commons.wikimedia.org/wiki/File: Perceptron_moj.png where it was made available under a CC BY-SA 3.0 licence. It is included within this book on that basis. It is attributed to Mayranna.

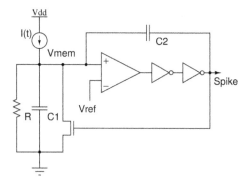

Figure 2.2. The original Mead neuron. Copyright 2004 IEEE. Reprinted, with permission, from [78].

between biological coverage of advanced neural networks and neuromorphic circuits. A main difference between neuromorphic circuits and the most biological neuromorphic models is the use of hardware for circuits versus software/mathematics for more detailed neuromorphic models.

The neuromorphic circuit field actually began with Cal Tech Professor Carver Mead's introduction to neuromorphic circuits followed by the notable collaboration between California Institute of Technology student Michelle Anne (Misha) Mahowald and Carver Mead [49], first with Mead's book [50] and then Mahowald's dissertation [42]. The original Mead neuron is shown in figure 2.2.

A number of researchers have designed, fabricated and tested artificial neurons, and now the trend is toward increasingly *biomimetic* neurons, neurons that mimic biology[2]. Others have used general-purpose computers to simulate neural networks. Schüffny *et al* provide a good survey of research performed up to 1999 [68]. By 2012, a very small number of projects aimed at construction of an entire artificial brain or cortical columns consisting of many neurons, either from general-purpose computers [46] or more specialized architectures such as cellular automata [15] or asynchronous ARM processors [34]. Finally, there were researchers that focused on

---

[2] Exactly how detailed models must be to be termed *biomimetic* is an ongoing discussion.

specific brain structures like the retina, or applications, like image recognition. While many neuron electronic circuits in the literature had some biomimetic features (e.g. [18, 19, 39, 55, 65]), the complete range of biological neural variations has not been implemented in a single neural electronics model or even in the variety of neuron models distributed throughout the research community.

Boahen, who studied with Mead, has also modeled retinal processing, including the visual cortex with electronic circuits ([4, 5]), as early as 1989 [6]. Many researchers describe analog neural circuits, with only a few describing mixed-signal circuits. The closest electronic models to biological neurons in early neuromorphic circuits include mixed-signal models, e.g. Liu and Frenzel's spike train neuron [39], Pan's bipolar neuron [57], the cellular neural network research by Chua et al [12, 13] and the research by Hasler (e.g. [19]) discussed in more detail in this text. Chiju et al extended the cellular neural network (CNN) work and tested their neural model on specific applications [76]. Sato et al [67] use stochastic logic to obtain analog behavior from digital circuits. Chen and Shi [11] use pulse width modulation. Linares-Barranco et al [38] describe a CMOS implementation of oscillating neurons. Fu et al [22] present thin-film analog artificial neural networks. Early research that is continuing is performed by Indiveri started in 1992 [62]. Between these researchers, there are hundreds of publications on neuromorphic circuits.

A basic CMOS neuron with learning capabilities is found in Chao's MS thesis [10]. The basic neural structure, the Parker neuron, was designed by Parker, and the learning circuitry was researched by Chao. The original dendrite circuit was designed to match Shepherd's dendritic computation sketch, with an enhancement of the dendrite circuit to accept spike train inputs [58]. Figure 2.3 provides a layout of the Parker neuron with two inputs, excitatory and inhibitory, each containing an action potential and a synapse weight w. Each dendrite in the neuron contained two inverters and two capacitors composed of transistors. Synapses are not shown.

Other noteworthy neurons capable of learning were also proposed ([23, 27, 35, 40, 47, 60, 66, 75, 81]). Koosh and Goodman [35] put a digital computer in the loop for training, control and weight updates, and the neural network is analog, a style realized by several research groups. Commercial neural networks incorporating learning were available by 2006, albeit only weakly biomimetic, and were in use by the high-energy physics community.

A paper by Wells [79] proposed a neurocomputer architecture intended to solve the problems of interconnectivity, variable synaptic weights and learning; these were issues not solved completely by any electronic neuron models published by 2006. Moravec [54] made predictions of when inexpensive general-purpose computers would match the human brain in processing power, although his predictions seemed optimistic based on our own estimates. Finally, Jeff Hawkins, inventor of the PalmPilot, presented an eloquent if somewhat informal discussion of the brain [26] that motivated the biomimetic assumptions on the BioRC project.

Elias [18] had performed modeling of dendritic trees that were similar to the BioRC models. The primary difference involved his use of resistors and capacitors, and the BioRC group's use of transistors. In addition, his synapses involved single transistors, and BioRC's more complex dendritic trees account for variability in

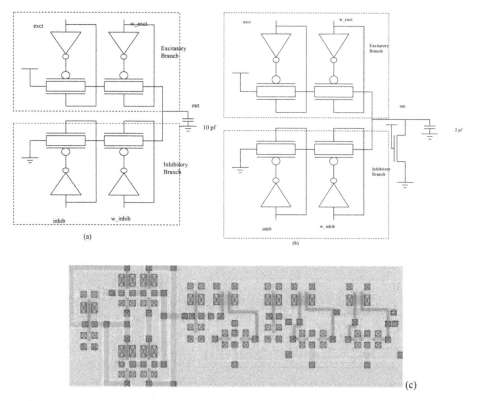

Figure 2.3. A basic Parker CMOS neuron dendrite. (a) The original dendrite circuit. (b) The dendrite circuit modified to accept spike train inputs. (c) Layout of Parker's original neuron.

neurotransmitter concentrations and learning. Elias' model was more analog than BioRCs, while BioRC's resembled a pulse and timing circuit. Elias' model will be discussed later in the text in chapter 7.

As technology has advanced in what has become the Golden Age of micro-electronics, futurists like Ray Kurzweil began to predict the construction of artificial brains that behaved like human brains in the near future. In 2006, Kurzweil wrote that 'We will have the requisite hardware to emulate human intelligence with supercomputers by the end of this decade' (2010) [36]. Kurzweil added that the required software would not be available to have the supercomputer pass the Turing test until the end of the 2020s. More recent comments by Kurzweil have moved this timeline to 2045.

Henry Markram, a well-known neuroscientist who published the first findings on spike-timing-dependent plasticity (STDP), became interested in modeling the human brain, and leads the Blue Brain project in the Brain Mind Institute at EPFL in Switzerland. 'A model that replicates the functions of the human brain is feasible in 10 years' (written in 2009), according to Markram. 'I absolutely believe it is technically and biologically possible. The only uncertainty is financial. It is an extremely expensive project and not all is yet secured' Markram commented in 2013. By 2015 Markram had secured funding from the European Brain Project but by 2019 the project structure had been rethought, and there was significant controversy over whether the neuroscience knowledge to build an artificial brain was complete enough to proceed with artificial brain construction. While Markram had modeled the details of ion channels in the biological neurons of a mouse brain in exquisite detail using Hodgkin–Huxley models, the connections between neurons were generated using statistical properties of the mouse brain, and at one point only about 10 000 neurons were modeled on an IBM Blue Gene multiprocessor with 8192 processing elements[3]. Since then other efforts have been undertaken to simulate more neurons with varying degrees of biological accuracy. The text will return to recent past history of attempts to model the brain, once it introduces more anatomy and physiology of individual neurons, the biological cells in the brain believed to carry out a primary role in processing information, learning and memory.

It is important to mention Karlheinz Meier and Johannes Schemmel of the BrainscaleS project [51], that will be described later in chapter 17, Shih-Chieh Liu, Bernabé Linares-Barranco, Tara Julia Hamilton, André van Schaik, Ralph Etienne-Cummings, Tobi Delbruck, Shih-Chii Liu, Piotr Dudek, Philipp Häfliger, Sylvie Renaud, Gert Cauwenberghs, John Arthur, Kai Hynna, Fopefolu Folowosele, Sylvain Saighi, Teresa Serrano-Gotarredona, Jayawan Wijekoon, and Yingxue Wang, all of whom coauthored [2].

2.2 Complexities of modeling the brain

While many researchers have focused on implementing simplified functions with artificial neurons, beginning with simplified models might not lead to more complex neurons as the circuits evolve, and might not result in brain-like behavior. Approaches to building even simplified neurons should consider the ultimate goals: intelligence, memory, reasoning and autonomous behavior, including self-awareness, consciousness, a moral compass and social responsibility. This 'end game,' if the discussion can use a chess analogy, must be taken into account, the earlier the better. Beginning a chess game without an understanding of where it is going to end up might lead to becoming trapped without a winning strategy. So even the simplest neurons must be constructed in ways that do not block future solutions to the hardest problems, the toughest challenges in modeling an artificial brain.

2.2.1 Introduction to the toughest challenges for artificial brains

The list of toughest challenges to modeling an artificial brain is quite brief, when each challenge is summarized. However, overcoming each challenge consists of dozens of sub-challenges. The major challenges neuromorphic circuit designers must tackle are:

---

[3] Interested readers can Google 'cat fight' or read more about the argument between Markram and Dharmendra Modha of IBM in IEEE Spectrum [1].

1. The **complexity** of each neuron and its synapses, including nonlinear neural computations;
2. Building artificial systems the **scale** of the human brain with 100 billion neurons and trillions of synapses;
3. Providing **dense interconnectivity** and the **immense parallelism** possessed by the biological brain;
4. Compensating for changes in **signal arrival timing** with planar and 2 1/2 D technologies;
5. Implementing **plasticity**, the changes in synapse strength and neural connectivity as learning occurs;
6. Implementing **interactions with glial cells**, in particular astrocytes;
7. Implementing various **spiking patterns** that make up *the neural code*;
8. **Gene expression** modifying neural structures and connections; and
9. Reducing overall **power consumption** of such a dense, powerful system so that it can be used in practice.

Many of these challenges interact; e.g. scale, interconnectivity, parallelism, power and density all interact. Satisfying one alone might cause the other parameters to change adversely, affecting the design. It is indeed a multiple-criteria optimization problem.

The BioRC project [59] has investigated the use of nanotechnologies to implement aspects of the neural circuits that have been designed, with the belief that a paradigm change in technology might be required to meet some, if not all of the challenges [74]. In parallel with these investigations, the use of CMOS circuits to model brain functions has continued on the BioRC project as well as on other analog circuit approaches to modeling the brain.

While this chapter provides some extended discussion of the details of these challenges, solutions will be found later in the text. At this point, the reader is being made aware of all these challenges, but details of the neuromorphic circuit solutions will be discussed in later chapters.

2.2.1.1 Challenge 1: implementing neural complexity

Individual neurons are complex computation engines hence, this is a lengthy section. *Excitatory* and *inhibitory* synapses respond to *action potentials* (voltages), signals sent from other neurons, with varying degrees of response in the form of positive and negative cell potentials (voltages), respectively. The varying response, called *synaptic strength*, changes under learning and over time. Even over a very short interval, repeatedly stimulating a synapse can cause a decrease in response, called *adaptation*. Potentials are summed, sometimes non-linearly. Potentials traveling along the dendritic arbor are attenuated and spread (like a low-pass filter). *Gap junctions*[4] between adjacent neurons (or between two astrocytes) are present, especially in developing neurons.

---

[4] Connections that allow charged particles, ions, to flow between two neurons.

A challenge involves the complexities of the synaptic connections, and variations in neural processing, not just in different regions of the brain but also in different types of neural cells involved in *proximal* (nearby) and *distal* (distant) processing [9, 70]. Modeling a complete list of neural complexities and variations is probably not required for good emulation, but major features that contribute to differences in neural behavior in some significant way must be considered. First, the text considers some complexities that are found in most brain neurons, and then examines some variations between neurons that are significant to behavior at the cellular level. These complexities can be categorized into chemical variations, synaptic structural variations, and dendritic structural variations. Most of these variations are discussed in reference [70].

At the synapse, action potentials (spikes) traveling down the axon cause *neurotransmitters* (chemical messengers) to be released. These transmitters cross the *synaptic cleft*, the space between neurons, and cause ion channels in the postsynaptic synapse to open (figure 1.9). The resulting ion flow causes a voltage change in the postsynaptic neuron. In cortical neurons, synapses themselves vary widely, with *ligand*-gated (chemical) and voltage-gated ion channels that conduct charged particles. Ligand-gated channels are receptive to a variety of transmitters [70] that cause ion channels to open. These transmitters can also decrease or increase the excitability of the postsynaptic receptors in the synapse to stimuli by the presynaptic cells, possibly by altering cell membrane conductance. A further complication of transmitter function is via the *retrograde process* that directly or indirectly modulates transmitter release in the presynaptic junction, a form of extremely local feedback. Retrograde actions typically occur more slowly than presynaptic to postsynaptic activation. In addition, *adaptation* can cause synaptic responses to decrease when spiking occurs repeatedly.

Action potentials arriving at the synapses create postsynaptic potentials on the dendritic arbor that combine in a number of ways. Multiple action potentials in sequence at a single synapse cause multiple postsynaptic potentials to sum, called *temporal summation*. Transmitters acting on secondary messengers can have short- or long-term effects on synaptic junction activation, referred to as short-term facilitation and depression, and long-term potentiation and long-term depression. Facilitation increases the likelihood of the neuron firing, and depression decreases the likelihood. The activation probability of a given synaptic junction is up- or down-regulated by the amount and timing of presynaptic and postsynaptic activity. A final transmitter complication involves the occurrence of multiple transmitters at a single synapse, sometimes providing conflicting messages of potentiation and depression. The neurotransmitter dopamine can convert short-term potentiation to long-term potentiation, and can strengthen synapses, depending on the situation.

Complex dendritic computations affect the probability and frequency of neural firing. These computations include linear, sublinear, and superlinear additions along with generation of dendritic spikes, and inhibitory computations that shunt internal cell voltage to resting potentials or decrease the potential, essentially subtracting voltage. Furthermore, some neuroscientists show evidence that the location of each synapse in the dendritic arbor is an important component of the dendritic computation [56, 61], essential to their neural behavior, and there is growing consensus among neuroscientists that aspects of dendritic computation contribute significantly to cortical functioning. Further, some propagation of potentials and other signaling is in the reverse direction, affecting first-order neural behavior (for example, see the reset mechanism affecting dendritic spiking plasticity in section 8.2) [41, 64]. The extent of the detailed modeling of dendritic computations and spiking necessary for brain emulation is an open question, but the behavior of neurons that can exhibit dendritic spiking does change when spiking is not suppressed.

Dendritic structural variations have a first-order impact on the behavior of individual neurons and neuronal circuits. The locations of excitatory and inhibitory synapses on the dendrite branches and spines determine the functions realized by the combinations of synaptic inputs [52]. In chapter 7, the text will illustrate a candidate electronic design for a dendritic tree that has functions dependent on the locations of the synaptic connections. Nonlinear dendritic summations (e.g. 8 mV + 7 mV = 40 mV) can occur on the postsynaptic potentials inside the neuron and dendritic spikes can occur, depending on the locations of the synapses. The dendritic spikes can be caused by different ions, like sodium and especially calcium entering the neuron, and the shapes of the spikes can be different. These spikes propagate more quickly and with less attenuation than most postsynaptic potentials, and can be strong enough to cause the neuron to spike at the axon hillock, depending on the specific dendritic spike voltage and rate of voltage change [3].

In the axon hillock, thresholds for spiking vary depending on the derivative of the membrane potential. The potential for spiking can vary (dendritic plasticity), and increase or decrease depending on the type of spike, circumstances, and whether the neural spike generated at the axon hillock back propagates to the dendrites, like the reflection of an electromagnetic wave[5]. The dendritic computations depend on whether the signals to be combined are on the same or different branches of the dendrite and whether the input signals are weak, medium or strong [53]. Figure 2.4 shows results of excitatory postsynaptic potentials (EPSP) summation at the soma of a layer-5 pyramidal neuron with respect to within-branch and between-branch stimulations. Between-branch EPSP summation is linear for weak and medium stimuli and slightly superlinear for strong stimuli. Within-branch EPSP summation is linear for weak stimuli, superlinear for medium stimuli and sublinear for strong stimuli.

Another complexity in computation in neurons is that they appear to exhibit stochastic behavior or chaotic behavior, including neurotransmitter release probabilities, and the variations in threshold required for firing [43, 44]. Neurons do not fire with certainty and sometimes spontaneously fire. While this property of biological neurons could be ignored to simplify modeling, it turns out to be useful when neurons are learning about themselves and their environments, and so it is helpful to incorporate neural variability [77]. Some neuroscience results indicate that the variability appears to be chaotic, that is, possessing a behavior that is highly

---

[5] Actually the spike propagates everywhere, in all directions, but the most noteworthy effects besides forward propagation are back propagation effects.

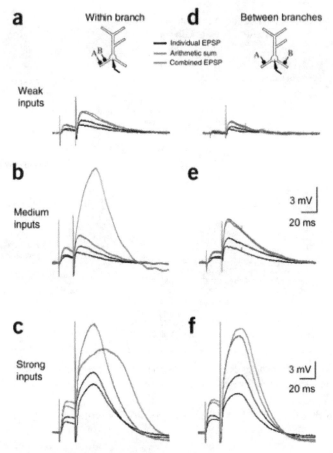

Figure 2.4. EPSP summation variations in pyramidal neurons, from Polsky. Reprinted from [61], copyright (2004), with permission from Springer Nature.

variable but determined by a chaotic equation, with outcome dependent on initial conditions. Other results indicate that stochastic mathematics matches biological neural behavior well. The text will explore this more deeply in chapter 9.

The retina, part of the brain, has a very different neural structure with most neurons non-spiking. The biological retina was summarized in section 1.8 and the neuromorphic retina will be discussed later in chapter 12.

2.2.1.2 Challenge 2: building to human brain scale

The prospects for building a human brain with CMOS technology seem limited. Figure 2.5 shows the progress of device scaling over time, taken from the International Technology Roadmap for Semiconductors (ITRS) Executive Summary 2014 [30] [6]. Analog circuits seem to convey efficiencies over digital circuits when performing approximate computations, even with CMOS, so they are

---

[6] The ITRS has been supplanted by the International Roadmap for Devices and Systems (IRDS) [29].

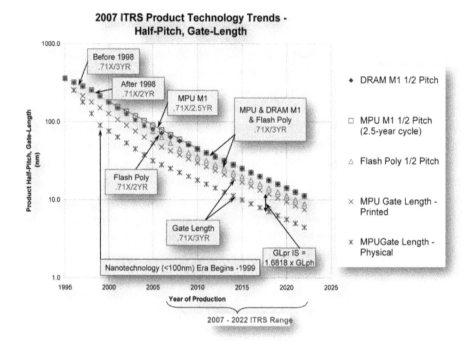

Figure 2.5. International Technology Roadmap for Semiconductors graph of expected transistor sizing over time. Reprinted from [30] with permission from SIA.

highlighted in this text. The use of nanotechnologies will greatly help in meeting this challenge.

2.2.1.3 Challenge 3: providing dense connectivity and immense parallelism

One of the most difficult of the challenges in modeling the brain is the massive interconnectivity. Cortical neurons possess an average of 10 000 and up to 100 000 synaptic connections [70] [7]. With approximately 100 billion neurons in human cortex, and approximately 60 trillion synaptic connections, connectivity in the artificial brain cortex will be a major challenge. Even in the cerebellum there are postulated to be 100 billion small granule cells, each with up to 100 synaptic connections [70]. While some connections originate in *proximal* (nearby) neurons, some originate in *distal* (distant) neurons, posing an interconnection problem for the candidate modeling technologies. One of the *foci* of the predictions on interconnection requirements is on possible interconnection strategies that support the massive synaptic connections of the cortex.

Connection-wise the mammalian cortex is 2D, albeit with six layers, folded around the sub-brain, with wrinkles, roughly into the shape of a sphere. The wiring

---

[7] There are between 10^4 to 10^5 distinct input connections to each neuron, and 10^4 output connections from each neuron.

is mostly two-dimensional, with the exception of the brain stem, thalamus, motor/sensory neurons to the spine, and the cerebellum. The brain's spherical shape minimizes the across-brain connection length and volume, although many connections are global. The surface of the brain is wrinkled, not a smooth sphere, so local connections are not necessarily minimized by the overall spherical shape. When this spherical shape is stretched into a plane, or stacked planes in a 3D technology like stacked CMOS dies, many long connections in the biological brain become even longer and perhaps indirect. Timing of neural behavior is exquisitely precise in the biological brain, as the text explores later, so indirect (networked) connections might become problematic. The dense brain interconnectivity is shown in figure 2.6, where each connection shown is actually a bundle of neurons called a tract. Recent research by Bassett *et al* [17] derives a *Rent exponent* for the biological brain that could be used to compute the quantity of connections emerging from a volume of brain tissue. Early indications are that this Rent exponent is sufficiently large (many distal connections) so as to cause connectivity problems with conventional CMOS electronics.

While Finfet technology has allowed scaling to continue, the number of layers of metal was predicted to be 12–13 by 2014 for Finfet technologies. This is not expected to change dramatically, so dense interconnections required for neuron–neuron connections (not even including astrocytes) would likely not be possible with CMOS circuits. Philip Wong at Stanford and TSMC [71] has shown layers of technologies, including thin-film nanotechnologies that likely will increase connectivity in neuromorphic circuits. So the scaling of the artificial brain to human proportions will likely require some form of nanotechnology.

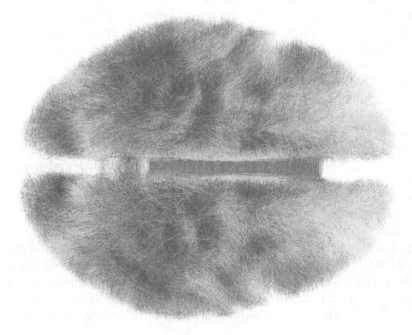

Figure 2.6. Tracts (bundles of neurons) in the human brain.

A very significant second complexity of neural structure is the existence of synaptic divergence (fan out in engineering terms) and convergence (fan in). A single axon can fan out to many presynaptic connections, or many synapses can form around a neuron with a single axon. Multiple synapses can converge (fan in) to a single postsynaptic terminal, either from a single oversized presynaptic terminal or from multiple presynaptic terminals. Axons can influence the activation of other axons directly, either by sharing ion flow, or by forming synaptic connections, axon to axon. Likewise, there can be dendrodendritic connections that act like synaptic junctions. Synaptic divergence can enhance the signal-to-noise ratio and hence is useful in constructing brain emulators that are fault tolerant, like the biological brain itself. A more subtle type of interconnection involves synchronization, where activity in one neural region influences activity in other regions.

Multiple connections, either fanning into or out of a neuron tend to support the same sign activities, either excitatory or inhibitory. Some synaptic connections have a low probability of firing. Multiple connections increase the probability of activation occurring, and therefore increase the 'safety factor' of the sub-circuit firing properly. Multiple synapses at the inputs to a single neuron that produce EPSPs or inhibitory postsynaptic potentials (IPSPs) can combine, or sum spatially or temporally to produce a potential that is a nonlinear summation of the single potentials. In addition, the action of the inhibitory potentials can depend on the type of inhibition. Modeling this nonlinear summation is considered important in capturing essential brain functioning.

A further complication in biological brains is imposed by feed-forward inhibition. Here excitatory synapses make direct connections from a presynaptic to postsy-naptic connection, while other synapses from the 'output' neuron connect through a relay neuron to the 'input' neuron through an inhibitory synapse. There is a delay through the relay neuron creating an excitatory–inhibitory sequence in the output neuron. Another neuronal behavior that might be important to capture is recurrent inhibition, where excitatory potentials in a neuron back propagate to dendrites on that neuron that activate other neurons through dendrodendritic junctions. Those neurons then inhibit the original neuron through inhibitory synapses that create IPSPs in the original neuron. Lateral inhibition also occurs. An EPSP in a neuron can activate IPSPs in neighboring neurons. Some feedback structures produce rhythmic activity or oscillations. Some neurons produce bursts of spikes with a single activation, while others produce a single spike. The periods and duty cycles of the spike trains are sometimes significant, and variations in frequency cause different responses.

The immense parallelism supported by the dense interconnectivity of the biological brain leads to a situation where 100 billion neurons are computing in parallel asynchronously: there is no clock. In the human brain, neuron-to-neuron communi-cation is over a spherical volume with longer connections tuned by oligodendrocytes for faster propagation. With conventional CMOS electronics, transistor-to-transistor communication is in parallel layers on a set of planes with longer connections that must be tuned for faster propagation; late signals will be ignored. We suspect that the level of parallelism and synchronization of the brain will be difficult to achieve with conventional electronics.

2.2.1.4 Challenge 4: signal timing

Because the brain is not clocked, biological signals arrive at synapses and are conveyed by neurons to other synapses in an asynchronous fashion. The timing of such signals is inexact. Signals arriving close together in time on nearby synapses can cause dendritic spiking and perhaps other forms of coincidence detection. Signals spaced further apart in time are unlikely to cause dendritic spiking or to act as coincidence detectors. Synchronous neuromorphic hardware requires rapid clocking to capture signals that arrive closely in time so that the impact of near coincidence can be detected even if the signals are not exactly coincident. Missing such near coincidence in clocked neuromorphic systems can cause loss of information. A reference to biological neurons and the need for precise timing is found in [80], where Yang shows that different cortical areas are sensitive to differences in neural timing.

2.2.1.5 Challenge 5: brain plasticity

New neural connections form within hours in the biological brain, often called *structural plasticity*, frequently to already connected neurons. However, connections between previously unconnected neurons can occur. Plasticity due to new neurons forming and propagating through the brain is rare, however new neurons form well into old age in humans in the hippocampus, the seat of memory activity. It is generally accepted that an emulated brain with static neural connections and neural behavior would not produce intelligence. Synapses must be 'plastic': the strength of the excitatory or inhibitory connection must change with learning, and neurons must also be able to create new synapses and hence new connections during the learning process. Research on the mechanisms by which biological neurons learn, make and break connections, and possess memory is ongoing, with hypotheses and supporting data appearing frequently. These studies have led to a basic understanding of synaptic and structural plasticity. For presynaptic neurons (the sending neurons) when facilitation or depression occurs, making the synapse stronger or weaker, more or fewer neurotransmitters are available/released. The postsynaptic neuron (the receiving neuron) can experience depression or potentiation continuously as more or fewer receptors respond to the neurotransmitters sent by the presynaptic neuron. Synaptic strengths thus vary depending on neurotransmitter availability (pre) and receptor (post) availability. The ability of dendrites to form small spikes is also plastic, and changes depending on circumstances.

Being able to reconfigure circuits on-line as needs change is important to plasticity. Nanotechnologies may play a role in such reconfiguration. Finally, astrocytes exert some control over synaptic strengths, as do neural experiences, leading to the next challenge.

2.2.1.6 Challenge 6: astrocytic interactions

In the last decade, attention has been given to the role of glial cells in neural behavior, glial cells being much more numerous in the brain than neurons. There are ten times as many glial cells (including astrocytes) as neurons in the brain. Astrocytic interactions (between neurons and astrocytes) affect neural behavior.

Glial cells in the biological brain control blood flow and propagation speed. Glial cells affect processing and memory, communicating neural activity, down regulating activity, encouraging new connections, synchronizing neurons, influencing synaptic strength, and repairing stroke damage. Figure 2.7 shows connections between astrocytes and neurons in the biological brain. Not shown here are the *gap junctions* that astrocytes use to connect to each other. The role of astrocytes, a type of glial cell, in learning and memory is being actively investigated (see [20, 21] for early publications). Neuromorphic circuits including astrocytes have been constructed, with an early BioRC paper beginning a series of dissertations and publications [33]. More publications will be provided in the chapter on astrocytes.

2.2.1.7 Challenge 7: power consumption

A CMOS (conventional electronic) brain is likely to consume megawatts of power. Even a carbon nanotube FET brain[8] could consume megawatts operating at subthreshold voltages unless attention is paid to low-power design. Markram's Blue Brain supercomputer is said to use 1 MW, while a human brain is thought to consume 20–40 W. Once again, nanotechnologies are sure to play a role in power

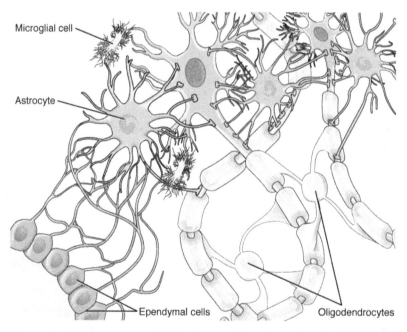

Figure 2.7. Connections between astrocytes (blue) and neurons (orange) are shown in this figure. Note that the astrocytes connect to the synapses, soma and axon of each neuron. Reproduced from [24] CC BY 4.0.

---

[8] Carbon nanotubes are nanostructures composed of carbon atoms arranged in a tube, 1 nm in diameter, that can act as a conductor or semiconductor. The first carbon nanotube synapse was announced in 2011 [32].

reduction. An example dendritic arbor is shown in section 16.5 and more low-power techniques are found in [45].

2.2.1.8 Challenge 8: the neural code

Spikes seldom travel alone in the biological brain. Multiple spikes are often sent by the presynaptic neuron. Occasional spikes just keep the connection active. Spacing and timing affect how the spikes are received. The neural code is more than just a rate code. The interspike interval patterns also contain information, as do spike shapes. One of the most complex behaviors in the human brain is the variety of spiking patterns. As the text discusses in the next chapter, Izhikevich has categorized these patterns and built software that is parameterized to generate a large variety of patterns [31]. This categorization is a good collection on which to construct a future *neural code*. The neural code is described more in chapter 13.

2.2.2 Reliability and fault tolerance in biological neurons

Neuronal networks are able to be fault tolerant. In biological neurons, there are often multiple synapses for presynaptic/postsynaptic neuron pairs, insuring that the information is received by the postsynaptic neuron. This will help ensure that the information is actually received because each synapse is not that reliable. When a designer builds a CMOS chip, the designer is confident that the majority of chips from a 'run' are going to work well, until the circuit is scaled down into nano-technological sizing. Transistors are increasingly unreliable with increased scaling (nanosizing). So, having multiple synapses that transfer the same message is a way to increase reliability of nanoscale neuromorphic circuits.

There is signal persistence in biological postsynaptic potentials so that signals can arrive early or late and still have an impact on the postsynaptic neuron. When a spike arrives at a neuron, it is going to translate into a PSP that stays around for a while, about ten times longer than the original spike. Because of this, spikes can arrive at various times, with possible delays, and can still sum and cause a neuron to fire. This is the kind of fault tolerance that does not rely on all signals arriving during a small clock period.

Superlinear responses in neurons to specific input combinations of actively responding synapses (dendritic spikes) allow a small number of presynaptic neurons to invoke firing in a postsynaptic neuron. Their specific input combinations cause tiny spikes near the synapses called dendritic spikes. The sharper the spike or the more prolonged voltage, the more strongly it will travel to the soma, causing the neuron to spike. This is fault-tolerant behavior because a few inputs that are really related to each other (close to each other in space as well), coming in, can cause a dendritric spike and can cause a neuron to spike. This way there is no need to count on a massive influx of spikes coming in to make a neuron fire. This is not at all like a simplified leaky-integrate-and-fire neuromorphic system where each input has impact independent of the other inputs. In biological neurons, more importance is given to closely related inputs. This leads to more reliable neurons and a compact way of performing computation. A dendritic spike, as we will describe later, is one of the most important events that happens in a neuron. The faster the slope of any voltage waveform in the neuron, caused by inputs arriving close together and dendritic spiking occurring, the more likely for neural spiking to happen. Fast slopes indicate the arrival of something important.

There are some spiking patterns that are designed to make sure that the synapses are responding. These spiking patterns help make the synapse more reliable. Spiking patterns are designed to insure postsynaptic response. There are redundancies in the neural networks so that identical pathways operate properly even when individual neurons fail. Also, neural networks provide quasi-redundancy, with multiple pathways arriving at a destination neuron through occurence of different but related computations. For example, recognition of a square shape could be performed by recognition of four edges at specific locations and orientations, or recognition of 90 degree corners at specific locations. Either approach could provide square recognition, while both in combination could provide recognition even when part of the square shape is occluded or the image is noisy. Multiple synapses in a neural circuit also provide redundancy that makes them more reliable [28]. Finally, astrocytes perform *homeostasis* (state preservation) when synapses fail, encouraging nearby synapses to strengthen [7, 72]. The BioRC project has exploited this mechanism in a circuit described in chapter 11 from Rebecca Lee's dissertation [63] and in a conference paper [37].

2.2.3 Other neuromorphic system and circuit surveys

Other surveys of brain emulation are worth referencing here. They provide a different perspective than ours. Sandberg and Bostrom [8] provide an excellent survey of the overall issues in brain emulation, although they do little discussion of actual brain emulation projects. They cover different levels of emulation, different neural models, computational requirements of emulation, and brain mapping technologies. De Garis, Shuo, Goertzel, and Ruiting [16] provided the most similar survey to ours, covering half of the historical projects mentioned here. This is a good reference for another perspective on these projects. It is part one of a two-part survey. The second part, written by Goertzel, Lian, Arel, de Garis, and Chen [25], surveys higher-level brain models aimed at producing intelligent behavior, inspired by human intelligence but not based on emulation of neural networks; this work is closer to classical AI.

More recent surveys include [14, 69, 73]. The article by Schuman contains extensive references. Also of note is [82]. An extensive survey of neuromorphic circuits [2] categorizes circuits in a table, with design styles listed in table 2.1, and then discussed in the text.

Table 2.1. Design styles from Indiveri. Reproduced from [2] CC BY 4.0.

Weak inversion	Strong inversion
Voltage mode	Current-mode
Non-clocked	Switched capacitor
Biophysical model	Phenomenological model
Real-time	Accelerated-time

In the Indiveri table, *weak inversion* refers to subthreshold transistor operation, and *strong inversion* refers to above threshold operation. *Voltage mode* and *current mode* refer to the forms of inputs and outputs. *Non-clocked* is essentially asynchronous behavior where charge flows, and *switched capacitor* moves charge when transistors are switched on/off. *Biophysical models* model the biology of the structure and *phenomenological models* (e.g. differential equations) model abstract behavior. *Real-time systems* approximate the timing of biological systems and *accelerated-time systems* model systems with timing significantly faster than biological systems. Many neuromorphic circuits are combinations of these design styles, complicating the behavior and analysis of the circuits. For a detailed analysis of circuits existing in 2011, refer to the extensive paper by Indiveri [2] that covers many examples.

2.3 Chapter conclusion

This chapter has provided a history of neuromorphic circuits, and a lengthy discussion of the complexities of modeling the human brain with electronics. A brief section discussed other surveys of neuromorphic systems and circuits.

2.4 Book outline

The next chapter provides an introduction to modeling neuromorphic circuits. Chapter 4 covers mathematical models of spiking neurons. Chapter 5 covers the spiking mechanisms in the neuron, chapter 6 discusses the synapse, and chapter 7 covers passive dendritic computations, with linear summation of PSPs. Active dendrites with dendritic spiking are covered in chapter 8. Variable neural behavior is presented in chapter 9, followed by learning and memory in chapter 10, covering systems that learn and strengthen synapses and neural pathways. Interactions with astrocytes, other brain cells that contribute to computations, are described in chapter 11. Modeling the retina is the subject of chapter 12. The neural code (meaning of the spike signals) is presented in chapters 13 and 14. Nanotechnology for neuromorphic circuits is covered in chapter 15, advanced topics are highlighted in chapter 16, including low-power design and neuromorphic systems is the final chapter (chapter 17).

2.5 Exercises

Why is building an artificial brain so difficult? Give the top three reasons to convince the public it is difficult.

References

[1] Adee S 2010 Cat-brain fever *IEEE Spectr* **47** 16–7
[2] Indiveri G *et al* 2011 Neuromorphic silicon neuron circuits *Front. Neurosci.* **5** 1–23
[3] Azouz R and Gray C M 2000 Dynamic spike threshold reveals a mechanism for synaptic coincidence detection in cortical neurons *in vivo Proc. Natl. Acad. Sci. USA* **97** 8110–5
[4] Benjamin B V *et al* 2012 A superposable slilcon synapse with programmable reversal potential *Proc. Annu. Int. Conf. IEEE Eng. Med. Biol. Soc.* 2012 771–4
[5] Boahen K 2005 Neuromorphic microchips *Sci. Am.* **292** 56–63

[6] Boahen K A *et al* 1989 A heteroassociative memory using current-mode MOS analog VLSI circuits *IEEE Trans. Circuits Syst.* **36** 747–55

[7] Boddum K *et al* 2016 Astrocytic GABA transporter activity modulates excitatory neuro-transmission *Nat. Commun.* **7** 13572

[8] Sandberg A and Bostrom N 2008 Whole brain emulation: a roadmap *Technical Report #2008-3* Future of Humanity Institute, Oxford University www.fhi.ox.ac.uk/reports/2008-3.pdf

[9] Calvin W H and Graubard K 1979 *Styles of neuronal computation The Neurosciences Fourth Study Program* ed O Schmitt and F G Worden (Cambridge, MA: MIT Press)

[10] Chao C 1990 Incorporation of learning within the CMOS neuron *MA Thesis* University of Southern California

[11] Chen L and Shi B 1991 Building blocks for PWM VLSI neural network *5th Int. Conf. Signal Processing Proc. WCCC-ICSP* **1** pp 563–6

[12] Chua I 1996 CNN Chips Crank up the Computing Power *IEEE Trans. on Circuits and Devices* **12** 18–27

[13] Chua I and Yang I 1988 Cellular neural networks: theory and cellular neural networks: applications *IEEE Trans. on CAS* **35** 1257–95

[14] Davies M *et al* 2021 Advancing neuromorphic computing with Loihi: a survey of results and outlook *Proc. IEEE* **109** 911–34

[15] De Garis H 1996 CAM-brain ATR's billion neuron artificial brain project—a three year progress report *Int. Conf. on Evolutionary Computation* 886–91

[16] De Garis H *et al* 2010 A world survey of artificial brain projects, part I: large-scale brain simulations *Neurocomputing* **74** 3–29

[17] Bassett D S, Greenfield D L, Meyer-Lindenberg A, Weinberger D R, Moore S W and Bullmore E T 2010 Efficient physical embedding of topologically complex information procesing networks in brains and computer circuits *PLOS Comput. Biol.* **6** e1000748

[18] Elias J, Chu H and Meshreki S 1992 Silicon implementation of an artificial dendritic tree *Proc. Int. Joint Conf. Neural Networks* 1 (Baltimore, MD: IEEE) 154–9

[19] Farquhar E and Hasler P 2004 A bio-physically inspired silicon neuron *2004 EEE Int. Symp. Circuits and Systems (IEEE Cat. No. 04CH3752)* 1

[20] Fields R D 2009 *The Other Brain: From Dementia to Schizophrenia, How New Discoveries about the Brain Are Revolutionizing Medicine and Science* (New York: Simon and Schuster)

[21] Douglas R 2002 Fields and Beth Stevens-Graham. New insights into neuron-glia communication *Science* **298** 556–62

[22] Fu C *et al* 1992 A novel technology for fabricating customizable VLSI artificial neural network chips *Int. Joint Conf. Neural Networks (IJCNN)*

[23] Gerstner W and Kistler W 2002 *Spiking Neuron Models* (Cambridge: Cambridge University Press)

[24] *Glial Cells* URL: https://courses.lumenlearning.com/wm-biology2/chapter/glial-cells/

[25] Goertzel B *et al* 2010 A world survey of artificial brain projects, part II: biologically inspired cognitive architectures *Neurocomputing* **74** 30–49

[26] Hawkins J and Blakeslee S 2004 *On Intelligence* (New York: Times Books)

[27] Haykin S 1999 *Neural Networks: A Comprehensive Foundation* 2nd edn (Englewood Cliffs, NJ: Prentice-Hall)

[28] Hiratani N and Fukai T 2018 Redundancy in synaptic connections enables neurons to learn optimally *Proc. Natl Acad. Sci.* **115** E6871–9

[29] *International Roadmap for Devices and Systems* 2020 URL: https://irds.ieee.org/

[30] *International Technology Roadmap for Semiconductors* 2015 URL: https://en.wikipedia.org/wiki/International_Technology_Roadmap_for_Semiconductors

[31] Izhikevich E M 2003 Simple model of spiking neurons *IEEE Trans. Neural Netw.* **14** 1569–72

[32] Joshi J *et al* 2011 A biomimetic fabricated carbon nanotube synapse for prosthetic applications *2011 IEEE/NIH Life Science Systems and Alications Workshop (LiSSA)* 139–42

[33] Joshi J, Parker A C and Tseng K-C 2011 An in-silico glial microdomain to invoke excitability in cortical neural networks *2011 IEEE Int. Symp. Circuits and Systems (ISCAS)* pp 681–4

[34] Khan M M *et al* 2008 SpiNNaker: mapping neural networks onto a massively-parallel chip multiprocessor *Neural Networks, 2008. IJCNN 2008.(IEEE World Congress on Computational Intelligence). IEEE Int. Joint Conf. IEEE.* pp 2849–56

[35] Koosh V F and Goodman R 2001 VLSI neural network with digital weights and analog multipliers *Proc. ISCAS '01* 2 233–6

[36] Kurzweil R 2006 *The Singularity Is Near* (Harmondsworth: Penguin Books)

[37] Lee R K and Parker A C 2019 An Electronic Neuron with Input-Specific Spiking *2019 Int. Joint Conf. Neural Networks (IJCNN)* 1–8

[38] Linares-Barranco E, Sanchez-Sinencio B, Rodriguez-Vazquez A and Huertas J L 1991 A CMOS implementation of FitzHugh-Nagumo neuron model *IEEE J. Solid-State Circuits* **26** 956–65

[39] Liu B and Frenzel J F 2002 A CMOS neuron for VLSI circuit implementation of pulsed neural networks *Industrial Electronics Society, IEEE 2002 28th Annual Conf. of the IECON'02* 4 3182–5

[40] Liu J and Brooke M 1999 Fully parallel on-chip learning hardware neural network for real-time control *Proc. ISCAS'99* 5 372–4

[41] Losonczy A, Makara J K and Magee J C 2008 Compartmentalized dendritic plasticity and input feature storage in neurons *Nature* **452** 436–41

[42] Mahowald M 1992 VLSI analogs of neuronal visual processing: a synthesis of form and function *PhD Thesis* California Institute of Technology URL: http://caltechcstr.library.caltech.edu/591/

[43] Mahvash M and Parker A C 2011 Modeling intrinsic ion-channel and synaptic variability in a cortical neuromorphic circuit *2011 IEEE Biomedical Circuits and Systems Conf. (BioCAS)* 69–72

[44] Mahvash M and Parker A C 2013 Synaptic variability in a cortical neuromorphic circuit *IEEE Trans. Neural Netw. Learning Syst.* **24** 397–409

[45] Mamdouh P 2019 Power-efficient biomimetic neural circuits *PhD Thesis* University of Southern California

[46] Markram H 2020 *Brain Mind Institute, EFPL* URL: http://bmi.epfl.ch/

[47] Mass W and Bishop C 1999 *Pursed Neural Networks* (Cambridge, MA: MIT Press)

[48] McCulloch W and Pitts W 1943 A logical calculus of the ideas immanent in nervous activity *Bull. Math. Biophys.* **5** 115–33

[49] Mead C and Mahowald M 1988 A silicon model of early visual processing *Neural Netw.* **1** 91–7

[50] Mead C 1989 Analog VLSI and Neural Systems *Computation and Neural Systems Series* (Reading, MA: Addison-Wesley)

[51] Meier K *et al* 2020 *Brainscales Project Overview* http://brainscales.kip.uni-heidelberg.de

[52] Mel B W and Schiller J 2004 On the fight between excitation and inhibition: location is everything *Sci. STKE* **2004** e44

[53] Mitchell J F, Stoner G R and Reynolds J H 2004 Object-based attention determines dominance in binocular rivalry *Nature* **429** 410–3

[54] Moravec H 1998 When will computer hardware match the human brain? *J. Evol. Technol.* **1** 10

[55] Murray A *et al* 1991 Pulse-stream VLSI neural networks mixing analog and digital techniques *IEEE Trans. Neural Netw.* **3** 193–204

[56] Otor Y *et al* 2022 Dynamic compartmental computations in tuft dendrites of layer 5 neurons during motor behavior *Science* **376** 267–75

[57] Pan D and Wilamowski B M 2003 A VLSI implementation of mixed-signal mode bipolar neuron circuitry *Neural Networks, 003. Proc. Int. Joint Conf.* **2** 971–6

[58] Parker A C, Friesz A K and Pakdaman A 2006 Towards a Nanoscale Artificial Cortex *Proc. 2006 Int. Conf. Computing in Nanotechnology (CNAN'06)* URL: http://scholar.google.com/scholar?q=%5C%E2%5C%80%5C%9CTowards+a+Nanoscale+Artificial+Cortex%5C&%5C#38;hl=en%5C&%5C#38;client=firefox-a%5C&%5C#38;rls=org.mozilla:en-US:official%5C&%5C#38;hs=jGF%5C&%5C#38;um=1%5C&%5C#38;ie=UTF-8%5C&%5C#38;oi=scholart

[59] Parker A C 2013 The biorc biomimetic real-time cortex project (University of Southern California) http://ceng.usc.edu/~parker/BioRC_research.html

[60] Perez-Uribe A 1999 Structure-adaptable digital neural networks *PhD Thesis* EPFL

[61] Polsky A, Mel B W and Schiller J 2004 Computational subunits in thin dendrites of pyramidal cells *Nat Neurosci.* **7** 621–7

[62] Raffo L *et al* 1992 A neural architectural model of simple and complex cortical cells *1992 1st Annual Int. Conf. of the IEEE Engineering in Medicine and Biology Society* **4** 1572–3

[63] Lee R 2018 Astrocyte-mediated plasticity and repair in CMOS neuromorphic circuits *PhD Thesis* University of Southern California

[64] Remy S, Csicsvari J and Beck H 2009 Activity-dependent control of neuronal output by local and global dendritic spike attenuation *Neuron* **61** 906–16

[65] Reyneri L 2002 On the performance of pulsed and spiking neurons *Analog Integr. Circuits Signal Process.* **30** 101–19

[66] Ros *et al* 2003 Post-synaptic time-dependent conductance in spiking neurons: FPGA implementation of a flexible cell model *IWANN'03: LNCS 2687* **2687** 145–52

[67] Sato S *et al* 2003 Implementation of a new neurochip using stochastic logic *IEEE Trans. Neural Netw.* **14** 1122–7

[68] Schuffny R *et al* 1999 Hardware for neural networks *4th Int. Workshop Neural Networks in Applications*

[69] Schuman C D *et al* 2017 A survey of neuromorphic computing and neural networks in hardware *ArXiv* abs/1705.06963

[70] Shepherd G M 2004 Introduction to synaptic circuits *Synaptic Organization of the Brain* ed G M Shepherd (Oxford: Oxford University Press)

[71] Shulaker M M *et al* 2014 Monolithic 3D integration of logic and memory: carbon nanotube FETs, resistive RAM, and silicon FETs *2014 IEEE Int. Electron Devices Meeting* 27.4.1–4

[72] Somjen G G 2002 Ion regulation in the brain: implications for pathophysiology *Neuroscientist* **8** 254–67

[73] Staudigl F, Merchant F and Leupers R 2021 A survey of neuromorphic computing-in-memory: architectures, simulators and security *IEEE Design Test* **39** 90–9

[74] *The BioRC Project Website*. URL: http://ceng.usc.edu/simparker/BioRC_research.html

[75] Upegui A, Pena-Reyes C A and Sanchez E 2005 An FPGA platform for on-line topology exploration of spiking neural networks *Microprocess. Microsyst.* **29** 211–23

[76] Vhiju C 2005 Analysis and performance of a versatile CMOS neural circuit based on multi-nested approach *7th IEEE Int. Symp. Signals Circuits and Systems* 417–20

[77] Waschke L *et al* 2021 Behavior needs neural variability *Neuron* **109** 751–66

[78] Wei D and Harris J G 2004 Signal reconstruction from spiking neuron models *2004 Int. Symp. Circuits and Systems (ISCAS)IEEE* 5 (Piscataway, NJ: IEEE) V

[79] Wells R B 2003 Preliminary discussion of the design of a large-scale general-purpose neurocomputer (MRC Institute The University of Idaho) https://webpages.uidaho.edu/rwells/techdocs/Preliminary%20Discussion%20of%20the%20Design%20of%20a%20GP%20Neurocomputer.pdf

[80] Yang Y and Zador A M 2012 Differences in sensitivity to neural timing among cortical areas *J. Neurosci.* **32** 15142–7

[81] Yao X 1999 Evolving artificial neural networks *Proc. IEEE* **87** 1423–47

[82] Yirca B 2020 A survey of emerging neuromorphic devices and architectures enabled by nanomaterials https://phys.org/news/2020-03-survey-emerging-neuromorphic-devices-architectures.html

IOP Publishing

Neuromorphic Circuits
A constructive approach
Alice C Parker and Rick Cattell

Chapter 3

Approach to neuromorphic circuits

Alice C Parker

This chapter covers the evolutionary approach to neuromorphic circuits taken by the BioRC project, starting with simplistic structures that model individual elements of electronic neurons. An introduction to analog transistor behavior is given to provide background for the remaining chapters. Basic analog circuits are introduced and the chapter discusses the rationale for using analog circuits for neural modeling.

3.1 Introduction

The primary approach to neuromorphic circuits described in this text is using analog and mixed-signal circuits to model neuronal behavior. Indiveri and Sandamiskaya, in a recent paper [2], make a strong argument for analog and mixed-signal circuits in neuromorphic systems because computation and memory are integrated into the circuits in a manner not done in traditional computing. State memory is contained in transistor capacitances, integrated with the transistors performing synaptic and neural functions. Also, circuits are not time-multiplexed, but systems perform massive computations in parallel, asynchronously, on individual neuromorphic circuits. In addition, as the neural signals flow through the electronic neurons there is passage of time similar to that occurring in biological neuronal networks, without synchronizing circuits to keep track of time as is done in digital neuromorphic systems. Neuromorphic systems using analog and mixed-signal circuits are compact, adaptive and event-driven. Indiveri says eloquently 'analog neuromorphic circuits use the physics of silicon to directly emulate neural and synaptic dynamics.' Reading at least the first few pages of this recent paper are recommended to set the stage for this text.

This text is designed to take an evolutionary approach towards solving the artificial brain problem—to show how fundamental structures can be built that mimic the brain in a simplistic manner, and to show how such structures can evolve to incorporate more complexities as the knowledge about the brain increases. Parts of the neuron are covered first, then entire neurons and small systems of neurons are

doi:10.1088/978-0-7503-5097-6ch3

presented. As the mechanisms modeled become more complex, the neuron parts become more complex, neurons themselves are more complicated, and neuronal networks are more extensive.

Creating neuromorphic analog electronic circuits can take one of two approaches. For the first approach, the field of computational neuroscience contains many mathematical models of neurons. Computational neuroscientists build mathematical models of neurons, synapses and neuronal networks, models that can be quite intricate, detailed and accurate. Engineers can match the circuit behavior to the mathematical models. Matching circuit behavior to differential equations is straightforward electronic engineering—circuit designers do not need to understand the mechanisms that control neural behavior.

However, there is a different approach where the designers approximate neural behavior with circuit elements that have behavior that in some way is analogous to neural behavior. Analog neuromorphic circuit engineers often build more-approximate models of neurons and neuronal networks, and the modeling language used is the language of transistor physics. Matching analog circuit elements and circuitry to transistor behavior is more complex than matching to mathematical models. Designers must understand some basics of neuroscience. The circuits might not be so elegantly described mathematically, and the elements are usually simpler and more intuitive. The second approach can be called *approximate neural design*. This approach uses voltages, charge and/or currents to represent ions and neurotransmitters and uses transistors to control how charges flow. Gate capacitance and parasitic capacitances (interconnections and diffusions) are often used to create low-pass filters to delay responses to input signals, shaping neural waveforms Channel resistances combine with these capacitances to create RC time constants in the signals. In some cases, especially when timing should match biological timing, fabrication of on-chip capacitors is used to create rise/fall times similar to biological neurons. Note that neurotransmitters and ions are all modeled with charge, current and voltage in the circuits we present here.

It is important to note that transistor physics is often described in differential equations, the language many computational neuroscientists use. However, transistor physics descriptions are used in complex simulation packages like SPICE so that circuit simulations of transistor circuits can be performed by analog designers, who do not manipulate the differential equations directly. So, in a manner, analog neuromorphic circuit engineers craft elaborate mathematical models of neurons and networks, using differential equations encapsulated in circuit simulations to model transistor circuits as the basis for the mathematical models. Due to the complexity of these differential equations, they will not be described further here.

The axon hillock circuit introduced in chapter 5 is a combination of both approaches presented in this text, but the focus of the text is on electronic models of neural mechanisms, the second approach. The text focuses on the design of neuromorphic circuits that are the product of the BioRC (BIOmimetic Real-time Cortex) research group at the University of Southern California [4], with other contributions included for contrast and recognition of early and unique contributions.

The central goal in the BioRC research is to demonstrate electronic circuits that mimic the intelligence, learning and memory capabilities of the brain through the use of analog electronic circuits forming neuromorphic systems of networked neurons. While fabrication of integrated circuits is the long-term goal of the BioRC project, the circuit models themselves provide significant insight into simplified models of the biological mechanisms modeled.

BioRC researchers use an analog approach to build novel custom circuits that exploit the resistive and capacitive properties of transistors rather than using standard analog blocks. Analog circuits offer several advantages and share a similar physical environment to that experienced by the nervous system, e.g., they can be susceptible to noise and highly unreliable, for which careful design skills are required. They allow for emulation of biophysical characteristics with fewer transistors than their digital circuit counterparts, and offer higher-speed perform-ance at lower energy cost. Specifically, the BioRC approach generally follows the original approach of Carver Mead [6], taking advantage of the similarity of transistors and the elementary functions found in the brain.

BioRC uses NMOS (n-channel metal-oxide semiconductor) and PMOS (p-channel metal-oxide semiconductor) transistors as the main computational circuit elements and focuses on their resistances and capacitances to represent the time constants of biological computations. Voltages and currents are used to represent the chemical elements involved in the computations. Each input to a transistor is used to represent a biological event. BioRC circuit designs of individual or a few neurons operate at an *accelerated* time, several orders faster than real-time biology. Once the circuits scale to larger portions of a biological brain, with many more synapses per neuron, speeds decrease due to the larger capacitances of the circuits, and perhaps approach biological neural delays. The focus of the BioRC work is on fundamental research and as such we are concerned with finding ways to represent biological processes using circuits. At this point we are not evaluating the power or speed constraints in BioRC circuits, although a later chapter in this book has a section that focuses on ultra-low power design. Certainly subthreshold circuits (to obtain biological potentials) also result in slower circuits. Note that BioRC circuits in this book represent simulation models that may need more circuit components to complete the system before being implemented as fabricated chips. Capacitances and resistances may need to be modeled with transistor characteristics to achieve voltage scaling and biological delays.

One of the main challenges we face in neuromorphic designs is finding the trade-off on the level of biological details to be incorporated in our circuits for an accurate representation while keeping the circuits as simple as possible. This is a daunting task and an ill-posed problem. To explain this briefly we could think of modules that perform computations (e.g. synapses) to be used repeatedly in a network, where unnecessary details in each synapse could drastically increase the overall circuit overhead. This could downgrade computational performance by limiting the number of functions embedded on a chip. To minimize circuit overhead, we take the approach of customizing BioRC designs with focus on specific and well-chosen biological functions implemented with a small number of transistors for approximate modeling rather than on mathematical models. This implies that BioRC researchers design their own circuit topologies rather than using standard analog blocks such as analog amplifiers, OTAs (operational transconductance amplifiers), and other common analog circuits. The BioRC circuits capture first-order interactions and as such aim to describe biological principles of computations while minimizing circuit complexity/overhead. BioRC researchers focus on exploiting the properties of transistors, using their resistive and capacitive intrinsic functions so that biological time constants can be modeled without the need for discrete elements that often take a large portion of the silicon area.

Interconnectivity between blocks is important as blocks will be used as part of a large system where a variety of configurations will be tested. Therefore, we provide this capability and guarantee that circuit modules can be connected in a plug-and-play fashion. Current mirrors are used in places to avoid loading between circuit blocks. However, when summing potentials or dealing with axonal fan-out, current mirroring is not used as it isolates circuits from summed capacitances. BioRC circuits are designed to be robust and stable over a wide range of inputs. *Monte Carlo* simulations are used to simulate circuits with parametric variations, determining the range of operation of each circuit as parameters are varied.

BioRC has a library of circuits with main circuit components such as synapses, dendrites, and axon hillocks, among others, that are covered in this text. This text has also introduced new modules of computations to emulate astrocyte functions and their communication with neuronal cells. Tunability of specific features allows us to test different biological functions in neuronal networks. There are many control inputs in the neuromorphic circuits that we produce; in actual implementations those control inputs would be common to many neurons or would be generated internally on chip, based on the state of the circuit as execution progresses. Here, we show them as inputs into the circuit to illustrate the level of control the designer and user have over the behavior of each circuit. In an integrated neural circuit, such inputs would be produced by additional circuits found in the final chip modeling biological mechanisms. The use of control knobs (voltages on transistor gates) to modulate transistor behavior allows a broad range of neural behaviors with a simple, single-transistor mechanism. For example, *reuptake* control, is a control for the reuptake rate, where reuptake is a technical term for 'the reabsorption by a presynaptic nerve ending of a neurotransmitter that it has secreted'. One way of controlling an input signal, let us say the reuptake input, is by assigning a DC bias voltage that could be common to many synapses to control the reuptake rate of neurotransmitters in a static manner. Another way could be to control the synapses in a dynamic manner where the input reuptake could be used to increase the rate of neurotransmitters taken back from the cleft through a feedback mechanism. Additional modeling may be required to capture the biomimetic aspects of a dynamic mechanism.

A hypothetical example could be as follows: consider that an increase in the reuptake input voltage would cause a faster discharge in the cleft node and thus a faster excitatory postsynaptic potential (EPSP) decay. Assuming the spike rate arriving at the presynaptic side increased, an increase in the neurotransmitter release could be observed by the change in the average voltage in the cleft node; this in turn may be sensed by feedback circuitry causing an increase in the voltage at the reuptake node which thus decreased the discharging time constant in the node, emulating a faster reuptake of neurotransmitters. This would have impact on the temporal dynamics of the EPSP node in the circuit as the EPSP node is dependent on the cleft node.

The proposed circuits contain parasitic capacitances along with transistor channel and interconnection resistances. In many BioRC circuits, we utilize such non-linearities to avoid using discrete elements such as resistors and capacitors. While small example BioRC circuits are quite fast, the performance would be slowed significantly when the massive fan-in and fan-out proportional to biological neurons were implemented, due to capacitive loading and interconnect resistance, a major challenge due to the massive interconnections in the brain. The existence of synaptic divergence (fan-out in engineering terms) and convergence (fan-in), causes significant delays in electronic circuits. Therefore, while small example BioRC circuits work at nanosecond (CMOS) speed, these circuits, when incorporated into large networks with thousands of synapses per neuron, would slow down significantly due to wiring interconnection capacitances. Thus the relative timing differences between BioRC electronics and the biological waveforms would be significantly reduced.

BioRC circuits have evolved from a small handful of transistors modeling a simple synapse or axon hillock to many transistors, modeling noisy behavior, astrocyte interaction, spiking variations and long-term memory. The basic neural structures have evolved to be more complex, while still retaining fundamental models tested a decade earlier. This evolutionary approach to neuromorphic circuit design has shown to provide rapid development of novel circuits as the understanding and impact of neuroscience knowledge has increased.

3.2 Introduction to electronic modeling of neurons

Basic transistor operation underlies analog electronic models of neurons. There are N-Type and P-Type transistors that refer to the types of impurities that are used to create the transistors. In N-type transistors, the majority carriers of current are electrons and in P-type transistors, the majority carriers are holes (positive charge, the absence of electrons). N-type majority carriers flow from the source to the drain. P-type majority carriers flow from the drain to the source.

Most of the transistors discussed in this text are MOS transistors, with either N-type or P-type impurities. Positive current direction for NMOS transistors (N-type impurities) is from drain to source. For NMOS transisors, I_{DS}, the drain to source current, is positive.

P-Type majority carriers are holes. Holes are the absence of electrons; instead of the electrons flowing, the electrons move from hole to hole and the holes appear to move in the opposite direction, taking much more energy than electron flow, as shown in figure 3.1. PMOS transistors are not as efficient as NMOS transistors because energy is expended moving the electrons from hole to hole. In PMOS

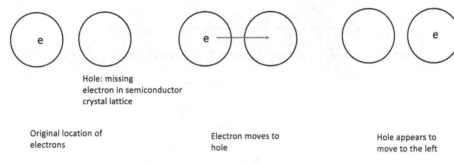

Figure 3.1. Hole flow in semiconductors.

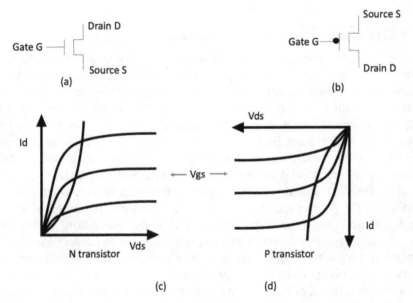

Figure 3.2. Transistor symbols and IV characteristic curves for NMOS and PMOS transistors. (a) Is NMOS and (b) is PMOS.

transistors, I_{SD} is positive. The transistor symbols and IV curves are shown in figure 3.2(a)–(d). Note that current can flow in the NMOS transistor when the voltage between the gate and source is non-zero and positive (above a threshold), and in the PMOS transistor when the voltage between the gate and source is non-zero and negative (below a threshold). In summary, for NMOS transistors $V_{gsn} = V_{gn} - V_{sn}$.

For PMOS transistors, if $V_{gsp} > V_{tp}$, the PMOS transistor is OFF.

If $V_{gsp} \leqslant V_{tp}$, the PMOS transistor is ON.

For NMOS transistors, if $V_{gsn} \geqslant V_{tn}$, the NMOS transistor is ON.

If $V_{gsn} < V_{tn}$, The NMOS transistor is OFF. A number line showing the relationships between all these quantities is shown in figure 3.3.

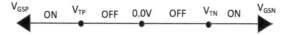

Figure 3.3. Number line showing the quantities used in the inequalities in the text.

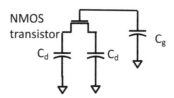

Figure 3.4. Device capacitances in an NMOS transistor. Note that the capacitor sides grounded here, not tied to the transistor, could be tied to supply voltage or another node in the circuit. C_g is gate capacitance, and C_d is diffusion capacitance.

3.2.1 *RC* (resistance–capacitance) time constants

In analog neuromorphic circuits, signals are usually shown as waveforms with rise and fall times that vary, depending on the meanings of the signals and their locations. MOS transistors are useful circuit components in analog neuromorphic circuits because they contain several capacitances that modulate rising and falling signals in the circuit in which each transistor is embedded. Some analog neuro-morphic circuits, like most BioRC circuits, are designed to perform as pulse and timing circuits. Transistor sizing changes channel resistance as well as gate and diffusion capacitances, so that the waveform rise and fall times vary. Circuits containing multiple transistors have complex signals with varying rise and fall times, depending on the regions the transistors are in. Exact computations of waveforms are difficult, and not usually performed except by simulation. Approximating waveforms by varying resistances and capacitances can be done. Waveforms can be estimated using a technique analogous to Elmore delays in digital circuits [3] [1].

Transistor gate capacitances are proportional to gate area. For planar MOS transistors, this is usually computed using the product of channel length and channel width. Diffusion capacitances (source and drain capacitances) are more complex to compute, but an approximation can be performed[2]. These gate and diffusion capacitances vary in practice depending on the voltages applied to each transistor in operation, but can be assumed to be constant in estimating waveform shapes and delays. Figure 3.4 illustrates the major capacitances associated with an NMOS transistor. Sizing each transistor can control, to some extent, the shapes of the waveforms associated with the transistor. The width of each transistor is inversely proportional to resistance R and the channel length of each transistor is proportional to resistance R. Each RC time constant contributes to the rising or falling

---

[1] [3] is an excellent reference for CMOS circuit analysis and circuit design.
[2] VLSI design textbooks typically compute diffusion capacitance as proportional to the sum of the sidewall capacitance times the perimeter of the diffusion, plus the area of the diffusion floor times the capacitance of the diffusion floor per unit area.

exponential signal delay in a transistor circuit where capacitance and resistance are both proportional to delay.

3.2.2 Basic neural models

To introduce neural modeling, figure 3.5(a) shows modeling of a *neuron* in a simplified fashion, as a simple circuit receiving a spike and transmitting it. A more detailed model shows the connections between neurons modeled as a synapse between two neurons in figure 3.5(b). In the simplest case, the synapse receives a spike, an action potential (AP), and produces a *membrane potential (MP)* that is a voltage internal to the neuron. That voltage summed with other membrane potentials causes an *AP* or a voltage spike to be produced by the spiking circuit. Note that the neuron shown contains portions of synapses, and the boundary between two neurons is the synapse itself. Some circuitry within the neuron is considered part of the synapse itself. The sending neuron contains part of the synapse and the receiving neuron contains the other part. The receiving neuron is considered postsynaptic and the sending neuron is considered presynaptic.

We begin this introduction to neural modeling by introducing circuit fragments (portions of circuits) then combine them to create neural circuits. These fragments assume the transistors are in the linear mode of operation, and behave like voltage-controlled resistors, where the voltage controlling the channel resistance is the voltage between the gate and source of the transistor. The current through the resistor is the drain current of the transistor being modeled. The simplest neuron circuit fragment contains a simple ion-channel electronic model of multiple ion channels acting in parallel that uses a single transistor acting as a voltage-controlled resistor with diffusion capacitances at either end of the resistor. Figure 3.6 shows an ion channel electronic circuit fragment. The ion channels are found in the synapse, elsewhere in the neuron, and in the axon initial segment, where spiking occurs. The fragment shown in figure 3.6 shows the flow of positive ions into a neuron through all parallel ion channels, charging up the potential in the cell by charging the capacitance shown. Note that the capacitance at the top end of the transistor is not shown since it is connected on both sides to the supply voltage (represented by a horizontal bar), hence does not have an effect on the circuit.

Similar ion channels using a single NMOS transistor model the flow of positive charges out of the neuron. Figure 3.6 shows the ion channel controlled by the

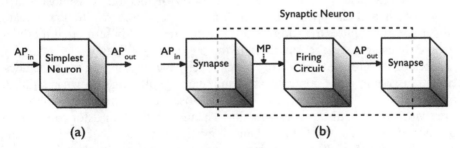

Figure 3.5. Block diagrams of simple neuron circuits. Credit: Evan Clark.

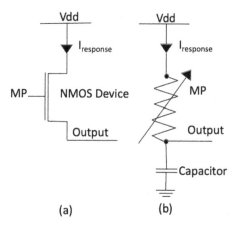

Figure 3.6. The ion channel circuit. (a) The ion channel electronic circuit with a single MOS transistor. (b) The equivalent circuit. *MP* (membrane potential) is the control voltage applied to the gate of an NMOS transistor that causes current flow in parallel ion channels.

membrane potential, the voltage inside the neuron and the output is being pulled up, in this case towards the supply voltage. Other ion channels could pull the voltage down towards ground or a negative voltage. Still other ion channels are controlled by the concentration of *ligands* (chemicals) that attach to the ion channel's receptors, opening the ion channel.

To add a second set of ion channels, the circuit can be modified to add a second transistor in parallel to the first ion-channel transistor. For example, calcium ions can flow in parallel with sodium ions. Calcium ions increase the charge more quickly than sodium ions because calcium ions have two positive charges instead of one. However, the biological mechanism by which calcium ions flow is different, and the flow is slower, so the comparison between sodium and calcium channels is not so straightforward, but the flows can be adjusted by adjusting resistances of the two channels in a circuit model. So, sodium and calcium ions can be added together, at a node, using current addition to create a total current.

Certain channels called *NMDA channels* are different because voltage, along with a ligand, can control whether to open an NMDA channel or not, making the NMDA channel a voltage-gated and ligand-gated channel. So, the input to the ion channels in this case must be some combination of membrane voltage and the presence of a ligand that opens the channels in order for the current to flow. Creating complex control requires the addition of a second transistor in series that modulates the ion flow using a voltage representing the presence of a ligand.

Therefore, to modulate a set of ion channels, the circuit fragment includes a second transistor in series, controlled by a modulating voltage, as shown in figure 3.7. Note that the ion channel transistor could be closer to or further from the voltage source with minimal effect on the behavior. The modulating transistor could be used more as a switch to control the ion channel, much as channels that are both voltage V_m and *ligand* gated. If sets of ion channels are primarily ligand-gated, the

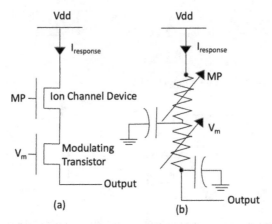

Figure 3.7. (a) Voltage-gated ion channel with series transistor that modulates the ion-channel transistor and (b) the equivalent circuit. MP is the membrane potential.

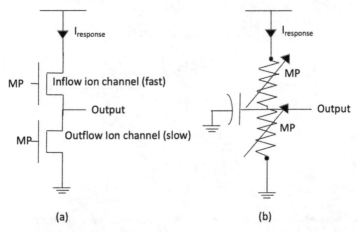

Figure 3.8. (a) Two sets of ion channels in opposition, one charging parasitic diffusion capacitances, and one discharging capacitances. Note that both capacitances are lumped into a single capacitor in the figure. (b) Shows the equivalent circuit. While technically the PMOS diffusion capacitance is between the *output* and V_{dd}, it is shown as lumped with the NMOS diffusion capacitance between the *output* and Gnd.

modulating transistor could have more effect on the output variation than the voltage-gated channel controlled by membrane potential.

Two ion channel sets in opposition could be handled as shown in figure 3.8. The transistor tied to V_{dd} could represent the Na$^+$ (sodium) channel, and the transistor tied to ground could represent the K$^+$ potassium channel. A designer could also insert feedback to limit the rise or fall of the output. This is done usually to limit the MP but could be used anywhere ion channels are present, as shown in figure 3.9. The techniques described here, and shown in the figures, can be combined into more complex circuits. Consider two transistors, one of them is increasing the voltage across (pulling up) some capacitance and the other is decreasing the voltage across (pulling down) the capacitance. The idea is to create some sort of a waveform that

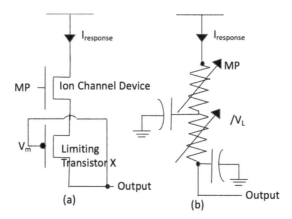

Figure 3.9. Limiting transistor used to limit the rise of the output of the ion channel circuit.

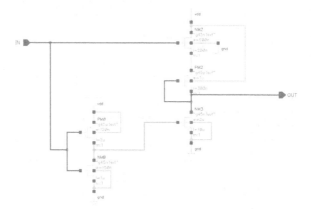

Figure 3.10. Circuit containing two ion channel NMOS transistors and a limiting PMOS transistor. The NMOS transistor tied to ground is driven by an inverter.

rises and falls, modulating the voltage rise and fall depending on the requirements. There may be no requirement to have a voltage rise to V_{dd} or fall to 0.0 V.

The circuit can contain a PMOS transistor X near the capacitor, as shown in figure 3.9. The control (gate) voltage of this transistor can be used, as it's rising, to turn off transistor X. Initially transistor X is on and current is flowing, but as the voltage output rises, eventually the output turns off transistor X and limits the output voltage V rising. After V reaches a limit it will stop rising, limiting the output. Modulation by using transistors that can be turned off and on as the voltages change can be used throughout a neural circuit to change the way it behaves. To limit the output voltage falling, the above method could be used in the *pull-down* circuit connected to ground. As the output voltage falls, the *pull-down* transistor's gate voltage falls, turning off the *pull-down* transistor. The basic techniques described here are used throughout the neuromorphic circuits described in this text. Figure 3.10 combines figures 3.8 and 3.9 in a simulated circuit. Transistor sizes

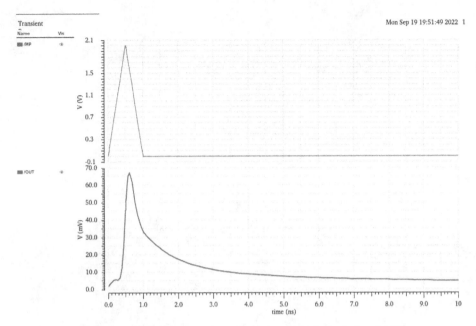

Figure 3.11. Simulation waveforms from the circuit shown in figure 3.10.

are shown. The simulation waveforms for this circuit are shown in figure 3.11. Note that the waveforms are not smooth, a side effect of the simulation software used. Physicists have constructed simplified learning neural networks with interconnected networks of variable resistors, reminiscent of the simple synapse models we are proposing here [5]. While most biological mechanisms are absent from this learning model, it provides a basis for a crude neural network built of variable resistor models built with MOS transistors.

In addition, neural circuit designers use some classical analog circuit techniques, including *current mirrors, differential pairs, single-transistor amplifiers, voltage-to-current converters, current adders, self-resetting circuits,* and *one-shot circuits,* along with digital *inverters* and other techniques introduced here that will be used in the chapters that follow.

3.3 Basic analog circuits

The first circuit introduced is the differential pair, shown in figure 3.12. This circuit adds two currents, I_1 and I_2, that result in I_b.

The second analog circuit used frequently is the current mirror (figure 3.13). The circuit parameters are adjusted so that the output current matches current flowing in transistor *M1*. The terminal attached to *M2* is also attached to the output circuit, and changes in that circuit structure and behavior will not alter the current flow in *M2*, I_{out}, in essence avoiding loading the current mirror. Transistors *M1* and *M2* are both kept in saturation (active mode). Note that for *M1*, $V_d1 = V_g1$, forcing saturation. The current flowing through *M1* and *M2* are forced to be the same if

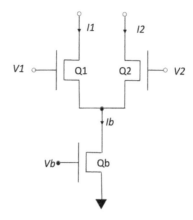

Figure 3.12. A Differential pair circuit.

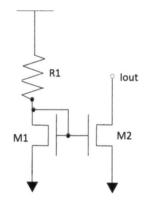

Figure 3.13. A current mirror circuit.

the transistors are the same width and length. An excellent introduction to current mirrors is found in Wikipedia.

Analog voltage adders are rarely used besides the BioRC project, since current addition is much simpler to implement with a differential pair circuit. A basic voltage adder by Chaoui is shown in figure 3.14 [1]. Differential pairs and a current mirror are used in the circuit. Note that transistors M2 and M6 correct for nonlinearities, and V_{ss} is negative, allowing the voltage adder to add negative voltages.

A monostable timing (*one-shot*) circuit shown in figure 3.15(a) is used to produce signals of different duration. The purpose of this circuit is to generate a single output pulse when it is triggered by the input. This fourth analog circuit useful for neuromorphic circuits is also called the *monostable multivibrator*. At the beginning, both V_{IN} and V_{OUT} are low, and the internal nodes V_1 and V_2 are at V_{DD}. When a spike arrives, V_1 drops to *GND* that leads V_2 to start dropping. Once V_2 drops below the switching point of the inverter (*X*1, *X*2), it causes V_{OUT} to rise to V_{DD}. Whenever V_{OUT} stays at V_{DD}, V_1 remains low. V_2, however, falls since the voltage across the

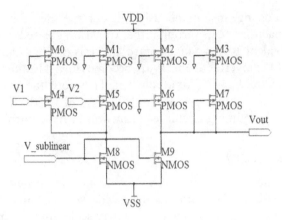

Figure 3.14. Chaoui voltage adder.

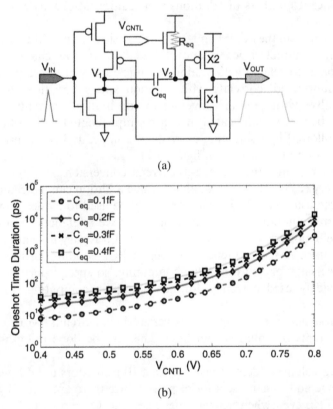

(a)

(b)

Figure 3.15. Monostable *one-shot timing* circuit and its characterization. (a) *One-shot timing* circuit: this circuit is used to generate a prolonged output from a short pulse input. The time period is regulated by the $R_{eq} \cdot C_{eq}$ time constant. (b) Monostable one-shot timing circuit characterization. The voltage control modulates the output pulse duration. The time duration shown here ranges from 8 ps to 120 ns given the two parameters, C_{eq} and V_{CNTL}.

capacitor does not change instantaneously, but starts to rise again due to the current charging the capacitor, C_{eq}, through the transistor biased with V_{CNTL}. This transistor is equivalent to a voltage-controlled resistor R_{eq}. Once V_2 reaches the switching point of the inverter again, V_{OUT} becomes low. The time it takes to charge V_2 is determined by the $R_{eq} \cdot C_{eq}$ time constant. Therefore, the prolonged duration is controlled by these two parameters R_{eq} and C_{eq}. Figure 3.15(b) shows the characterization of the one-shot timing circuit as a function of the control input, V_{CNTL}.

3.3.1 Why analog circuits?

Many neuromorphic researchers use analog and/or *pulse and timing* circuits to model neural signaling. These circuits may scale voltages and currents to match technology or biology. Likewise, the circuits may scale timing to match technology or biology. There is some motivation to use analog circuits versus digital circuits or software. Depending on the precision required, a minimum number of transistors in a full adder for digital sum + carry is at least 4 transistors/bit[3]. Neural computations involve significant numbers of additions and multiplications, as well as other non-linear operations.

Analog circuits, on the other hand, use few transistors. Individual MOS transistor current/voltage characteristics mimic charge flow in ion channels in neurons. Multiplication is correlated with analog amplification, while voltages and currents, added and subtracted, correlate with addition and subtraction. Analog current addition involves wiring circuits together to add multiple currents. While voltage addition can be more complicated, it can be implemented with voltage-to-current conversion followed by combining currents at a node, and reconverting current to voltage at the output, as shown in figure 3.14.

Transistors perform the voltage-to-current conversion and current-to-voltage conversion very easily. However, analog voltage addition can use significant power. Adding charge using switched capacitors could be used to reduce power consumption in dendritic computations, as the reader will see references to in section 16.5.

One of the major advantages of software is that it is easy to change connectivity. The disadvantage is speed. General-purpose CPUs contain hardware complexity that is unnecessary for neuromorphic computing, so special purpose or simplified CPUs are widely used currently for neuromorphic computing, as described in chapter 17.

Why do designers use analog circuits versus digital circuits? Most neural circuits must add currents or voltages somehow. This can be done using analog voltage adders.

For analog voltage adders, it takes at least 10 transistors to add two real values. Analog voltage adders can use a lot of power since there are generally connections from V_{DD} to V_{ss}, even when neurons are quiescent. Currents can be added just by connecting wires. Adding charge involves switching capacitors. It is comparatively easier to do some functions with analog circuits than with digital circuits, using

---

[3] http://3.14.by/en/read/BarsFA-4T-full-adder

fewer transistors. But there are many other factors that make building analog circuits much more complicated than building digital circuits. (In the research world some researchers are building analog circuits to model the brain. In the commercial world engineers are building digital circuits.) In cases where you might be able to build large scale systems like an entire brain, analog circuits will be able to give some size advantages over digital circuits.

However, the brain is said to make new connections every hour. How do you do that with MOS circuits? Once CMOS circuits are fabricated. the circuit structure is frozen, unless you put in an elaborate switching mechanism. There's no easy way to deal with this problem. Something that might work would be a solution built with nanocomponents, where the connections could be changed. In some nanotechnologies one might be able to make and break connections on the fly and real time, online, while the system is in operation.

With simple analog circuits, currents can be added, voltage can be added (possibly by adding currents), a simple single-transistor amplifier can be built and one can build a self-resetting circuit.

3.4 Chapter summary

This chapter covered an approach to constructing electronic neurons using CMOS transistors. Neural structures implemented in circuits were shown, and analog transistor behavior was summarized. The text continues here with a discussion of mathematical models in chapter 4.

3.5 Exercises

1. The ion channel circuit shown in figure 3.9 (mark all correct answers):
    (a) Limits the rise in membrane potential;
    (b) Has two ion channels;
    (c) Modulates the output membrane potential;
    (d) Contains a PMOS transistor.

References

[1] Chaoui H 1995 CMOS analogue adder *Electron. Lett.* **31** 180–1
[2] Indiveri G and Sandamirskaya Y 2019 The importance of space and time in neuromorphic cognitive agents *IEEE Signal Process. Mag.* **36** 16–28
[3] Kang S, Leblibici Y and Kim C 2014 *CMOS Digital Integrated Circuits Analysis & Design* (New York: McGraw-Hill)
[4] Parker A C 2013 The biorc biomimetic real-time cortex project (University of Southern California) URL: http://ceng.usc.eduparker/BioRCresearch.html
[5] Stern M *et al* 2021 Out of equilibrium learning dynamics in physical allosteric resistor networks *Fourth Workshop on Machine Learning and the Physical Sciences (NeurIPS 2021)*
[6] Mead C 1989 *Analog VLSI and Neural Systems* (Addison-Wesley)

IOP Publishing

Neuromorphic Circuits
A constructive approach
Alice C Parker and Rick Cattell

Chapter 4

Mathematical models

Alice C Parker, Yilda Irizarry-Valle, Rebecca Lee and Suraj Chakravarthi Raja

There are a wide variety of mathematical neuronal models, also known as spiking neuron models, that can be expressed in the form of ordinary differential equations (ODEs), including the Integrate-and-Fire (I&F) model and its different model variations (i.e. the leaky I&F model, the adaptive I&F model, etc), the Hodgkin–Huxley (H&H) model [10], and the Izhikevich model [12].

This chapter presents mathematical models of spiking neurons, with emphasis on the Izhikevich model, examining the two dozen neuro-computational models that Izhikevich presents for biological spiking neurons. We also look at a historical model, leaky I&F, and the classic H&H model is summarized. We examine and compare the computational cost of these computational models. The H&H model is very accurate, but by far most expensive computationally. The Izhikevich model is two orders of magnitude less expensive arithmetically, and achieves acceptable accuracy on all of the cases we examine.

4.1 Izhikevich's spiking model

In Izhikevich's 2003 paper, he presents different biological neural spiking patterns, representing the output firing patterns coming from a neuron. Izhikevich shows a variety of spiking variations for biological neurons (these are all human). Some animals don't have all these varying spiking patterns. Izhikevich said that it's inaccurate to reduce a spiking pattern to binary (0 or 1). Spiking patterns are important because there might be some information that could be used. Izhikevich makes a statement in his paper that inappropriate choices of spiking model may lead to results having nothing to do with information processing by the brain. So using an appropriate spiking model is crucial in his opinion, especially when modeling the brain.

This chapter focuses on Izhikevich's mathematical model that produces a variety of spiking patterns and the Leaky I&F model used widely in neuromorphic circuits. However, a few other models are more than worthy of mention.

4.1.1 Izhikevich's spiking patterns

Figure 4.1 shows Izhikevich's patterns.

Izhikevich provides mathematical models of spiking that illustrate the circumstances when a neuron decides to spike, but does not explain how the inputs are processed in biological neurons to produce the current or voltage inside a neuron to cause spiking. Synapses and the dendritic arbor are not included in the model, but the catalog of spiking variations is useful to show the range of neural behaviors possible. This range of behaviors may contribute to the *neural code*, as described in section 1.9.

Figure 4.1(A) shows *tonic* spiking, where spiking continues as long as current is injected. There are three variations of tonic spiking, where spike rate is repeated while the input current is injected in *regular spiking* (RS) excitatory neurons, *FS (fast spiking)* inhibitory interneurons where the spike rate increases with the same current injection, and *LTS (low threshold spiking)* inhibitory interneurons where the spiking occurs at a lower threshold of current as current is injected. *Interneurons* are simpler neurons that connect the more complex neurons in a biological neuronal network. *Inhibitory* interneurons inhibit or stop the neurons they impinge on from spiking, or at least lower the probability of spiking.

Figure 4.1(B) shows *phasic spiking*, where the neuron produces one spike at the onset of current injected. This illustrates sporadic spiking that typically has no result downstream in the succeeding neurons.

Figure 4.1(C) illustrates *tonic bursting*, periodic *bursts* of spikes, also called *chattering*. A *burst* of spikes is a cluster of spikes that rides on a DC component of the spike train. The value of bursting is that a burst may overcome transmission failure, reduce neuronal noise, transmit importance (saliency) and transmit to frequency-selective neurons. Inter-burst frequency (between bursts) <50 Hz may contribute to gamma oscillations in the brain.

Figure 4.1(D) shows phasic bursting, where one burst occurs at the beginning of current injection. Figure 4.1(E) shows a mixed mode where a burst is followed by tonic spiking. A variation of tonic spiking is shown in figure 4.1(F), where spike frequency adaptation occurs and spike frequency decreases. This first produces a burst, followed by gradual decreasing frequency of regular spikes. This can occur in RS neurons and also LTS interneurons that tend to spike more frequently. This adaptation is partly because of the limited chemical sources in the neuron. This also occurs in LTS interneurons. Sometimes it's called a *depressing synapse* that runs out of resources. When the synapse has spikes impinging, it starts to produce the actual output spikes, after a point of time, it starts depleting it's resources and spikes become less frequent.

Bursting is a cluster of spikes. Bursting results in the neuron being more likely to transmit its signal because bursting is reducing the occurence of noise. This overcomes transmission failure. A burst can also mean that the neuron is more likely to produce a spontaneous spike as well. But a spontaneous spike might not trigger anything downstream because usually the receiving neuron is also responsive to a burst of spikes. Frequency-selective and pattern-sensitive neurons don't always

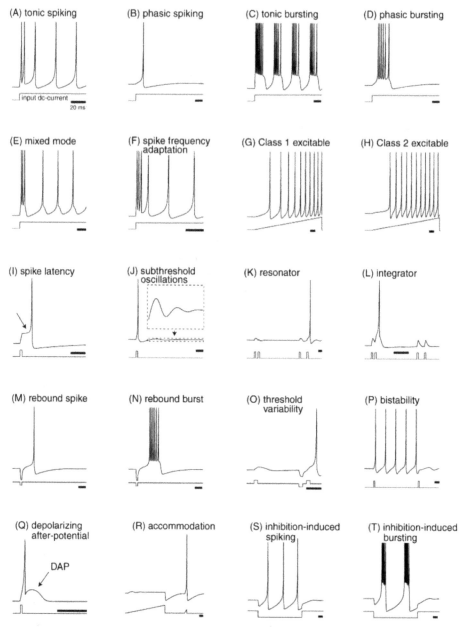

Figure 4.1. Summary of the neuro-computational properties of biological spiking neurons taken from [12]. Shown are simulations of the same model given in [12] (1) and (2), with different choices of parameters. Each horizontal heavy black bar denotes a 20 ms time interval. There are two traces in each diagram A-T. The lower one is the input stimulus and the upper one is the output voltage. The MATLAB file generating the figure and containing all the parameters, as well as interactive MATLAB tutorial program can be downloaded from the Izhikevich's website. This figure is reproduced with permission from http://www.izhikevich.com, where an electronic version of the figure and reproduction permissions are freely available.

respond to the same signal. Neurons sending bursts can transmit to both these types of neurons. Figure 4.1(G) and (H) show two major classes of excitability. Class 1 neurons shown in G spike depending on strength of input 2–200 Hz (e.g. RS neurons). Increased current produces increased frequency of spiking at the output. In figure 4.1(H) Class 2, quiescent or fixed frequency spiking (e.g. 40 Hz) is shown. It does not matter how fast the inputs to the neuron are arriving; spiking does not depend on the strength of the input.

Spike latency, shown in 4.1(I), occurs with spiking where delay can be inversely proportional to the strength of the input signal. So, the weaker the signal, the longer the delay. For example, spike latency can be around 10 ms for RS neurons. After spiking, neurons can oscillate at subthreshold amplitudes, as shown in 4.1(J). These neurons can act as band pass filters, where lower and higher frequency signals are blocked from passing through the filter. Figure 4.1(K) shows frequency preference and resonance, where neurons can act as resonators, responding to specific frequencies of stimulation. There might not be spikes in the output but some oscillations may be present. This can act as a band pass filter.

Neurons can also act as integrators and coincidence detectors, spiking when stimuli arrive close together in time (figure 4.1(L)). Consider that there are two closely spaced spikes arriving. If you have them spaced a certain distance apart, a spike is obtained at the output. So, it's always sensitive to certain frequencies of spiking. Consider two spikes that arrive quickly and two spikes that arrive more slowly. Faster input spikes are more likely to produce a spike at the output. Two overlapping postsynaptic potentials (PSPs) rise high enough, pass the threshold and produce a spike at the output. If these PSPs are separated a little bit more in time, then that threshold might never be crossed. This can be modeled using a synapse powered by a capacitor with a charge on it instead of V_{DD}. When a spike comes along and the neuron responds, the capacitor is discharged. If the next spike comes along too quickly, the neuron cannot respond now because of the discharged capacitor. After some time, the capacitor is slowly charged externally, then when a spike comes along, it responds.

Rebound spikes, shown in figure 4.1(M), appear after the current goes negative. This is the opposite of the previous spiking pattern. Alternately, figure 4.1(N) shows a rebound burst due to a negative current. There are also different shapes of spikes. Figure 4.1(M) shows a *rebound spike* which can create a membrane potential (MP) (voltage) decreasing by an injected current decreasing and when the current rises again, it triggers the spike. If there is a slightly different kind of neuron then, instead of causing a single spike, an entire *rebound burst* can be produced as a result of the rising current, as shown in (N).

Spiking is shown in figure 4.1(O) if and only if there is low enough threshold voltage. Some neurons can be bistable (figure 4.1P)), spiking in a tonic manner if the injected current is in phase with the spiking, or quiescent, if the current is out of phase. Shown in figure 4.1(O) and (P), a small current blip doesn't cause spiking to happen, but a larger rise in current, that results in fast rise in voltage, can cause the output to spike. The explanation for this is *threshold variability*, a decrease in spiking threshold due to a rapid rise in input current. So, the spiking threshold depends on how fast the MP in the neuron is rising. Bistability depends on the time when the current is injected. If the current is injected at the right time, the neuron spikes, as shown in figure 4.1(P).

Many neurons display *accommodation* (figure 4.1(R)), where the threshold for spiking is inversely proportional to the slope of input current stimulation. After a neuron spikes, it may *hyper polarize*, meaning the voltage may go lower than the resting potential and then rise, as shown in (R), possibly due to potassium currents, or it may produce a little extra rising bump after the spike, called *depolarizing*, possibly due to calcium currents, as shown in figure 4.1(Q).

Inhibition-induced spiking and bursting is shown in figure 4.1(S) and (T). (S) and (T) show spiking and bursting caused by negative current, due to inhibition, the opposite of what might be expected. This is the result of *presynaptic* spikes arriving at inhibitory synapses, resulting in *postsynaptic* spiking or bursting, instead of inhibition of spiking.

4.1.2 Mathematics of Izhikevich's spiking model

Izhekevich' mathematical models do not include the synapses or the dendritic arbor; they just cover the spiking circuit, the axon initial segment. These models are not necessarily formal closed-form mathematical models. Some are piecewise models.

The Izhikevich mathematical model consists of two equations (4.1) and (4.2). Despite the lack of any biophysical meaning compared to H&H model, it is an excellent mathematical model because it is as simple as the I&F model, yet it can produce many of the cortical neuronal behaviors based on four parameters a, b, c, and d [12]. The model is based on the mathematical theory of bifurcation and the phase portrait. Bifurcation theory states that '*In dynamical systems, a bifurcation occurs when a small smooth change made to the parameter values (the bifurcation parameters) of a system causes a sudden 'qualitative' or topological change in its behavior. Generally, at a bifurcation, the local stability properties of equilibria, periodic orbits, or other invariant sets changes*' [7].

$$v' = 0.04v^2 + 5v + 140 - u + I, \text{ if } v \geqslant 30 \text{ mV, then } v \leftarrow c \qquad (4.1)$$

$$d\rho(v, T) = \rho_v(T)dv = \frac{8\pi K_B T}{c^3}v^2 dv. \qquad (4.2)$$

where v represent the neuron's MP, u is the recovery variable, I represents the input current, and a, b, c are dimensionless parameters describing the time scale of u, the sensitivity of u, and the after-spike reset value of the MP, respectively. Details of the model and dimensionless parameters and how the parameters change with different spiking patterns are found in [12]. A comparison between other neuron spiking models is shown in table 4.1, where the complexity of a model is measured based on the number of floating points (FLOPS) operations [11]. Figure 4.1 shows various action potential (AP) patterns that can be generated using Izhikevich's mathematical spiking model.

Table 4.1. A comparison between different spiking models. FLOPS is the number of floating point operations. Copyright 2004 IEEE. Adopted, with permission, from [11].

Models	biophysically meaningful	tonic spiking	phasic spiking	tonic bursting	phasic bursting	mixed mode	spike frequency adaptation	class 1 excitable	class 2 excitable	spike latency	subthreshold oscillations	resonator	integrator	rebound spike	rebound burst	threshold variability	bistability	DAP	accommodation	inhibition-induced spiking	inhibition-induced bursting	chaos	# of FLOPS
integrate-and-fire	-	+	-	-	-	-	-	+	-	-	-	-	+	-	-	-	-	-	-	-	-	-	5
integrate-and-fire with adapt.	-	+	-	-	-	-	+	+	-	-	-	-	+	-	-	-	-	+	-	-	-	-	10
integrate-and-fire-or-burst	-	+	+		+	-	+	+	-	-		-	+	+	+	-	+	+	-	-	-		13
resonate-and-fire	-	+	+	-	-	-	-	+	+	-	+	+	+	+	-	-	+	+	+	-	-	+	10
quadratic integrate-and-fire	-	+	-	-	-	-	-	+	-	+	-	-	+	-	-	+	+	-	-	-	-	-	7
Izhikevich (2003)	-	+	+	+	+	+	+	+	+	+	+	+	+	+	+	+	+	+	+	+	+	+	13
FitzHugh-Nagumo	-	+	+	-		-	-	+	-	+	+	+	-	+	-	+	+	-	+	+	-	-	72
Hindmarsh-Rose	-	+	+	+		+	+	+	+	+	+	+	+	+	+	+	+	+	+			+	120
Morris-Lecar	+	+	+	-		-	-	+	+	+	+	+	+	+		+	+	-	+	+	-	-	600
Wilson	-	+	+	+		+	+	+	+	+	+	+	+	+	+	+		+	+				180
Hodgkin-Huxley	+	+	+	+		+	+	+	+	+	+	+	+	+	+	+	+	+	+			+	1200

u is the membrane recovery variable that accounts for the activation of K^+ ionic currents and inactivation of Na^+ ionic currents, and provides negative feedback to v[1].

If v skips over 30, then first v is reset to 30, and then to c so that all spikes have equal magnitudes (threshold is -70 to -40 mV, resting is -70 mV)[2]. 13 floating point operations are required. The parameters are set as follows:

- $a = 0.02$ typically;
- $b = 0.2$ typically but can vary;
- $c = -0.65$ m mV typically;
- $d = 2$ typically.

A neural network simulation was performed by Izhikevich, using 10k neurons and 1 M random synaptic connections, with random thalamic inputs. Some parameters a–d were selected using random numbers to get heterogeneous neurons. Izhikevich assigned each excitatory neuron c and d and assigned each inhibitory neuron a and b, based on a random variable r_i. More details are found in the 2003 Izhikevich publication [12] (figure 4.2).

---

[1] Note that there is no I (current) in the u model.
[2] Actually this means that there is a ceiling function that limits v to 30 mV.

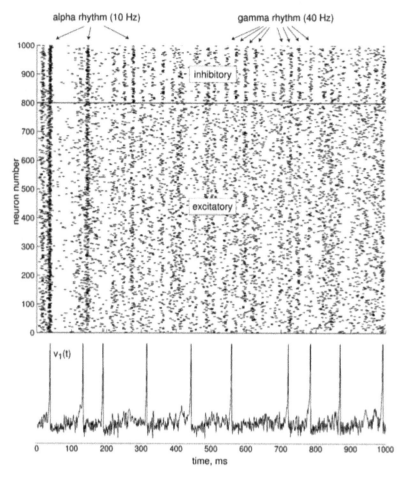

Figure 4.2. Simulation of a network of 1000 randomly coupled spiking neurons. Top: spike raster shows episodes of alpha and gamma band rhythms (vertical lines). Bottom: typical spiking activity of an excitatory neuron. All spikes were equalized at 30 mV by resetting $v - 1$ first to +30 mV and then to c. Copyright 2003 IEEE. Reprinted, with permission, from [12].

4.2 Leaky integrate-and-fire spiking model

The I&F model is one of the most widely used neuron spiking models. It is the simplest neuronal spiking model. The model describes a neuron as an integrator where a neuron integrates its synaptic inputs and then compares the result with a threshold value. In the I&F model, a neuron generates a spike only when the neuron's specific threshold value is exceeded. Despite the appeal of the model's simplicity, it does not appear to be as computationally useful as other models as it fails to explain many of the cortical neuronal behaviors, and it does not provide any biophysical meaning. The equation describing the I&F model is shown in equation (4.3).

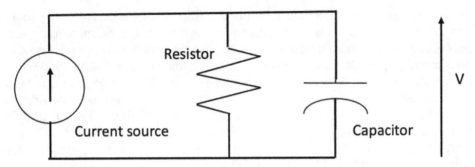

Figure 4.3. Leaky I&F equivalent circuit. V is the difference in voltage between the inner neuron and the space outside the neuron, or the MP. The capacitance is shown polarized since the voltage across the capacitor (the MP) is never negative.

$$v' = I + a - bv, \text{ if } v \geqslant v_{\text{thresh}}, \text{ then } v \leftarrow c \qquad (4.3)$$

where v_{thresh} represents the neuron's threshold for spiking, v represents the MP, I represents the input current (stimulus), and a, b, c are the parameters describing the peak and the resting potential of the generated spike. t is time in ms, and I is input current. $-bv$ is the leaking charge. This neuron is *class I* excitable, with tonic spikes of a constant frequency. The model acts as an integrator and is piecewise. The integration continues if and only if $v < V_{\text{threshold}}$. Otherwise, v is reset to c (cell membrane resting potential), a spike is output and the voltage v is set to the resting potential. Izhikevich states each iteration can be implemented in software, to perform numerical integration, using an integration time step of 1 ms. He states that 'the iteration takes only four floating-point operations (additions, multiplications, etc) plus one comparison with the threshold.' This simple model cannot be used for phasic spiking, bursting, or rebound. The threshold is usually fixed in this model. The equivalent circuit model for this is a current source with capacitor and resistor in series, as shown in figure 4.3. From the Izhikevich paper, numerical integration for simulation purposes can be performed as follows: he sets the time period to 1 ms, but it could be smaller. $v(t + \tau) = I + a - bv(t)$ is executed repeatedly.

If $b = 0$, the neuron is not leaky. The model does not cover phasic spiking, bursting, rebound, threshold variations, bistability, autonomous dynamics, random dynamics pr chaotic dynamics, some of which will be covered later. It also does not support changes in initial conditions.

4.3 The Hodgkin–Huxley model 1952

The H&H model for neural spiking was first published in 1952. It describes how APs in neurons are initiated and propagated down the axon. The model consists of a set of nonlinear differential equations that is a continuous-time model. Hodgkin and Huxley were awarded the Nobel prize in 1963 for this research.

The H&H model [9], is one of the essential neuronal spiking models. Hodgkin was the first to experiment with the dynamic bifurcation concept before the actual development of the mathematical bifurcation theory was published. The model consists of many parameters describing the activation and deactivation of ion channels and other biophysical dynamics. Despite the complex representation of the H&H model, it provides biophysical meaning describing neuronal behaviors. Hence, it is a widely used model in the field of computational biology. Besides, the H&H model describes the neurons as dynamical systems by which the model classifies the neuron behaviors into three classes according to their excitability through studying the frequency to the current relationship (Class 1, Class 2, and Class 3). In Class 1 excitability, the neuron's spiking frequency increases with the increase of the injected current's amplitude [8]. In Class 2 excitability, the neuron generates spikes at a small range of frequencies independent of the injected current amplitude [8]. In Class 3 excitability, the neuron spikes with a single spike corresponding to a pulse of injected current, and, at a very high pulse of current, a neuron may exhibit tonic spiking. An equivalent circuit for the model is shown in figure 4.4. The voltage difference between the extracellular medium and the intracellular medium is about $-70\,\mathrm{mV}$ when the neuron is resting, and there is about a $+110\,\mathrm{mV}$ AP, resulting in a peak

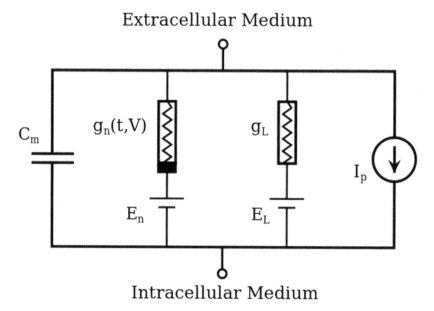

Figure 4.4. Equivalent circuit used in the H&H model. The extracellular medium is outside the neuron and intracellular medium is inside the cell. C_m represents the membrane capacitance modeling the lipid (fatty) membrane, g_n represents ion channel conductance (inverse of resistance), g_L is the leaky membrane conductance. The electrochemical gradients driving the flow of ions, batteries (E) (also called electromotive force) depend on the ratio of ions of the channel's type inside and outside the cell. E_n is the electromotive force that moves ions in the reverse direction of the ion concentration gradient. In the detailed model, E_n is replaced with E_{Na} for sodium and E_K for potassium. This File:Hodgkin-Huxley.svg has been obtained by the authors from the Wikimedia website, where it is stated to have been released into the public domain. It is included within this book on that basis.

potential of about 40 mV. I_p is the pump current that restores the MP to the resting potential by moving ions in the reverse direction.

The H&H model contains a differential equation with four state variables: $v(t)$, $m(t)$, $n(t)$, and $h(t)$, that change with respect to time t. The MP is V_m. The current flowing through the membrane $I_c = c_m dV_m/dt$ and the charge stored in the membrane capacitance $Q_c = C_m V_m$. The current flowing through the ith ion channel is $I_i = g_i(V_m - V_i)$ where V_i is the *Nernst (reversal) potential* of the ith ion channel, the potential across the membrane at which there is no net current flow. The Nernst equation indicates how much force there is on the ions depending on their concentrations outside and inside the cell, called the *electromotive* force. Outside the neuron there exists higher concentration of sodium than inside. Inside the neuron there exists a higher concentration of potassium than outside. So, the Nernst equation tell us how the ions are to diffuse between the input and output depending on the Nernst equation or the Nernst potential.

The Nernst equation is the following:

$$E_x = \frac{RT}{F} \ln \frac{[C_x]_o}{[C_x]_i} \qquad (4.4)$$

where C_x are the ion concentrations inside (i) and outside (o) the neuron. R is the universal gas constant: $R = 8.314\,472(15)$ in joules per kelvin per mole. T is temperature in kelvins. F is the Faraday constant, the number of coulombs per mole of electrons.

Note that the ion channel properties are denoted by the type of ion in the channel. g_K and g_{Na} are the potassium and sodium conductances per unit area, V_K and V_{Na} are the potassium and sodium reversal potentials, and g_l and V_l are the leak conductance per unit area and leak reversal potential. The time-dependent elements of this equation are V_m, g_{Na}, and g_K, where the last two conductances depend explicitly on voltage as well. Note that the sodium and potassium ion channels are in parallel, from cell interior to cell exterior. The Nernst potentials are 55 mV for sodium and −70 mV for potassium. Resting potential can be computed using the Goldman equation below, and is −60 mV.

$$V_{rest} = U_T \ln \frac{P_K[K^+]_o + P_{Na}[Na^+]_o}{P_K[K^+]_i + P_{Na}[Na^+]_i} \qquad (4.5)$$

Since biological spikes primarily depend on sodium and potassium ion channels, the total current I through the neural cell membrane can be computed as follows:

$$I = \text{capacitance current} + \text{ion channel currents} + \text{leak current} \qquad (4.6)$$

$$I = C_m dV_m/dt + g_K(V_m - V_k) + g_{Na}(V_m - V_{Na}) + g_l(V_m - V_l)$$

Hodgkin and Huxley experimentally determined the current equation to be a function of *mean* conductances.

The entire H&H model shown below includes the current equation above, modified with the addition of parameters n, m and h, and the means of the conductances.

$$I = C_{\mathrm{m}}\frac{dV_{\mathrm{m}}}{dt} + \bar{g}_{\mathrm{K}}n^4(V_{\mathrm{m}} - V_{\mathrm{K}}) + \bar{g}_{\mathrm{Na}}m^3h(V_{\mathrm{m}} - V_{\mathrm{Na}}) + \bar{g}_{\mathrm{l}}(V_{\mathrm{m}} - V_{\mathrm{l}}) \qquad (4.7)$$

and three differential equations for the dimensionless parameters n, m and h, shown below in equations (4.8), (4.9), and (4.10).

$$\frac{dn}{dt} = \alpha_n(V_{\mathrm{m}})(1 - n) - \beta_n(V_{\mathrm{m}})n \qquad (4.8)$$

$$\frac{dm}{dt} = \alpha_{\mathrm{m}}(V_{\mathrm{m}})(1 - m) - \beta_{\mathrm{m}}(V_{\mathrm{m}})m \qquad (4.9)$$

$$\frac{dh}{dt} = \alpha_h(V_{\mathrm{m}})(1 - h) - \beta_h(V_{\mathrm{m}})h \qquad (4.10)$$

α and β are rate constants for the ion channels that depend on voltage but not on time. There are many computations possible for α and β. A specific computation is used for membrane current I:

$$I = \frac{a}{2R}\frac{\partial^2 V}{\partial x^2} \qquad (4.11)$$

There are some issues related to the H&H model, or for that matter, any mathematical model. In general, when adding biological features, the model must be amplified or changed. For example adding calcium currents to the H&H model would involve an additional term in the current equation, an additional differential equation and an additional rate constant. Finally, there is no model here of variable behavior that is chaotic or stochastic, a hallmark of biological neuronal networks.

4.4 Other spiking models

The FitzHugh–Nagumo model is similar to and preceded Izhikevich's model. There is no reset and no stochastic or chaotic behavior. Here are the basic equations for this model:

$$v' = a + bv + cv^2 + dv^3 - u \qquad (4.12)$$

$$u' = \varepsilon(ev - u) \qquad (4.13)$$

Izhikevich provides a comparison of spiking models, although the comparison is somewhat dated. His comparison is shown in figure 4.5.

There are numerous mathematical models of spiking neurons in the literature. Most models cover a single spiking pattern, the *phasic spike*. However, the situation becomes more complicated when other spiking patterns are used. While it would be possible to construct electronic neurons by curve-matching electronic circuit behaviors to these mathematical models, the circumstances surrounding the spiking patterns may differ due to anatomical differences in neurons, along with different input (presynaptic) spiking patterns. The text discusses many of these variations

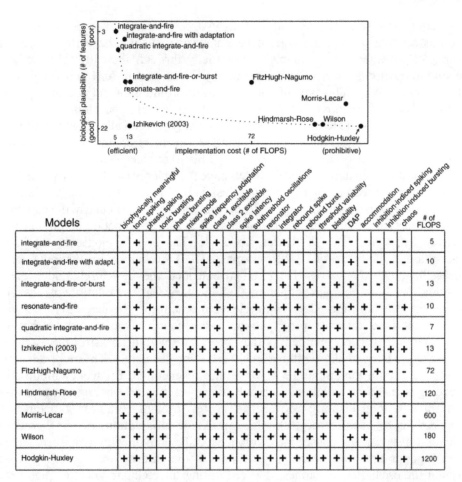

Figure 4.5. This figure shows comparison of the neuro-computational properties of spiking and bursting models; see figure 4.1. '# of FLOPS' is an approximate number of floating point operations (addition, multiplication, etc) needed to simulate the model during a 1 ms time span. Each empty square indicates the property that the model should exhibit in principle (in theory) if the parameters are chosen appropriately, but the author failed to find the parameters within a reasonable period of time. Copyright 2004 IEEE. Reprinted, with permission, from [11].

throughout the book. It would be useful to capture variations in spiking due to input and anatomical variations, as the text discusses later. At this point, the text focuses on the most basic leaky I&F model that is used widely in neuromorphic circuits, and the Izhikevitz model, due to its wide variety of spiking patterns.

4.5 Astrocyte mathematical models

Mathematical models have been developed to study the modulation of amplitude, frequency, or both in astrocytic calcium waves and their correlations with neuronal activity. In astrocytes, the intensity of stimulation, i.e. the number of neuro-transmitters that bind astrocytic receptors, is known to establish the level of interaction between astrocytes and neurons. Astrocytes can communicate with a few neurons sending a local message, if calcium waves do not have the strength to propagate to other microdomains or eventually through the entire glial cell and beyond to other glial cells. Global communication may occur only under high levels of neuronal activity. This type of communication would allow all neurons spanned by the astrocyte synctium (cluster of connected astrocytes) to be contacted. Calcium waves could propagate to other astrocyte cells in a syncytium allowing them to reach neurons far away and thus establish an indirect form of communication between neuronal paths that otherwise would not be able to contact each other.

In the last decade mathematical models have focused on: (1) the description of the mechanisms that lead to the generation of calcium waves in astrocytes; (2) the use of these models to incorporate neuro-astrocyte interactions, particularly the capability of astrocytes to facilitate neuronal firing; and (3) the gap-junction communication between astrocytes. The Li–Rinzel model [15] has been a pioneer work in the description of the Insositol 1,3,4 triphosphate (IP3) mechanism for the induction of intracellular calcium waves. De Pittà [4] extended the Li–Rinzel model [15] to account for more complex signaling that includes Ca^{2+} regulation by the IP3-dependent calcium-induced calcium-release mechanism[3]. In his study, De Pittà shows that long distance propagation of regenerative waves (waves that are generated and then regenerated as they propagate within an astrocyte) is closely related to the intracellular (within the cell) encoding of calcium. The more calcium is present, the more the amplitude of waves are regenerated. Frequency modulation encoding of calcium oscillations with pulsating dynamics induces regenerative waves that travel a long distance between astrocytes through nonlinear gap junctions (connections between astrocytes), while amplitude modulation encoding produces calcium waves that are constrained within a specific domain within an astrocyte. De Pittà suggests that nonlinear gap junctions, in the case of weak coupling, could explain the oscillation dynamics observed during intercellular calcium wave propagation in astrocyte networks [3].

The gatekeeper model [24] introduces the ability of astrocytes to reduce the calcium flux by means of presynaptic mGluR channels, using the Li–Rinzel model [15] for the calcium dynamics. In the gatekeeper model, a phenomenological variable has been used to account for the finite amount of glutamate in the astrocyte. Astrocytes release glutamate that binds presynaptic neural terminals, activating neural mGluR channels, causing the decrease of calcium influx into the presynaptic neuron, and reducing the probability of evoked transmitter release. The gatekeeper model shows that the amplitude of excitatory and inhibitory postsynaptic currents in the neuron is decreased due to the astrocytic control over the calcium influx into the presynaptic neuron mediated by glutamate.

The Nadkarni [16, 17] model is the first to incorporate the astrocyte's capability to modulate a neural synapse using the Li–Rinzel model for the calcium dynamics. Amiri [2] constructed a minimal neuronal network of two Morris–Lecar neuron

---

[3] As well as IP3 dynamics resulting from PLC-mediated synthesis and degradation by IP3 3-kinase (3K) and inositol poly phosphate (IP) 5-phosphatase (5P) [4].

models. This work includes dynamics between astrocytes and neurons which follows Nadkarni's model [16]. Amiri provides a theoretical analysis establishing that a healthy astrocyte increases the threshold value of synchronization and thus has the potential to induce desynchronization in neurons.

Di Garbo [6] developed a biophysical model for the calcium dynamics that describes experimental results [19]. The model is able to show the adnosine triphosphate (ATP)-evoked biphasic (two phase) calcium response in the astrocyte. This response is described by the transient phase, evoked by the release of calcium from the endoplasmic reticulum (ER) in the astrocyte, and the sustained phase that is dependent on the influx of extracellular calcium into the astrocyte mediated by P2X purinoreceptors that regulate communication between neurons and glia [13]. Di Garbo also developed a biophysical model for a minimal network consisting of a single astrocyte, pyramidal neuron, and an interneuron [5]. The model shows the modulation properties of astrocytes on both the pyramidal neuron and interneuron by the release of glutamate from the astrocyte. Following experimental results, Di Garbo shows the role of astrocytic released ATP in the modulation of the ability of the interneuron to fire. Di Garbo's results also show that the increase in intracellular calcium in the astrocyte leads to a decrease in the calcium oscillations, which is in agreement with experimental data [14, 20, 21]. Di Garbo shows that the reduction of calcium influx from the ER to the cytoplasm does not result in calcium oscillations, which is also in agreement with experimental data [18]. Moreover, it was also shown that the increase of intracellular calcium leads to a decrease in the period of the calcium oscillations, in agreement with experimental results [20].

A main difference found in Di Garbo's results compared with the experiments in [1, 20, 22] is that, while in these experiments the inhibition of SERCA-pumps leads to a decrease in the frequency and amplitude of the calcium oscillations, the Di Garbo model [5] shows an increase in the frequency of calcium oscillations, while the amplitude of the oscillations is in agreement with the previous studies. In an effort to reveal the dynamics and effect of slow inward currents (SICs) on neuronal synchrony, Wade [25] formulates a mathematical model that describes the astrocyte-neural interactions for the induction of SICs into neurons. Unlike other mechanisms of astrocytes, such as calcium waves, there is no current biophysical model that details the steps in the generation of SICs. In an effort to capture the empirical relationship between neurotransmitter release from the synapse, calcium oscillations, and SIC generation, Wade has combined biophysical models of neuron (leaky I&F model), synapse (Tsodyks's model [23]), astrocyte calcium waves (Li–Rinzel and the Nadkarni and Jung model [15–17] along with an empirical model of SICs. Wade presents an early empirical model of SICs that captures important aspects of the process.

Calcium oscillations are generated by the Li–Rinzel biophysical model, as it is a versatile model with amplitude modulation (AM), frequency modulation (FM) and a mixed AM–FM modulation, allowing the encoding of the levels of IP3. IP3 allows for the sensing of synaptic activity. SICs in Wade's model are triggered when coincidental events occur. These events include a presynaptic stimulus that arrives within a 100 ms time window along with calcium oscillations crossing from below a defined calcium threshold. Empirical observations show that glutamate released by astrocytes only binds NMDA receptors, however, activation of NMDA receptors requires a coincidental independent stimulus that allows the opening of AMPA channels. As there is no clear evidence on how AMPA receptors are activated, Wade assumes that a presynaptic stimulus is the independent depolarizing signal that serves for the activation of AMPA channels. The total current applied to the postsynaptic side is a function of the synaptic weight and the presynaptic release of transmitters as well as the astrocyte-driven SICs. Wade's model allows for tuning of the SIC amplitude and time constant to match the kinetics of experimentally observed SICs. Wade takes SIC activity a step beyond to show how astrocytes play a role in long-term potentiation/long-term depresssion. Wade's model shows how dynamic coordination in the brain is influenced by the bidirectional communication between neurons and astrocytes. A detailed description of the model can be found in [26].

4.6 Chapter summmary

This chapter surveyed major mathematical models used to describe neural behavior. A fundamental model, the H&H model, was described in some detail. The focus of the chapter was on the Izhikevich neural model that forms the basis for multiple modern neuromorphic systems.

The next chapter begins coverage of neuromorphic circuits implementing the neural spiking mechanism, identified as the *axon hillock* or the *axon initial segment*.

4.7 Exercises

1. What do the variables u and v represent in Izhekevich's spiking neuron model?
2. Leaky integrate-and-fire neurons (mark all correct answers):
   (a) Have dendritic spikes;
   (b) Allow the positions of synapses to affect computation;
   (c) Sum all synaptic inputs;
   (d) Have a model that incorporates spike timing-dependent plasticity.
3. The spike pattern shown in figure 4.1(L) is called:
   (a) Tonic;
   (b) Burst;
   (c) Integrator;
   (d) Class 2 excitable.
4. Which Izhekevich spiking pattern shows spiking frequency that depends on the strength of the inputs?
5. Izhikevich's differential equations describe (mark all correct answers):
   (a) Current flow in the upper right quadrant in the spiking circuit;
   (b) Membrane potential and the membrane recovery variable;
   (c) Potentials in the sodium and potassium channels;
   (d) Hodgkin and Huxley's channel conductances.

6. Many different spiking patterns can be obtained with Izhikevich's differential equations:
   (a) By changing the initial conditions of u and v;
   (b) By changing the signs of some terms in the differential equations;
   (c) By changing the values of the parameters in the differential equations;
   (d) By changing voltage to current in the equations.

References

[1] Aguado F *et al* 2002 Neuronal activity regulates correlated network properties of spontaneous calcium transients in astrocytes *in situ J. Neurosci.* **22** 9430–44

[2] Amiri M, Montaseri G and Bahrami F 2011 On the role of astrocytes in synchronization of two coupled neurons: a mathematical perspective *Biol. Cybern.* **105** 153–66

[3] Cornell-Bell A H *et al* 1990 Glutamate induces calcium waves in cultured astrocytes: long-range glial signaling *Science* **247** 470–3

[4] De Pittà M *et al* 2009 Glutamate regulation of calcium and IP3 oscillating and pulsating dynamics in astrocytes *J. Biol. Phys.* **35** 383–411

[5] Di Garbo A 2009 Dynamics of a minimal neural model consisting of an astrocyte, a neuron, and an interneuron *J. Biol. Phys.* **35** 361–82

[6] Di Garbo A *et al* 2007 Calcium signalling in astrocytes and modulation of neural activity *Biosystems* **89** 74–83

[7] Faye G 2011 An introduction to bifurcation theory *NeuroMathComp Laboratory* (ENS Paris, France: Laboratory, INRIA, Sophia Antipolis, CNRS)

[8] Hodgkin A L 1948 The local electric changes associated with repetitive action in a non-medullated axon *J. Physiol.* **107** 165

[9] Hodgkin A L and Huxley A F 1952 A quantitative description of membrane current and its application to conduction and excitation in nerve *J. Physiol.* **117** 500

[10] Hodgkin A L, Huxley A F and Katz B 1952 Measurement of current-voltage relations in the membrane of the giant axon of Loligo *J. Physiol.* **116** 424

[11] Izhikevich E M 2004 Which model to use for cortical spiking neurons? *IEEE Trans. Neural Netw.* **15** 1063–70

[12] Izhikevich E M 2003 Simple model of spiking neurons *IEEE Trans. Neural Netw.* **14** 1569–72

[13] Koizumi S, Fujishita K and Inoue K 2005 Regulation of cell-to-cell communication mediated by astrocytic ATP in the CNS *Purinergic Signal.* **1** 211–7

[14] Lavrentovich M and Hemkin S 2008 A mathematical model of spontaneous calcium (II) oscillations in astrocytes *J. Theor. Biol.* **251** 553–60

[15] Li Y-X and Rinzel J 1994 equations for InsP3 receptor-mediated $[Ca^{2+}]$ i oscillations derived from a detailed kinetic model: a Hodgkin-Huxley like formalism *J. Theor. Biol.* **166** 461–73

[16] Nadkarni S and Jung P 2004 Dressed neurons: modeling neural-glial interactions *Phys. Biol.* **1** 35

[17] Nadkarni S and Jung P 2007 Modeling synaptic transmission of the tripartite synapse *Phys. Biol.* **4** 1

[18] Nett W J, Oloff S H and Mccarthy K D 2002 Hippocampal astrocytes *in situ* exhibit calcium oscillations that occur independent of neuronal activity *J. Neurophysiol.* **87** 528–37

[19] Nobile M *et al* 2003 ATP-induced, sustained calcium signalling in cultured rat cortical astrocytes: evidence for a non-capacitative, P2X7-like-mediated calcium entry *FEBS Letters* **538** 71–6

[20] Parri H R and Crunelli V 2003 The role of Ca^{2+} in the generation of spontaneous astrocytic Ca^{2+} oscillations *Neuroscience* **120** 979–92

[21] Sneyd J *et al* 2004 Control of calcium oscillations by membrane fluxes *Proc. Natl Acad. Sci.* 101 1392–6

[22] Tashiro A, Goldberg J and Yuste R 2002 Calcium oscillations in neocortical astrocytes under epileptiform conditions *J. Neurobiol.* **50** 45–55

[23] Tsodyks M, Pawelzik K and Markram H 1998 Neural networks with dynamic synapses *Neural Comput.* **10** 821–35

[24] Volman V, Ben-Jacob E and Levine H 2007 The astrocyte as a gatekeeper of synaptic information transfer *Neural Comput.* **19** 303–26

[25] Wade J *et al* 2012 Self-repair in a bidirectionally coupled astrocyte-neuron (an) system based on retrograde signaling *Front. Comput. Neurosci.* **6** 76

[26] Wade J J *et al* 2011 Bidirectional coupling between astrocytes and neurons mediates learning and dynamic coordination in the brain: a multiple modeling approach *PLoS One* **6** e29445

IOP Publishing

Neuromorphic Circuits
A constructive approach
Alice C Parker and Rick Cattell

Chapter 5

The axon and the spiking mechanism

Chih-Chieh Hsu and Alice C Parker

The axon and the neural spiking mechanism are described here, beginning with a classic spiking circuit by Farquhar and Hasler, and followed by Armstrong and Hsu's spiking circuit, then covering multiple variations of Hsu's spiking circuit that followed. The chapter concludes with a brief discussion of neuromorphic modeling of axonal propagation.

5.1 Introduction

In biological neurons, the *axon hillock*, where the axon begins, conveying signals to other neurons, is adjacent to the *axon initial segment*, the neuronal spike initiation region. The hillock is enriched with sodium and potassium channels that are responsible for generating and shaping the action potential (AP). A fast sodium influx followed by a slow potassium outward current, causes the membrane potential adjacent to the axon hillock to rise rapidly and return to resting potential when equilibrium of the inward and outward currents is reached. The axon compartment containing the axon hillock and the axon initial segment, closest to the soma, has the highest density of sodium channels, resulting in the lowest threshold to initiate an AP. It is believed that the spikes originate just beyond the axon hillock in the axon initial segment (AIS) that connects to the axon of the neuron. Early publications from the *BioRC* group referred to the spiking circuit as the axon hillock itself. This text refers to the spiking circuits as the axon hillock, AIS circuits, or just simply spiking circuits.

Although it is generally believed that cortical neurons integrate their synaptic inputs and fire APs when the threshold is reached, some evidence has supported the theory that the threshold to fire an AP spike of cortical neurons *in vivo* depends on both the amplitude and the rate of membrane potential depolarization [3]. This reference showed that higher input synchronization, i.e., spikes from different presynaptic neurons arriving at the same time, induces lower spike threshold[1].

---

[1] Rate of membrane depolarization can also change due to dendritic spiking, as described in section 1.4.

This mechanism suggests that cortical neurons favor coincident inputs by generating reliable and precisely-timed AP spikes. Therefore, we present two types of axon hillock circuits, amplitude-sensitive and slope-sensitive, in this chapter. We characterize the spike threshold for both circuits: *constant spike threshold* for the former and *dynamic spike threshold* for the latter. Spiking circuits with varying spiking rates have been introduced by Hsu [5], earlier by Farquhar and Hasler [4] and others. This chapter mainly covers the two examples of neuromorphic spiking circuits, one from the dissertation by Ethan Farquhar, supervised by Hasler and one from the BioRC project. The second spiking circuit, from the BioRC group, later incorporated into Hsu's dissertation [5], was initially designed by Bradley Armstrong based on a self-resetting circuit in a student paper, and included in [6], unpublished. The origins of the use of self-resetting circuits for spiking neuromorphic neurons appear to be from Mead's book [10], discussed by Indiveri *et al* [1].

Example circuits will be shown here. In addition to Hsu's single regular-spiking model, we present Hsu's burst firing axon hillock model in section 16.2 that characterizes the depolarizing potential and the inter-spike interval in the burst output. Hsu's thesis presents much more information, including an equivalent RC model for Hsu's spiking circuit to characterize the activation and inactivation mechanisms of the voltage-gated ion channels involved in the generation of an AP.

It is worthwhile to mention once again the impressive catalog of spiking varieties collected by Eugene Izhikevich [7], that will be presented in chapter 13 and a variety of circuits producing spiking variations will be covered. Other researchers have modeled these spiking varieties in neuromorphic spiking circuits, including the recent work by Alzahrani and Parker [2].

5.2 Farquhar and Hasler's spiking circuit

One of the smallest (in terms of transistor count) spiking circuits described in the literature, Farquhar and Hasler's spiking circuit [4], was designed to directly mimic biological neurons, both in terms of voltage and timing. As such, it contained large capacitors to slow the waveforms, and was subthreshold, to match biological potentials (voltages). Figure 5.3 shows Farquhar's approach to the spiking circuit. The circuit was designed with MOS transistors acting in the subthreshold region. Note that the transistor, even in the subthreshold region, where digital designers traditionally consider the transistor to be cutoff, can behave in a linear or a saturation fashion, with current measured on a log scale. With subthreshold operation, power is low, and current flows in the transistor saturation region, allowing the transistor to act as a current source. V_{ds} can vary over a wide range.

In the subthreshold region, the NMOS transistor does not form an inverted channel of electrons. Some holes remain unfilled, and there are a few electrons beginning to form the channel, as shown in figure 5.1.

Subthreshold current flow magnitude is exponential to the gate-to-source voltage and thus there is exponential nonlinearity in the transistor operation. Designers sometimes call this **log domain** operation. Note there are two exponentials in the equation. The first, and most important, is the exponential relationship between V_{gs}

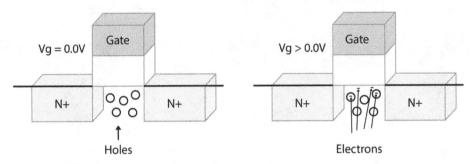

Figure 5.1. NMOS Transistor in the OFF region (when $V_g = 0.0$ V) and subthreshold region (when $V_g > 0.0$ V).

and drain current I_d, and the second is the weak exponential relationship between V_{ds} and the drain current I_d. We can consider the subthreshold current equations for the NMOS transistor to be modeled by the following equation, where N is a calculated constant, k and q are constants, and T is temperature.

$$i_{D(\text{sub-threshld})} \approx \frac{W}{L}\mu_e C_{ox}^*\left(\frac{kT}{q}\right)^2(n-1)e^{q\{v_{gs}-V_T\}/nkT}(1 - e^{-qv_{ds}/kT})$$

Using subthreshold operation reduces power consumption, and having operation in the saturation region allows the transistor to act as a current source. V_{ds} can vary over a wide range, and the nonlinearity is exponential.

A rudimentary spiking circuit could be constructed with two transistors, along with an inverter, one controlled by the AP, and one controlled by the inverted action potential, /AP. The inverter adds a delay to the circuit so that rise and fall of the output occur in sequence. Both transistors are driven by an amplified membrane voltage. Farquhar's spiking circut roughly follows this simple circuit, as shown in figure 5.2.

Farquhar uses a step voltage input for his spiking circuit, with input V_{mem} a step function rising from 0.0 V to 60 mV (although his conference paper shows different values for the step function). V_{mem} is the potential inside the cell membrane with respect to the potential outside the cell. There are two portions of the circuit, one mimicking sodium ion (Na$^+$) flow, and one mimicking potassium ion (K$^+$) flow. The sodium part of the circuit acts like a band-pass filter of high frequency, and the potassium part of the circuit acts like a low-pass filter (LPF) of the voltage V_{mem}. The cell membrane itself is assumed to act like a capacitor. Farquhar uses the Nernst potential to get current to flow to mimic the spiking circuit in a neuron. As long as the diffusion current is greater than the drift current (random motion of these ions), the current will keep flowing. There comes a point where the current stops flowing, that depends on both potassium and sodium ion concentrations. So, current flow depends on how permeable (ease of flow of an ion) the medium is to both potassium and sodium. Resting potential can be computed using the Goldman equation, -60 mV, as for the Hodgkin–Huxley model. Filtering a step function is shown in figure 5.4, with results of low-pass and band-pass filtering shown.

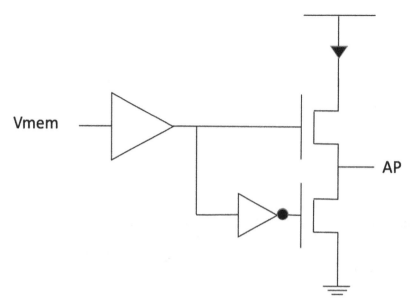

Figure 5.2. A rudimentary spiking circuit.

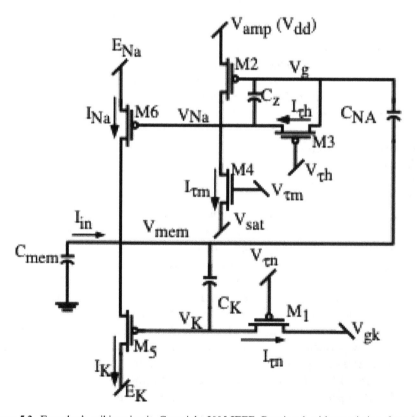

Figure 5.3. Farquhar's spiking circuit. Copyright 2005 IEEE. Reprinted, with permission, from [4].

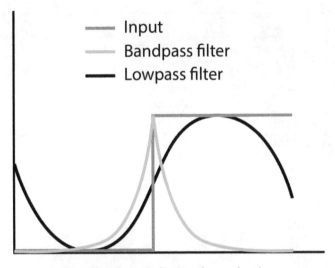

Figure 5.4. Example filtering of a step function.

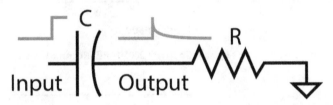

Figure 5.5. Behavior across a capacitor when a step function is applied to one side.

Note that the capacitors shown in Farquhar's circuits are quite large to increase delays in the circuit to biological speed in ms. Transistor capacitances are not sufficient for this delay unless quite large transistors are used. Some technologies have thin oxide between metal layers to support large capacitors, but most modern technologies do not.

To understand Farquhar's circuits from a simple circuit perspective, the behavior of a capacitor when presented with a step function potential at one side is important. The capacitor shows the output mirroring the input, then the output returns to the original potential, as shown in figure 5.5.

The discussion centers on the low-pass filter first. Note that the potassium current, shown in figure 5.6, rises slowly when a step function is applied to V_{mem}, acting like a low-pass fiter.

The potassium circuit is shown in figure 5.7. E_K is the Nernst potential of potassium, -70 mV. The location of transistor sources might be helpful in understanding this circuit. At the beginning of operation, the *source* of transistor M_K is connected to V_{mem}. The gate is connected to V_K, and V_K is initially low, since current is flowing through transistor M_{rn}. $V_{mem} = 0.0$ V in Step 1. Assume that V_{mem} rises from 0.0 V to 60 mV in Step 2. The voltage across capacitor C_K cannot change

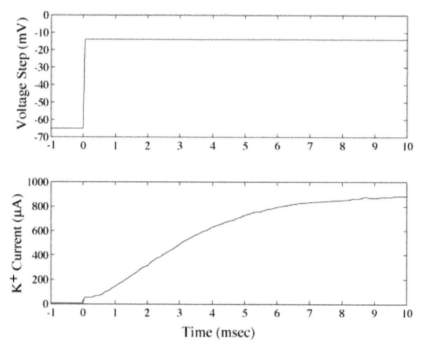

Figure 5.6. Potassium current: slower response. Copyright 2005 IEEE. Reprinted, with permission, from [4].

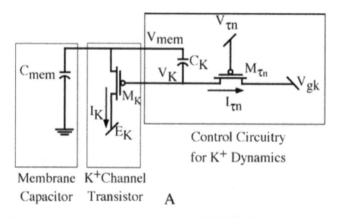

Figure 5.7. Farquhar's potassium channel circuit. Copyright 2005 IEEE. Reprinted, with permission, from [4].

instantaneously so V_K also rises to 60 mV. C_K acts as a short circuit. Current flow in transistor M_K is reduced since V_{gsp} is smaller in magnitude (closer to zero). Then, V_K starts falling in Step 3 and the capacitor C_K acts like an open circuit. More current flows in M_K. The time constant governing the fall of V_K is $C_K * R_{channel}$ (transistor $M_{\tau n}$).

The sodium current for Farquhar's spiking circuit is shown in figure 5.8. The sodium channel circuit is shown in figure 5.9. There is a capacitor that's holding the

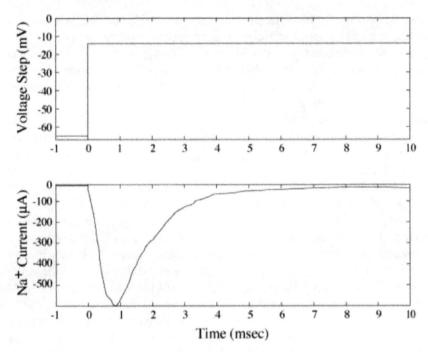

Figure 5.8. Sodium current: response looks like a band-pass filter, fast response. Copyright 2005 IEEE. Reprinted, with permission, from [4].

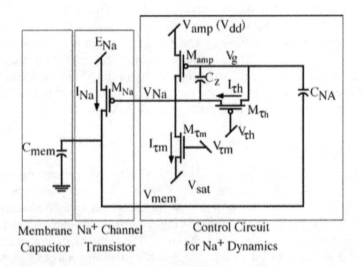

Figure 5.9. Farquhar's sodium channel circuit. Copyright 2005 IEEE. Reprinted, with permission, from [4].

membrane voltage C_{mem} and there is a sodium/ion channel. The sodium channel circuit has a slightly more complicated control circuit necessary to create a band-pass filter than the potassium channel circuit. The band-pass filter consists of two capacitors, one for falling I_{Na} current (C_{Na}) and the other for rising I_{Na} current (C_z).

Between the two time constants, the circuit causes a rise and fall in sodium current magnitude because Farquhar's circuit implements sodium current that's falling (from 0 to more negative value) and then it's rising. These two capacitances are essential to understanding how the circuit works. When one side of a capacitor voltage is a step function, the other side of the capacitor follows, but returns to its original voltage depending on the resistance of the circuit.

Initially E_{Na} is about 50 mV. That's the Nernst potential for sodium. V_{mem} is 0,0 V (Step 1). When V_g is 0 V and V_{amp} is V_{dd}, the *source* of M_{amp} is the transistor end that is connected to V_{amp}. The values of V_{sat} and V_{Na} are considered small. Initially V_g will be 0 mV. Then V_{mem} rises in a step function to 60 mV (Step 2). When it rises instantaneously, consider the two capacitors as short circuits. Now V_{mem} is 60 mV. Then V_g will rise to 60 mV. Across capacitor C_z V_{Na} rises to 60 mV. When V_g is 0 V initially, M_{amp} is ON. When the voltage on the gate of M_{amp} rises due to V_{mem} rising, the current that's flowing through this transistor will fall as the transistor is turning off. Now moving to the sodium channel, initially the voltage V_{Na} is very low but rises to 60 mV. as a result of V_{mem} rising, and it's then going to fall lower as the voltage V_{Na} discharges. This turns on M_{Na}, and the magnitude of the sodium current rises. At this point the sodium current is negative. Initially the source of M_{Na} is the end of the transistor that's connected to E_{Na}. The voltage of its gate is at subthreshold and it is negative. Now the source of M_{Na} will move when V_{Na} falls and V_{mem} increases to 60 mV. So, the M_{Na} transistor turns ON and the current will start to flow in the negative direction. As soon as the two capacitors have transferred their voltages (step function allows the voltage to transfer), then they are considered open circuits and out of the picture for the continued analysis. This makes it a bit easier to understand the circuit. Now, V_g continues falling, and current through M_{amp} increases (Step 3). This increases V_{Na} and I_{Na} decreases in magnitude (Step 4). The two time constants involve both transistors, but the resistances are more complicated to compute. The time constant for I_{Na} increasing in magnitude is a function of the channel resistance of $M_{\tau m}$ and the time constant for I_{Na} decreasing in magnitude is a function of the series channel resistances of both $M_{\tau h}$ and $M_{\tau m}$[2].

5.3 Hsu's spiking circuit

Hsu's spiking circuits are shown in this section[3]. The experiments presented in this section are HSPICE simulations with CNFET (carbon nanotube field-effect transistor) SPICE (simulation program with integrated circuit emphasis) models [8, 9]. The CNFET device parameters and characteristics are summarized as follows. The nominal power supply voltage is 900 mV. The transistor channel length is 10–100 nm. For a 32 nm CNFET device, the gate effective capacitance is approximately 4 aF and on-current is about 26 μA. The on-current ratio of an n-type CNFET over a p-type CNFET is about unity. The FO1 (fanout of 1) inverter gate delay is about 2.26 ps. Even though the CNFET shares a similar I–V curve to the MOS FET, the

---

[2] For a discussion of how the circuit works in terms of poles and zeros, refer to the original paper by Farquhar.
[3] Unless stated otherwise, all figures in this section are found in [5].

Table 5.1. Biological and electrical potential and timing scaling for AP. Reproduced from [5].

Parameter	Biological	Electrical
AP half-width	1 ms	5 ps
AP amplitude	110 mV	900 mV
AP spike threshold	−55 mV	163 mV
Resting potential	−75 mV	0 V (Ground)
θ frequency	5–10 Hz	1–2 GHz
AP burst frequency	330 Hz	66 GHz

electrical and physical properties of CNFET devices are far more complicated. The device resistance is primarily due to the quantum resistance at the junction between the doped nanotubes and metallic contacts, caused by energy-level differences of electrons between the two materials. The strength (conductance) of the transistor is typically modulated by the number of parallel carbon nanotubes per gate. The drive current increases when the number of tubes increases, but not in a linear relationship. However, when the number of tubes is larger than 10, the increasing inter-CNT charge screening effect limits the drive current. Therefore, the current flow through the transistor's drain and source terminals is in a limited range and is more difficult to control than with CMOS circuits.

Hsu scales the potential level and time of her spiking circuits to meet the carbon nanotube transistor's operating potential and speed. The potential level and timing parameters for the biological neuron and her electronic neuron are summarized in table 5.1. Essential parameters related to the neural signal AP are its duration, amplitude, spike threshold, membrane resting potential, frequency firing rate, and the high frequency burst firing rate. The timing parameters in her CNT (carbon nanotube) circuits are eight orders of magnitude faster than the biological ones. The potential levels are eight times larger than the biological ones.

5.3.1 The regular-spiking circuit

The circuit implementation of the axon hillock at the transistor level is shown in figure 5.10. The function of this circuit is that if the input V_{SOMA} is above a certain threshold, the output generates a spike. The pull-up transistor (X8) models the fast inward sodium current while the pull-down transistor (X7) models the slow outward potassium current. To mimic a fast rising phase due to the rapid increase of the Na$^+$ (sodium) channel conductance and a slower falling phase due to the slow increase of the K$^+$ (potassium) channel conductances of an action potential, Hsu adjusted the channel conductances of transistors X8 (P-type) and X7 (N-type) by placing more nanotubes in parallel to increase conductance.

The color-shaded segments mimic the activation and inactivation phases of the sodium and potassium channels as well as the delay time for the sequence of events that define the dynamics of an AP. First, Na$^+$-activation segment (X1, X2) turns on Na$^+$ channels rapidly. Transistor X8 is set to be less resistive to mimic the fast rise in AP.

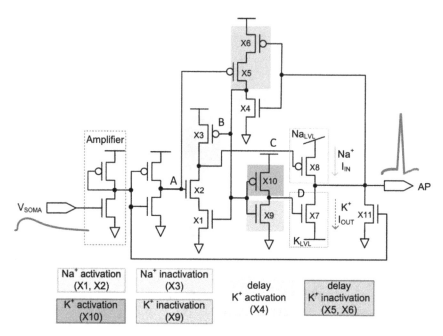

Figure 5.10. The Axon hillock circuit at the transistor level. The single-stage amplifier is used as a voltage interface between V_{SOMA} and the inverter threshold. The inverter is used to generate a full swing from GND to V_{DD} for the spiking circuit. First, the Na^+-activation segment (modeled by X1, X2) turns on Na^+ channels (X8) rapidly. After some delay (X4), Na^+-inactivation (X3) then turns off Na^+ channels. This portrays the gradual inactivation of Na^+ channels when the action potential reaches a depolarizing state. After some more delay (X4), K^+-activation (X10) turns on K^+ channels (X7). K^+-inactivation (X9) turns off K^+ channels after a longer delay (X5, X6 in series). The delay is controlled by adjusting the strengths of transistors. We use the resistive and capacitive properties of the transistors to achieve the desired time constants. X11 is used to pull the AP back to its resting potential. Reproduced from [5].

After some delay (X4) Na^+-inactivation (X3) then turns off Na^+ channels. This portrays the gradual inactivation of Na^+ channels when the action potential reaches a depolarizing state. K^+-activation (X10), after some more delay (X4), turns on K^+ channels. Transistor X10 is designed to be more resistive than X3 in order to mimic the biological behavior such that K^+-activation occurs a short period of time after Na^+-inactivation begins. K^+-inactivation (X9) turns off K^+ channels after a longer delay (X5, X6). The delay is controlled by adjusting the strengths of transistors, where decreasing transistor channel width increases delay, as does increasing channel length. We use the resistive and capacitive properties of the transistors to achieve the desired time constants.

The timing of signals changing in Hsu's axon hillock is shown in figure 5.11. While signal values and timings are approximated, depending on transistor sizing, this diagram assists the reader in understanding the behavior over time of the axon hillock. Signal transitions are numbered in order. Transition 6 occurs before 6+ but the timing between the two is not exact. Note that A falling is an external condition, resulting in B rising, and D falling.

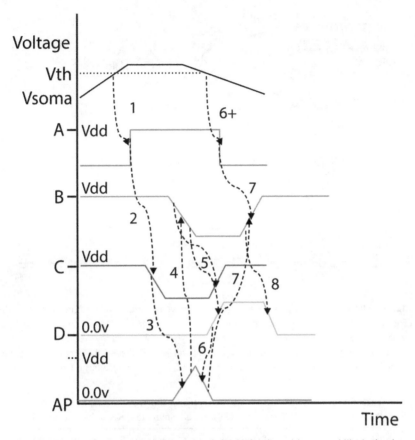

Figure 5.11. Sequencing and timing of signals in the level-sensitive axon hillock circuit.

The circuit implementation used in the axon hillock simulation is shown in figure 5.12(top). The dendritic arbor in this configuration is simplified to sum only four unitary excitatory postsynaptic potentials (EPSPs) that are activated at the same time. The simulation waveform is shown in figure 5.12(bottom). The time course of the unitary EPSP is prolonged to approximately six times the AP duration. The input AP is designed to have a fall time to rise time ratio of 1.63 and a spike half-width of 4.76 ps. Here the rise time is defined as the time for the signal to rise from 10% V_{DD} to 90% V_{DD} and the fall time is defined as the time for the signal to fall from 90% V_{DD} to 10% V_{DD}. The spike width is defined as the width of the signal rising-falling or falling-rising at 50% V_{DD}. The simulated output AP has a falling phase about 1.61 times slower than the rising phase and the error is within 2%. The simulated output has a spike half-width of 4.8 ps that is less than 1% mismatch. The peak potential of a unitary EPSP is set to be less than 5% of the amplitude of AP. This is controlled by the input voltage of the transistor that models neurotransmitter release in the excitatory synapse circuit (figure 6.5). The peak of V_{SOMA} shown here is at the threshold of AP initiation, therefore an output AP is generated (table 5.2).

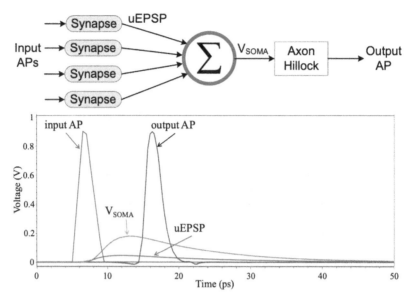

Figure 5.12. Simulated *axon hillock* circuit showing the relative potential level and time course of the neural signal. (Top) a hypothetical neuron configuration to simulate the *axon hillock* circuit. Four of the unitary excitatory postsynaptic potentials, *uEPSPs*, are summed at the soma with an *average-amplify* module (shown as the Σ symbol). The synapse and the summation circuit will be presented in the next chapter. (Bottom) the relative potential and time course of the neural signals: EPSP and AP. Reproduced from [5].

Table 5.2. AP and EPSP characteristics in the CNT circuit. The characteristics of the AP spike and EPSP from the CNT circuit simulation. Reproduced from [5].

Characteristics	Input AP	Output AP	unitary EPSP
Half-width (ps)	4.76	4.8	19
Fall/rise ratio	1.63	1.61	9.42
Amplitude (mV)	900	900	41.7

5.4 Variations in Hsu's axon initial segment

Hsu produced axon hillocks with variations. including one with slope-sensitive thresholds, and one with burst firing. A biomimetic *slope-sensitive axon hillock* circuit is shown in figure 5.13. We augment the original BioRC *axon hillock* module shown in figure 5.10 with a differentiation circuit component at the input stage. The *slope-sensitive axon hillock* circuit at the transistor level is shown in figure 5.13. The objective is to emphasize the temporal changes at the input, therefore we use a differentiator to filter out slowly varying input patterns. In equation (5.1), if the slope (dV/dt) on the left side of the equation is small, it results in a small V_2. Hence it makes the *axon hillock* less likely to fire spikes. For example, two somatic potentials, V_{SOMA1} and V_{SOMA2}, have the same amplitude but different slopes i.e., the rate of depolarization. If the slope of V_{SOMA1} ($\frac{dV_{SOMA1}}{dt}$) is much greater than the slope of

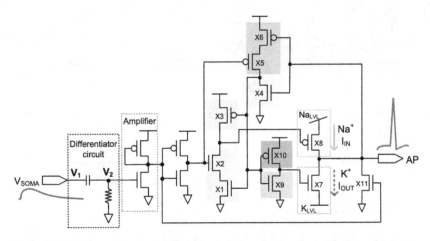

Figure 5.13. Slope-sensitive *axon hillock* circuit at the transistor level. Reproduced from [5].

V_{SOMA2} ($\frac{dV_{SOMA2}}{dt}$), then the spike threshold for V_{SOMA1} is lower than that for V_{SOMA2}. Therefore, the *slope-sensitive axon hillock* circuit has a dynamic threshold dependent on the input amplitude and slope, while the original *axon hillock* circuit has a constant threshold. Figure 5.10 shows the voltages V_1 and V_2 and the differential equation represented by the circuit.

$$\frac{d(V_1 - V_2)}{dt} = \frac{V_2}{RC} \tag{5.1}$$

The color-shaded segments mimic the activation and inactivation phases of the sodium and potassium channels as well as the delay time for the sequence of events that define the dynamics of an AP. The sequence of events has been previously described.

First, Hsu investigates the scenario when the spike threshold changes with synaptic input slope. Figure 5.14 demonstrates the simulation results by testing the BioRC *slope-sensitive axon hillock* circuit with different somatic potential amplitudes (V_{SOMA}) and rise times (t_r). It is observed that when the V_{SOMA} rise time increases, the amplitude of the V_{SOMA} required to evoke AP spikes increases as well. For example, when t_r is 100 ps, it fails to evoke spikes when V_{SOMA} is 160 mV, but it evokes spikes when V_{SOMA} rises to 180 mV. Hsu compared her CNT circuit simulation result to the computational model Azouz *et al* [3] proposed and found a similar inverse correlation between the spike threshold and the input synchronization. Azouz shows the dynamic spike threshold as rise time of V_{SOMA} increases and suggests when the multiple synaptic inputs are synchronous, the PSP rises more quickly, threshold falls, and fewer synapses are needed to evoke an AP spike. The inverse correlation between the spike threshold (y) and the synaptic input slope (x) measured with the CNT simulation can be fitted to equation (5.2).

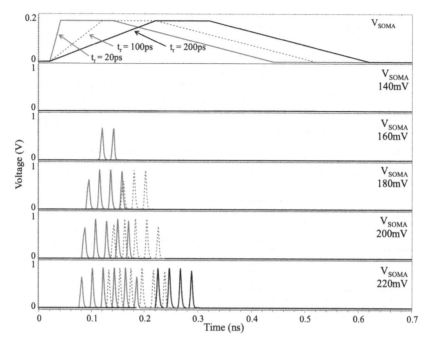

Figure 5.14. AP spike threshold is sensitive to both slope and amplitude of the somatic potential. Spike threshold under different rise time (t_r) and amplitudes of the somatic potential V_{SOMA}. When the input rises fast, i. e., $t_r = 20$ ps, it requires lower potential to generate a spike, i. e., 160 mV. However, when input rises relatively slowly, i. e., $t_r = 200$ ps, it requires higher potential to generate a spike, i. e., 220 mV. Reproduced from [5].

$$y = a + b \cdot e^{-x/c}$$
$$x = dV/dt$$
$$a = 160.2, \ b = 400, \ c = 1.526$$

(5.2)

5.5 Modeling axonal propagation

Spikes travel in all directions from the AIS. Most of the propagation is passive, and there is reduction in amplitude and introduction of delay in passive directions. Along the axon, however, those degraded signals meet the nodes of Ranvier that regenerate the initial spikes, acting as repeaters. A simple model of axonal propagation is shown in figure 5.15. The resistance R and Capacitance C are adjusted depending on the technology, axon length and amount of enwrapping by the oligodendrocytes.

5.6 Chapter summary

This chapter covered neural spiking circuits, with a detailed discussion of two spiking circuits, one by Farquhar and Hasler, and one by Hsu and Parker. Some variations in Hsu's spiking circuit are described, and there is a short discussion of Hsu's model of axonal propagation.

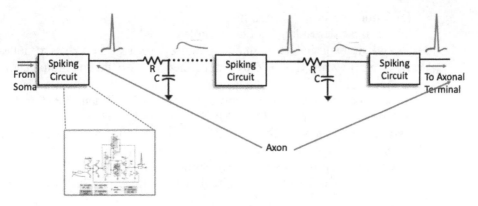

Figure 5.15. Axonal propagation circuit, with *RC* delays and nodes of Ranvier spike regeneration. The spike regeneration circuits are modeled with spiking circuits like those shown in figure 5.10.

The next chapter describes a major interface between neurons called the synapse. Indiveri's mixed-signal synapse is covered first, followed by the BioRC synapse. Some variations in the BioRC synapse to control strengths are introduced, and a short section covers Joshi's and Yue's contributions to synapse strength. An introduction to silent synapses concludes the chapter.

5.7 Exercises

1. When Farquhar's axon hillock circuit (figure 5.3) is triggered by a step function at V_{mem} (voltage rises instantaneously), what happens to the voltage across the capacitor C_{Na}? Show a simple waveform and a quick explanation that involves the capacitor C_{Na}.

2. In Farquhar's spiking circuit, figure 5.10, locate the voltages that indicate the electromotive forces for sodium and potassium (the forces that cause currents to flow in the ion channels). Show on the diagram. Sketch the shape of the input current Iin or the voltage V_{mem}.

3. The capacitance(s) contributing to the sodium spike timing in Farquhar's spiking circuit are:
   (a) C_z;
   (b) C_z and C_{Na};
   (c) C_K;
   (d) None of the above.

4. In Farquhar's spiking circuit (Figure 5.3), the transistor forming the potassium ion channel is:
   (a) M1;
   (b) M3 and M4;
   (c) M5;
   (d) M6.

5. The voltages and timing in Farquhar's spiking circuit (figure 5.3) are:
   (a) Matched to biological time;
   (b) V_{dd} and ns in his CMOS technology;

    (c) Similar to Hsu's carbon nanotube circuits;

    (d) Variable depending on the technology used.

6. Hsu's spiking axon hillock is shown in figure 5.10. List the values at nodes A, B, C and D when $V_{soma} = 0.0$ V, and when $V_{soma} =$ the maximum soma voltage.

7. Hsu's spiking axon hillock is shown in figure 5.10. When $A = B = V_{dd}$, what happens to C and D? Does AP change as a result?

8. In Farquhar's spiking circuit, figure 5.3, locate the voltages that indicate the electromotive forces for sodium and potassium (the forces that cause currents to flow in the ion channels). Show on the diagram.

9. Initial conditions in Hsu's spiking circuit (axon hillock), figure 5.10, assume that:

    (a) X3 and X4 are on;

    (b) X5 and X6 are on;

    (c) X1 and X2 are on;

    (d) X7 and X8 are on.

10. The falling time of the AP in Hsu's axon hillock, figure 5.10, depends on:

    (a) The falling time of the input, V_{soma};

    (b) How fast outputs of transistors in the axon hillock rise and/or fall;

    (c) How fast the sodium channel is activated;

    (d) How fast the action potential has risen.

References

[1] Indiveri G *et al* 2011 Neuromorphic silicon neuron circuits *Front. Neurosci.* **5** 1–23

[2] Alzahrani R A and Parker A C 2021 Neuromorphic autonomous spiking encoding *2021 IEEE Int. Symp. Circuits and Systems (ISCAS)* 1–5

[3] Azouz R and Gray C M 2000 Dynamic spike threshold reveals a mechanism for synaptic coincidence detection in cortical neurons *in vivo Proc. Natl Acad. Sci.* 97 8110–5

[4] Farquhar E and Hasler P 2005 A bio-physically inspired silicon neuron *IEEE Trans. Circuits Syst. I: Regular Papers* **52** 477–88

[5] Hsu C-C 2014 Dendritic computation and plasticity in neuromorphic circuits *PhD Thesis* University of Southern California

[6] Hsu C-C *et al* 2009 A carbon nanotube neuron with dendritic computations (unpublished)

[7] Izhikevich E M 2003 Simple model of spiking neurons *IEEE Trans. Neural Netw.* **14** 1569–72

[8] Wong H-S P and Deng J 2007 A compact SPICE model for carbon-nanotube field-effect transistors including nonidealities and its application—Part I: model of the intrinsic channel region *IEEE Trans. Electron Devices* **54** 3186–94

[9] Wong H-S P and Deng J 2007 A compact SPICE model for carbon-nanotube field-effect transistors including nonidealities and its application—part II: full device model and circuit performance benchmarking *IEEE Trans. Electron Devices* **54** 3195–205

[10] Mead C 1989 Computation and neural systems series *Analog VLSI and neural systems* (Reading, MA: Addison-Wesley)

IOP Publishing

Neuromorphic Circuits
A constructive approach
Alice C Parker and Rick Cattell

Chapter 6

Neural input circuits—the synapse

Chih-Chieh Hsu, Jon Joshi and Alice C Parker

The synapse circuit can be a complex part of the neuromorphic circuitry that models neuronal networks. This chapter contains a brief introduction to a basic synapse, the single-transistor synapse, followed by two other synapse circuit families that are markedly different from each other, one implementing current-mode processing (example from Indiveri's group in Zurich), and one implementing voltage-mode processing (example from the Parker BioRC group). The chapter concludes with coverage of neuromorphic circuits implementing *Spike Timing Dependent Plasticity* and the *Silent Synapse*.

6.1 Single-transistor synapse circuit

Some neuromorphic circuit designers use a single transistor as a synapse. An example circuit is shown in figure 6.1, where M1 acts as the synapse and M2 returns the output voltage to the resting potential. In order to force the synapse to appear biological, with *excitatory postsynaptic potential (EPSP)* about .1 magnitude of the action potential (AP), and with about 10 times the duration of the AP, the channel resistance of M1 should be about 0.1 of the channel resistance of M2, and both resistances should be large enough to slow the rise and fall of the EPSP. The two transistors M1 and M2 act as a voltage divider when both are on, and M2 is acts as a resistance to ground when only M2 is on and there is no AP.

Some neuromorphic engineers replace the transistor with a memristor to model synaptic strength. A memristor is a two-terminal device that changes resistance as current flows between the two terminals. Memristors can return output voltages to their resting potential as current flow changes, so no additional devices are required, simplifying the circuit. This modification will be mentioned later when nano-technological solutions are presented in chapter 15.

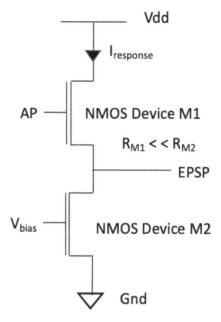

Figure 6.1. Single transistor synapse circuit.

6.2 Indiveri's synapses

Indiveri, his colleagues, and his students have used *current-mode* subthreshold complementary metal oxide semiconductor (CMOS) circuits to model neurons and synapses [2, 6, 7]. These circuits assume transistors are in saturation. Voltages, since the transistors are subthreshold, are comparable to biological voltages, and time constants are similar to biological time. The transconductance (ratio of output current to gate-to-source voltage V_{gs}) of the transistors is linear with respect to the gate-to-source voltage of the transistors.

An early Indiveri synapse circuit found in the paper by Giacomo Indiveri, Elisabetta Chicca and Rodney Douglas [6] is shown in figure 6.2. This Indiveri paper was one of the early ones on adaptive silicon synapses, synapses built with MOS transistors that adapt to different outputs depending on current state and different inputs. Indiveri's 2003 synapse circuit uses some structures that are *differential pairs*, where current can be added. This circuit also contains *current mirrors*. When all the transistor characteristics are properly tuned in a current mirror, then $I_{in} = I_{out}$, displaying a successful current mirror. Once the current is isolated with a current mirror, other structures can be included at the current mirror output without loading the input circuit being isolated. The dV_{dd} label stands for digital V_{dd}, which the designers kept separate from the analog V_{dd} to minimize noise on the analog part of the circuit. If you look carefully, you will notice that dV_{dd} is connected to transistors operating in the digital domain.

This adaptive silicon synapse is based on current-based computation rather than voltage-based computation. The paper shows short-term plasticity, a way to modulate synaptic strength. They use an *address event representation* or *AER*, a

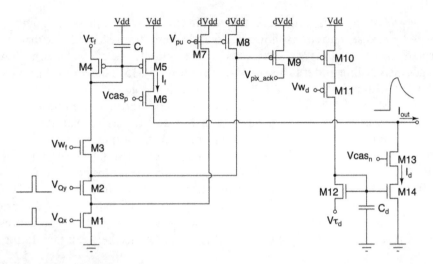

Figure 6.2. Early Indiveri synapse showing two differential pair integrators implemented with transistors M4–M6 (facilitating the synapse) and transistors M12–M14 (depressing the synapse). Copyright 2003 IEEE. Reprinted, with permission, from [6].

way for neurons to communicate with each other via a network, primarily in digital systems that may be connecting analog neurons [4]. Indiveri's original synapse uses two current mirror integrators including capacitors[1]. One current mirror performs facilitation that strengthens the synapse as spiking continues and the other current mirror performs depression that weakens the synapse with continuous spiking. It combines two currents together (I(facilitation)–I(depression)). The circuit uses digital switches to activate the synapse.

The circuit has two inputs, X and Y. These two inputs supply voltage at V_{qx} and V_{qy}, to turn on transistors M1 and M2. As a result, the X and Y form an XY address that selects the synapse. Transistors M1 and M2 provide current to the differential pair integrator performing facilitation formed by M4–M6 when the two pulses on the lower left select the XY position of the current synapse. They also provide a current path for the depressing differential pair integrator formed by transistors M12–M14 through transistors M10 and M11.

Other transistors in Chicca and Indiveri's early synapse play more utilitarian roles. Capacitor C_t is discharged when the faciliting part of the synapse is activated and C_d is charged when the depressing part of the synapse is activated. When X and Y both go high, voltage C falls, turning on transistor M9 when the input pulses arrive to provide an acknowledgement signal that the synapse has been activated. This is the networking part of the system, the AER signaling[2]. M3 is set as a weighting function.

---

[1] The current mirror is found in chapter 3 and discussed extensively on Wikipedia.
[2] Note that biological neurons do provide a type of acknowledgement across the synapse that flows in a *retrograde* fashion (backwards), so that the presynaptic side of the synapse continues to transmit across the synaptic cleft. This is how the synapse gets activated and responds.

Once the synapse is activated, the facilitating current mirror is going to be activated because current is flowing now through transistor M4. Current gets mirrored into transistor M5 that goes to the output. As current starts flowing, voltage starts falling and it turns on M4, that turns on M5. Then more current starts to flow. The more voltage A falls, the more it's going to turn on the mirror transistors M4 and M5. Then more current will flow through the output. M6 is a *cascode* transistor, connected in series with M5 and it acts to bias the system to control current flow, regulating the current flow to the output.

There is a weight (V_{wd}) that controls synaptic depression. The voltage across capacitor C_f is falling, so transistor M10 will turn on. Current is going to flow all the way from V_{dd} to M12, where the current will get mirrored to transistor M14. This results in depressing current that is lowering the amount of response. So, I_f current is flowing in from the facilitating synapse and I_D is flowing from the depressing synapse, resulting in the response I_{out} that is the difference between facilitating and depressing currents.

The dV_{dd} supply in the original synapse is a digital power supply, separate from V_{dd} that is the analog supply, to minimize digital noise.

The analog circuits used in Indiveri's current synapses are *differential pair integrators*, *current mirrors*, *log-domain low pass filters*, and *tau cell* circuits. The publications analyze the circuits by applying the *translinear principle* that traces a chain of transistors, with the sum of gate voltages proportional to the product of the currents flowing in the transistors. A good explanation of how the basic differential pair integrator synapse works is found in [2] as shown in figure 6.3. There, to paraphrase Bartolozzi, the n-channel metal-oxide semiconductor (NMOS) transistors are a differential pair, the M_t p-channel metal-oxide semiconductor (PMOS) transisor acts as a constant current source, and the M_{post} PMOS transistor is providing input current into the neuron I_{psc}. An input pulse to the synapse turns on M_{pre}, I_w begins to flow, and the capacitor C_{syn} discharges. V_{syn} falls, turning on the output transistor M_{post}, and causing current I_{psc} (not shown, but the voltage excitatory postsynaptic potential (EPSC) is shown) to flow through M_{post}. M_{post} is isolated from the synapse so the synapse cannot be loaded by what is connected to I_{psc} since M_{post} and M_{in} form a current mirror. When the input pulse falls, M_{in} turns off and M_t again charges the capacitor, decreasing I_{syn}.

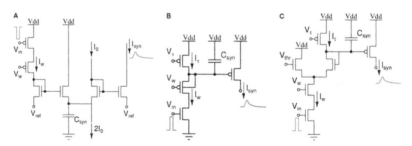

Figure 6.3. Indiveri's differential pair synapse. Reproduced from [24] CC BY 4.0.

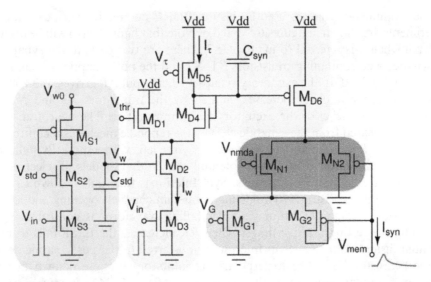

Figure 6.4. Indiveri's present synapse. The yellow highlights the differential pair integrator. The green highlights the short-term depression block, NMDA voltage-gated channels are highlighted by the red block, and conductance-based voltage dependence transistors are highlighted in blue, as found in [7], copyright 2014 IEEE, reprinted with permission.

In the present Indiveri synapse, the differential pair integrator plays a central role as shown in figure 6.4. In this synapse [7], there are two locations for the pulse representing the input AP, the gates of MD3 and MS3. The output is a current that has exponential rise and fall. The temporal dynamics are implemented by the differential pair integrator. V_τ controls the circuit time constant while the EPSC amplitude depends on V_{w0} and V_{thr}. To build a depressing synapse, the left pulse reduces the charge on C_{std}, lowering V_w. C_{std} is eventually charged back to a resting potential if no more pulses arrive over a period of time. V_w controls the current flow that is mirrored to the output, with V_w proportional to the current that is mirrored to the output. *Short-term facilitation* is achieved by altering V_{thr} to temporarily increase the output current.

6.3 The BioRC synapses

The BioRC project models synapses using voltage-mode circuits, similar to the modeling of biological synapses by many computational neuroscientists that considers potentials (voltages) in computational models. The first BioRC synapse was designed in 2006. This synapse is a little bit more complicated than the single-transistor synapse that was discussed before but it's less complicated than Indiveri's for a variety of reasons that are discussed later in this section. The original BioRC synapse was published as a carbon nanotube transistor circuit [16, 17], although many prior publications used a different synapse circuit based on an unpublished CMOS design. Hsu's thesis [9] models synapses as well as neurons using carbon nanotubes.

The biomimetic synapses used by Hsu in BioRC circuits for various simulation experiments are shown in figures 6.5 and 6.6. Note that figure 6.5(b) will be discussed in detail when it is referred to in chapter 7. There are two parts to the synapse, the presynaptic side containing transistors X1–X7 and the postsynaptic side containing transistors X8–X10. In the excitatory synapse, when input AP arrives, the voltage at Syn. Cleft (synaptic cleft) increases, limited by the transistors X3 and *NTe* that model the release level of the excitatory neurotransmitters. The neurotransmitters then will be cleared from the synaptic cleft by the reuptake mechanism controlled by another input *ReU*. The voltage increase at Syn. Cleft will temporarily pull up the voltage at Syn. Interior close to the potential at ECh that models the electromotive force across the sodium ion channels. Syn. Interior is then pulled down to resting potential by the transistor X10 modeling potassium channels opening and lowering Syn. Interior voltage. The timing of the falling waveform is controlled by *RR* (modeling the resting return); that is when *RR* increases, the EPSP falls to resting potential faster. Voltage at Syn. Interior is transferred to the postsynaptic dendrite by the transistor X11. The hyperpolarizing inhibitory synapse (shown in 6.6(a)) works in a similar way except the *electromotive force (EMF)* is now a negative potential. The circuit representation of the shunting inhibitory synapse is shown in figure 6.6(b). A flow diagram showing overall operation is shown in figure 6.7, the stages of which are indicated in color blocks in figure 6.5.

6.3.1 Variations in BioRC excitatory synapses to control strengths

Synapses vary their strengths with learning. Changes in synaptic strength are also thought to underlie learning and storing of new memories. The first control over synaptic strength in the BioRC synapse is the variation of neurotransmitter concentration, involved in short-term synaptic strength (depression and potentiation). The more neurotransmitters there are (*NTe* increases), the more *NTe* turns on the transistor X7. This control will increase voltage at the cleft node more quickly, indicating that the synapse is stronger at the presynaptic side. Likewise, the synapse can be made stronger on the postsynaptic side in the short term by changing the number of receptors on the ion channels, called *AMPA* channels, modeled by adding a transistor in series with transistor X8 controlled with receptor concentration voltage. The more receptors, the faster the ion channel moves charges to Syn. Interior and the higher the voltage at Syn.Interior rises. As the receptor concentration is increased, the receptor control transistor turns on more. So, this voltage is going to rise faster and possibly higher as well, depending on when the pull-down circuit controlled by *RR* gets activated. These variations can be added just by adding transistors in series or parallel and result in a lot of different behaviors in the circuit. The available neurotransmitters and receptors can be varied. Because of these control voltages, there are two different controls over the strength of the synapse.

Biological synapses allow control over synaptic strengths by controlling both neurotransmitters and receptors. Joshi has added receptor control to the excitatory and inhibitory synapses, as shown in figures 6.8 and 6.9. Parts of the excitatory synapse circuit (figure 6.8) exhibit biomimetic behavior corresponding to biological

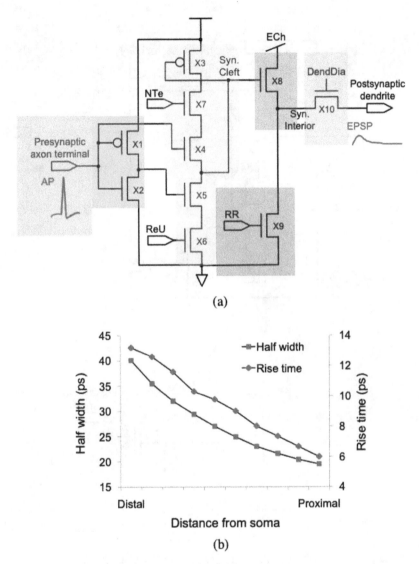

(a)

(b)

Figure 6.5. (a) A biomimetic excitatory synapse can be modulated by different neural mechanisms such as neurotransmitter concentration *NTe*, reuptake rate *ReU*, and rate of return to resting potential *RR*. (b) EPSP half width and rise time characterization. Distance from soma (*distal* to *proximal*) is modeled by *DendDia* control voltage, as discussed in chapter 7. Blue shows AP arrival, pink shows inhibition of neurotransmitter reuptake during excitation, yellow shows neurotransmitter release with limiting transistor, yellow-green shows reuptake of neurotransmitter, orange shows sodium ion flow into the synapse, purple shows sodium ions pumped back to the cell interior, and green shows a pass transistor connecting to the output of the synapse. Here, a current mirror could isolate the synapse circuit from neural computations occurring downstream. Reproduced from [9].

mechanisms. The AP impinges on two sections of the synapse, namely the neurotransmitter (presynaptic) section and a mechanism (*delay 1*) that delays the neurotransmitter reuptake. The pull-up transistor in the neurotransmitter section controls the neurotransmitter concentration in the synaptic cleft (the voltage at the synaptic

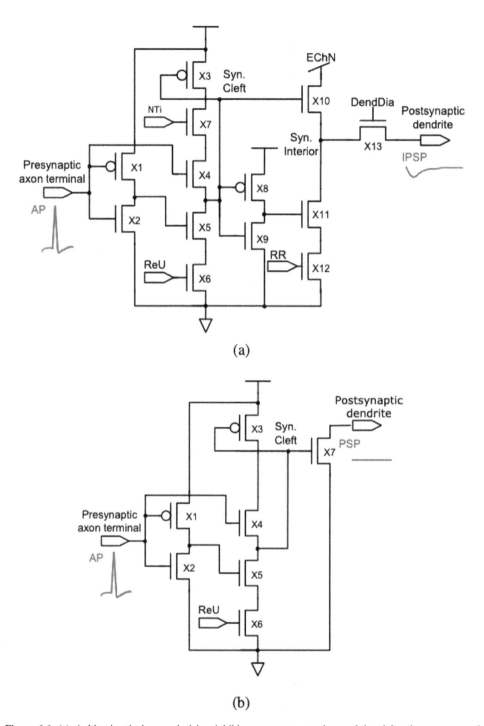

(a)

(b)

Figure 6.6. (a) A biomimetic hyperpolarizing inhibitory synapse can be modulated by the same neural mechanisms such as neurotransmitter concentration, reuptake, and ion pump. (b) A biomimetic shunting inhibitory synapse is active when an AP arrives and pulls down the potential at postsynaptic dendrite to ground (circuit resting potential), that is a negative voltage in biological neurons. Reproduced from [9].

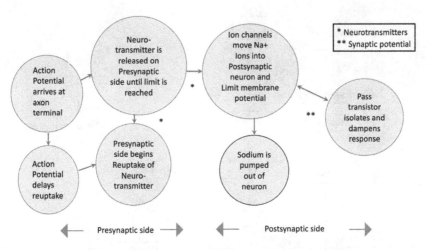

Figure 6.7. Flow diagram showing basic operation of the excitatory synapse shown in figure 6.5.

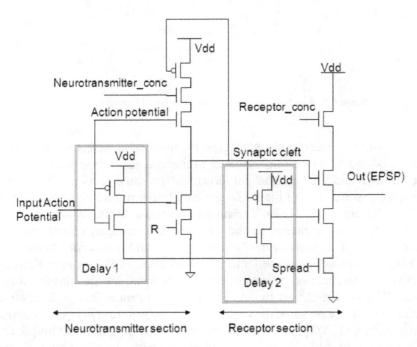

Figure 6.8. A carbon nanotube excitatory synapse with receptor modulation. Copyright 2009 IEEE. Reprinted, with permission, from [14].

cleft node) while the pull-down transistor models the reuptake mechanism that controls the drop in neurotransmitter concentration in the cleft. The reuptake delay is controlled by the rise time of the delay circuit, by varying the length of its PMOS transistor to indirectly control the falling RC time constant of the neurotransmitter

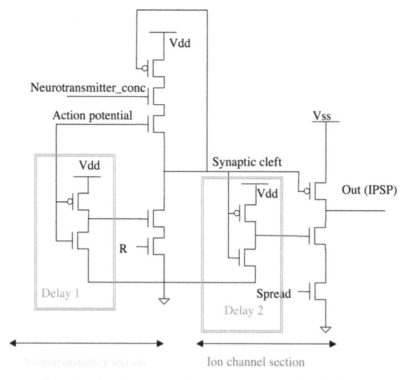

Figure 6.9. A carbon nanotube inhibitory synapse. Reprinted from [14].

concentration. The neurotransmitter release causes ion channels to open; depolarization is modeled by the pull-up transistor in the receptor section tied to V_{dd}. The fall of the EPSP is modeled by the pull-down in the same section. The time delay between the positive peak of the EPSP and its fall to ground is modeled by a second tuneable delay circuit (*Delay 2*). Variation in neurotransmitter concentration in the synaptic cleft causes a change in the EPSP peak amplitude, directly altering the synapse strength. The reuptake mechanism inputs R and *spread* control the spread of the EPSP, which modulates the temporal summation of the synapse EPSPs when successive APs impinge on a synapse or multiple synapses are stimulated at close intervals. The voltage across the gate labeled *Neurotransmitter_conc* controls the neurotransmitter release while the voltage across the gate *Receptor_conc* controls the receptor activation. Varying these two voltages controls the EPSP amplitude and provides a way to add circuits that exhibit plasticity. Joshi's inhibitory synapse presented here is based on the biomimetic behavior of a hyperpolarizing inhibitory synapse circuit designed to be compact, with correspondence between biological mechanisms and circuit structures. Synapse behavior is controlled by voltages on the gates of the transistors, acting as control knobs. The neurotransmitter concentration and the spread of the inhibitory postsynaptic potential (IPSP) (delay of return to resting potential) can be varied by controlling the neurotransmitter release and reuptake rates. The synapse also exhibits temporal summation of the IPSPs when APs impinge on the synapse at close intervals. This circuit models cell potentials and neurotransmitter concentrations with voltages, along with the correspondence between circuit elements and biological mechanisms.

Figure 6.9 presents the inhibitory synapse circuit that displays presynaptic as well as postsynaptic plasticity. The design is segmented into parts that facilitate biomimetic behavior corresponding to biological mechanisms. The AP impinges on two sections of the synapse as shown, namely the neurotransmitter section and a mechanism (*Delay 1*) that delays the reuptake of neurotransmitters. The pull-up transistor in the neurotransmitter section controls the actual neurotransmitter concentration in the synaptic cleft, modeled by the voltage at the synaptic cleft node, whereas the pull-down transistor models the reuptake mechanism that controls the drop in neurotransmitter concentration in the cleft. The chronological occurrence of reuptake is controlled by the rise time of the delay circuit, by varying the length of its PMOS transistor to indirectly control the falling RC time constant of the neurotransmitter concentration. The neurotransmitter release causes one or more ion channels to open; hyperpolarization is modeled by the pull-down transistor in the ion channel section tied to negative potential (V_{ss}). The ion flow responsible for the rise of the IPSP to the resting potential is modeled by the pull-up to ground in the same section. The time delay between the negative peak of the IPSP and its rise to ground potential is modeled by a second delay circuit (*Delay 2*) that is tuneable to vary the synapse properties. Variation in neurotransmitter concentration in the synaptic cleft causes a change in the IPSP negative peak amplitude thus directly altering the synapse strength [8]. Also, the reuptake mechanism R and *spread* input control the spread of the IPSP, which modulates the temporal summation of the synapse output when multiple successive APs impinge on the synapse or multiple synapses are stimulated at close intervals. The voltage across the gate labeled *neurotransmitter_conc* controls the current that models the neurotransmitter release while the voltage across the gate R controls the reuptake. Varying these two voltages controls the IPSP amplitude and the spread of the IPSP, respectively.

It might seem like the strength of the synapse is not that important to separate into two different strengths, but this separation shows some subtle effects like how the astrocytes are going to control the strengths of the synapses. Separating the presynaptic side and the postsynaptic side might be useful. In fact, it's shown that the astrocytes can change what happens at the synaptic cleft. How is this done? Astrocytes will take up neurotransmitters that weaken the synapse, and will release gliotransmitters that strengthen the synapse. So, the astrocytes can control something about the strength of the synapse by dealing with the concentration of neurotransmitters in the synaptic cleft itself, and the quantity of receptors to those neurotransmitters on the postsynaptic side of the synapse. Astrocytes will be discussed later in chapter 11.

Based on the average ratio of the excitatory and inhibitory synapses, i.e., 4:1, in the cortex, Hsu configured a hypothetical neuron to receive four excitatory synapses and one inhibitory synapse to test different scenarios shown in figure 6.10(a). The

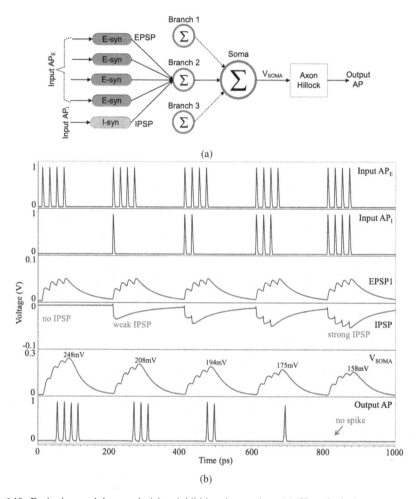

Figure 6.10. Excitation and hyperpolarizing inhibition integration. (a) Hypothetical neuron setup. The transistor-level circuits of *E-syn* and *I-syn* are shown in figure 6.5(a) and 6.6(a). (b) Different numbers of input AP spikes applied to the hyperpolarizing inhibitory synapse cause different strengths of IPSP. With stronger IPSP, the sum of PSP at the soma, V_{SOMA}, is not sufficient to evoke neuron firing; there is no output AP spike. Reproduced from [9].

unitary IPSP is configured to have the same amplitude (approximately 3% of the amplitude of an AP) but opposite sign of the unitary EPSP. In the first simulation (figure 6.10(b)), Hsu varied the number of input AP spikes to the inhibitory synapse and observed that with weak IPSP the neuron under test fires output AP spikes, however, when the IPSP is stronger the neuron becomes silent. In the second simulation (figure 6.11), we adjusted the neurotransmitter concentration in the inhibitory synaptic circuit (figure 6.6(a)) to generate weak IPSP and strong IPSP (with higher neurotransmitter concentration). We observed that the effective inhibition time window of the weaker inhibitory synapse is smaller compared to

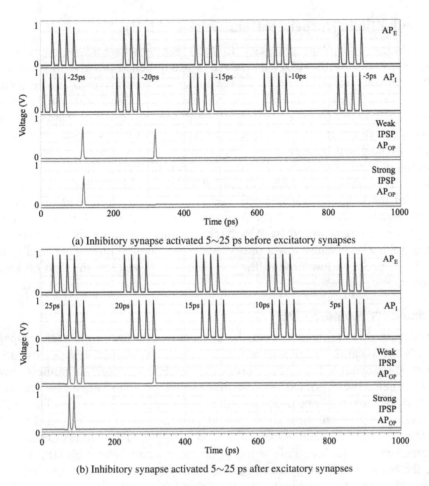

(a) Inhibitory synapse activated 5∼25 ps before excitatory synapses

(b) Inhibitory synapse activated 5∼25 ps after excitatory synapses

Figure 6.11. Effective hyperpolarizing inhibition time window comparison. A hyperpolarizing inhibitory synapse is activated (a) between 5 and 25 ps before and (b) between 5 and 25 ps after excitatory synapses. With weaker IPSP the effective inhibition window is less, between −15 ps and 15 ps while with stronger IPSP the effective inhibition window is larger, between −20 ps and 20 ps. Reproduced from [9].

that of the stronger inhibitory synapse. We defined the effective inhibition time window as that time window during which the inhibition still has effect to suppress the excitation even if they are not activated at the same time. This time window is defined as the difference between inhibitory input AP spike's arrival time and the excitatory input AP spike's arrival time, i.e., $t_{AP_I} - t_{AP_E}$. This result shows that an inhibitory synapse with different strengths can affect the final output response in two opposite states. When the IPSP is strong, it prevents the neuron from firing since the overall PSP is below the threshold, and an AP is generated otherwise in spite of the smaller IPSP. Therefore, strong IPSP induces a larger effective inhibition time window.

6.4 Spike timing dependent plasticity (STDP)

Spike timing dependent plasticity (STDP) strengthens and weakens synaptic response to APs. With STDP, a synapse is strengthened (long-term potentiation, LTP) when the presynaptic AP at a particular synapse preceeds the postsynaptic AP (the output of the neuron after the synapse). A synapse is weakened (long-term depression, LTD) when the postsynaptic AP preceeds the presynaptic AP or the presynaptic AP never existed. Thus, neurons modify their synaptic connections to adapt to changes in neural input. The ability of many neurons to modulate the strengths of their synaptic connections has been shown to depend on the relative timing of pre- and postsynaptic APs, called STDP. STDP has become an attractive model for learning at the single-cell level [15]. The temporal order of presynaptic and postsynaptic firing is a critically important aspect of STDP. The synapse is thought to be strengthened by APs back propagating along the dendrites along with depolarization caused by a previous action potential impinging on a synapse. The back propagation absent the previous AP weakens the future synaptic response.

Mechanisms behind STDP

Consider an AP that spikes from the postsynaptic neuron and back propagates towards the synapse. It allows the *NMDA* channels to open and positive ions to flow in. If the synapse has already produced a PSP using *AMPA* channels, then the *NMDA* channels are primed because they need both glutamate and voltage (from the AMPA channels opening) in order to cause them to open. The AP that propagates back, along with the glutamate, allows calcium to flow in through the *NMDA* channels. Calcium supercharges the synapse so that it has extra effect on the membrane potential. This is the basic mechanism behind STDP. So, by the time the back-propagating action reaches the synapse, if the synapse has already spiked, then the two incidents together could be enough to cause the *NMDA* channels to open. If the PSP is too late, when the AP propagates back, the *NMDA* channel is not going to open because the synapse excitation has disappeared. All the requirements for the channel to open are not being met. It's unclear what causes actual depression (weakening of the synapse) as a result but it appears to affect the presynaptic axonal terminal that connects to the synapse. It essentially means that the synapse is too late in contributing to a PSP or never contributed to the potential.

While *AMPA* channels in the postsynaptic density cause spiking to occur in the postsynaptic neuron, *NMDA* channels, both voltage- and ligand-gated (chemically gated), cause additional plasticity in the synapse, called LTP (strengthening the synapse) and LTD (weakening the synapse). *NMDA* channels are permeable to calcium, and the calcium flow into the synapse is largest when there is a back-propagating AP shortly after the synapse responds to a presynaptic spike. This calcium flow triggers potentiation. The *NMDA* channels open when there is strong depolarization of the synapse, when an AP is immediately followed by a back-propagating AP.

The *NMDA* channel has a magnesium block that is removed when the cell potential rises. This is the part of the *NMDA* channel that is voltage gated. Glutamate, the most common neurotransmitter, causes *AMPA* channels to open and also is the ligand-gated part of the *NMDA* channel. So the coincidence of a recent presynaptic spike with a back-propagating AP cause synaptic potentials to rise when glutamate is present. Opening the *NMDA* channels also causes some enzymes to be released, strengthening the *AMPA* channels. The enzymes employ phosphates that strengthen the *AMPA* channel receptors. Additional receptors that are calcium permeable can also be recruited. This process is reversible.

Henry Markram was one of the first people to disclose STDP and measure it in biological neurons [15]. He showed that the synapses are strengthened when a synapse is excited and then the neuron spikes. Synapses are weakened when the neuron spikes before a synapse is excited or when it is never excited. UCSD researchers Bi and Poo (1998) reported on this shortly after Henry Markram, showing STDP [3]. The STDP function shows the change of synaptic connections as a function of the relative timing of pre- and postsynaptic spikes after multiple spike pairings. The example in figure 6.12 shows that if the pre-spike arrives before the

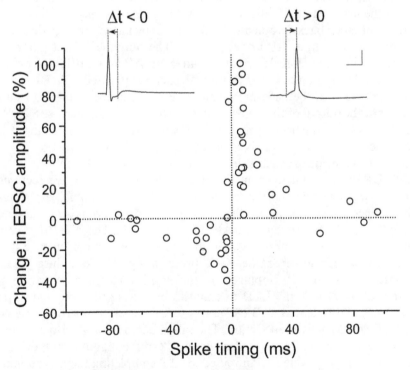

Figure 6.12. STDP and the difference between pre- and postsynaptic spike events with respect to synaptic strengthening. Reproduced from [3], copyright 1998 Society for Neuroscience.

post-spike, this leads to synaptic strengthening. But if the post- arrives before the pre-, it leads to synaptic weakening.

Arthur and Boahen [1] model CMOS synapses that correlate and store the pre-post synchronization using an SRAM-based approach. Work done by Tovar [25] models the STDP-based on Reichardt's correlation and uses the correlation towards inhibition and excitation of neighboring neurons. Tanaka demonstrates an STDP circuit based on digital gates and flip flops to store synchronization information [22]. Work by Huo [10] shows the role of membrane threshold in their STDP synapse as a part of an integrate and fire neuron. Similar circuitry has been reported on by Indiveri *et al* [11]. Sengupta reported ultra-low power neurons ($\approx$1.6 fJ per neuron per time step) and stochastic binary synapse designs with novel post-CMOS technologies, and showed simulation result of MNIST dataset recognition in STDP-based spiking neural network with over 99% accuracy rate [19]. Several works reported neuromorphic STDP designs incorporating metal oxide memristor devices [12, 13, 18, 21]. The neuromorphic STDP implementation with CMOS is explored thoroughly by [5, 20].

6.4.1 Joshi's STDP circuit

Joshi described an early BioRC STDP circuit in his dissertation (figure 6.13). The two inputs to the circuit are *input AP* and *back-propagating AP*. There are current mirrors in the first stage that basically act as delays. At the second block either the delayed input and back propagated AP are coincident, or the delayed back propagated AP and input AP are coincident. The output rise and fall is decided as previously discussed. Joshi's circuit has an input AP and a delay block to delay the input AP. The circuit also has as input a back-propagated AP. Together if the delayed input AP and the back-propagated AP are coincident, the high output of the inverter at the output of the upper-right current mirror can increase STDP. If the input AP arrives late, the back propagated AP will be delayed until the input arrives. Together they are viewed in the coincidence detector. If they occur roughly at the same time, the coincidence causes decrease in the synapse strength.

The STDP circuit, as shown in figure 6.13, is divided into five sections. The *receptor activation section* and the *magnesium block removal section* are responsible for coincidence detection when the presynaptic AP (input *AP*) precedes the postsynaptic AP (back propagating AP) to induce LTP. The *NMDA deactivation section* and the calcium channel section are responsible for coincidence detection when the input AP succeeds the back propagating AP to induce LTD. The presynaptic AP (input AP) impinges on the *NMDA* receptor activation section (transistor X2) to disable the LTD mechanism by raising the potential of point A and grounding the potential at B (X21) through the current mirror in the *NMDA* receptor (*NMDAR*) activation section. The raised potential at A also contributes to removing the magnesium block by turning on X8 in the magnesium block removal section. The back propagated AP impinges on X9 completing the magnesium block removal by pulling down point C through the inverting current mirror in the block removal section. The output of point C controls the pull-up of the Ca^{2+} level that

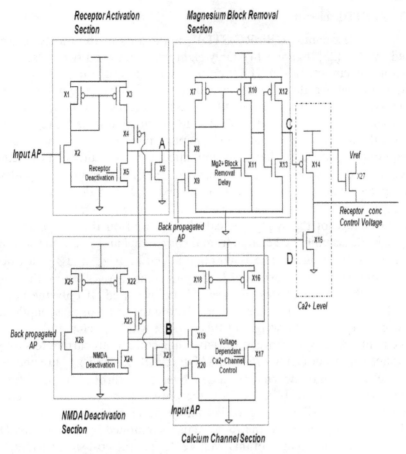

Figure 6.13. Joshi's STDP circuit. Reproduced from [14].

controls the receptor concentration, the signal labeled *Receptor conc* to induce LTP. The voltage across the gate of X5 (receptor deactivation) controls the duration of the time window for which the synapse has the receptors activated for LTP induction. The X11 gate voltage (*magnesium block removal delay*) controls the rise time for the *Receptor conc.* voltage. However, when the back propagated AP precedes the input AP it deactivates the NMDA channel by turning on X26 in the NMDA deactivation section causing the rise in potential at B that pulls the A potential to ground (X6) and turns on X19. The post-pre spiking on the calcium channel section (X19 and X20) raises the potential at point D, pulling down the *Receptor conc* control voltage to induce LTD. The voltage across the gate of X24 (NMDA deactivation) controls the timing of the window for that the synapse has the receptors deactivated for LTD induction. The voltage across the gate of X17 (voltage dependent Ca^{2+} channel control) controls the fall time for the final receptor control voltage.

Joshi's STDP circuit only sends a signal to strengthen or weaken synapse strength, and does not modulate that signal depending on the time difference between postsynaptic and presynaptic spikes.

6.4.2 Yue's STDP circuit

An additional less-complex BioRC STDP circuit used in the BioRC project was designed by Yue [23] (figure 6.14). Only eight transistors and two pulse generators are used in the circuit. In the STDP mechanism, the weight dynamics depend not only on the current weight, but also depend on the relationship between arrival times of the presynaptic and postsynaptic APs [15]. This means that, besides the synaptic weight, each synapse keeps track of the recent presynaptic spike history. In terms of Yue's STDP model, every time a presynaptic spike arrives at the synapse, the presynaptic spike will cause charge accumulation χ_{pre} in the diffusion capacitance of a transistor, and then the charge will decay gradually. Every time the postsynaptic neuron spikes, charge χ_{post} is also accumulated and then decays. When a postsynaptic spike arrives at the synapse due to back propagation from the axon hillock, the weight change of the synapse is calculated based on the presynaptic charges where χ_{pre} is the accumulated charge from the *pre* signal and χ_{post} is the accumulated charge from the *post* signal. The assumption is that both χ_{pre} and χ_{post} are decaying over time after rising high instantly. If the *post* signal arrives before the *pre* signal decays to 0, the weight of this synapse will be increased. If only the post signal arrives, that means the output neuron fires before the firing of presynaptic neurons that excite the synapse, the weight of this synapse will be decreased.

This circuit operates on charges, thus avoiding continuous current to save power. Each synapse in this design has its own STDP circuit. χ_{pre} and χ_{post} are analogous to electrical charges, and the charges decay over time through biasing transistors connected to the ground. If and only if the pre signal arrives first, the connected post-gated transistor will be charged. Then if the post signal arrives successively, the *Set* pulse will be triggered and the *Reset* signal is inhibited by discharging. One *Set* pulse will increase the strength of this synapse. If only the post signal arrives, the *Set* signal will not be triggered, because the pre-charging of the pre-transistor gate is absent, and the post signal will trigger the *Reset* pulse without discharging inhibition. One *Reset* pulse will decrease the strength of this synapse. All the charging nodes in Yue's circuit are discharged by a constant bias transistor to implement the differential timing factors. The amplitude of synapse weight change in the circuit implementation

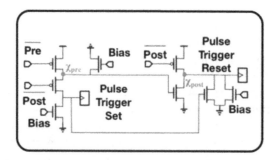

Figure 6.14. Yue's STDP circuit. Reproduced from [23].

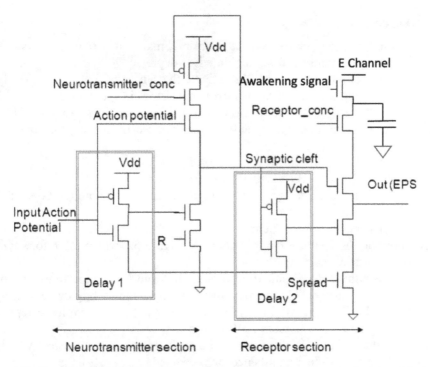

Figure 6.15. Silent synapse circuit formed from a conventional BioRC synapse circuit. Adapted from [14].

is a discrete value for each pulse. A positive-edge input will generate one current pulse output with fixed amplitude and duration.

6.5 The silent synapse

A basic silent synapse circuit can be formed from a BioRC synapse, as shown in figure 6.15. In this synapse, the *E Channel* voltage can be can be supplied by a circuit that only provides sufficient voltage when the synapse is to be awakened. Note that the receptor concentration control signal in this synapse can also be used to silence a synapse by setting the control voltage to 0.0 V, and can be awakened by setting it to V_{dd}.

6.6 Chapter summary

This chapter covered neuromorphic synapse circuits, beginning with a synapse designed by Chicca, Indiveri and Douglas. The chapter covered the BioRC synapse in some detail. Varying synaptic strengths was discussed, and a circuit mechanism for synaptic strength adjustment, the STDP circuit, was presented.

The next chapter covers circuit mechanisms for constructing a passive dendritic arbor. The chapter begins with Elias' dendritic arbor circuit, and a short introduction to voltage addition. The rest of the chapter covers Hsu's mechanisms for constructing a passive dendritic arbor.

6.7 Exercises

1. In the synapse circuit shown in figure 6.2, mark all correct answers:
   (a) The synapse can be facilitated or depressed;
   (b) Transistors M1 and M2 activate the synapse;
   (c) There are two current mirror integrators in the circuit;
   (d) Weight of the synapse is controlled by transistors M3 and M11.
2. Separating the presynaptic side of the synapse from the postsynaptic side (mark all correct answers):
   (a) Is found in the BioRC synapse;
   (b) Is found in the original Indiveri synapse;
   (c) Can separate synapse strengthening due to modulation of both neurotransmitters and receptors;
   (d) Is never done in neuromorphic circuits.
3. Show on the Indiveri synapse shown in figure 6.2 where inhibitory synapse strength is stored.
4. Why are there two inputs to transistors M1 and M2 on the Indiveri synapse shown in figure 6.2? Is this part of the synapse facilitating or depressing?
5. In the BioRC synapse in figure 6.15, the *synaptic cleft* voltage represents what quantity in the biological neuron?
6. In Joshi's STDP circuit, what two signals does he use to detect whether a synapse should be strengthened or weakened?
7. In the BioRC synapse in figure 6.15, there are two parts, on the left and right sides of the synapse. What do these two parts represent?
8. In Joshi's STDP circuit, what happens if the neuron spikes before its synapse is excited?
9. STDP (mark all correct answers):
   (a) Stands for synapse timing depression potentiation;
   (b) Weakens synapses strength if synapse excitation did not contribute to the generation of a postsynaptic AP;
   (c) Is the rule by which synapses are strengthened or weakened;
   (d) Does not rely on precise timing between presynaptic and postsynaptic spikes.

References

[1] Arthur J V and Boahen K 2005 Learning in silicon: timing is everything *Advances in Neural Information Processing Systems 18 (NIPS 2005)* pp 75–82
[2] Bartolozzi C and Indiveri G 2006 Silicon synaptic homeostasis *Brain Inspired Cognitive Systems BICS 2006*
[3] Guo-qiang B and Mu-ming P 1998 Synaptic modifications in cultured hippocampal neurons: dependence on spike timing, synaptic strength, and postsynaptic cell type *J. Neurosci.* **18** 10464–72
[4] Boahen K A 2000 Point-to-point connectivity between neuromorphic chips using address events *IEEE Trans. Circuits Syst.* II **47** 416–34
[5] Cameron K *et al* 2005 Spike timing dependent plasticity (STDP) can ameliorate process variations in neuromorphic VLSI *IEEE Trans. Neural Netw.* **16** 1626–37

[6] Chicca E, Indiveri G and Douglas R 2003 An adaptive silicon synapse *Proc. 2003 nt. Symp. Circuits and Systems, 2003. ISCAS'03I* 1 I

[7] Chicca E *et al* 2014 Neuromorphic Electronic Circuits for Building Autonomous Cognitive Systems *Proc. IEEE* **102** 1367–88

[8] 2001 *Synapses* ed W M Cowan, T C Sudhof and C F Stevens (Baltimore, MD: Johns Hopkins University Press) illustrated edition

[9] Hsu C-C 2014 Dendritic computation and plasticity in neuromorphic circuits *PhD Thesis* University of Southern California

[10] Huo J and Murray A 2005 The role of membrane threshold and rate in STDP silicon neuron circuit simulation *Artificial Neural Networks: Formal Models and Their Applications–ICANN 2005: 15th Int. Conf., Warsaw, Poland, September 11–15, 2005. Proc., Part II* (Berlin: Springer) pp 1009–14

[11] Indiveri G, Chicca E and Douglas R 2006 A VLSI array of low-power spiking neurons and bistable synapses with spike-timing dependent plasticity *IEEE Trans. Neural Netw.* **17** 211–21

[12] Indiveri G *et al* 2013 Integration of nanoscale memristor synapses in neuromorphic computing architectures *Nanotechnology* **24** 384010

[13] Hyun J S *et al* 2010 Nanoscale memristor device as synapse in neuromorphic systems *Nano Lett.* **10** 1297–301

[14] Joshi J 2013 Plasticity in CMOS neuromorphic circuits *PhD Thesis* University of Southern California

[15] Markram H *et al* 1997 Regulation of synaptic efficacy by coincidence of postsynaptic APs and EPSPs *Science* **275** 213–5

[16] Parker A C, Friesz A K and Tseng K-C 2009 Biomimetic Cortical Nanocircuits *Bio-Inspired and Nanoscale Integrated Computing* (Hoboken, NJ: Wiley) p 455

[17] Parker A C *et al* 2008 A carbon nanotube implementation of temporal and spatial dendritic computations *2008 51st Midwest Symp. Circuits and Systems* 818–21

[18] Antonio Pérez-Carrasco J *et al* On neuromorphic spiking architectures for asynchronous STDP memristive systems *Proc. 2010 IEEE Int. Symp. Circuits and Systems* (Piscataway, NJ: IEEE)

[19] Sengupta A *et al* 2016 Magnetic tunnel junction mimics stochastic cortical spiking neurons *Sci. Rep.* **6** 30039

[20] Seo J *et al* 2011 A 45 nm CMOS neuromorphic chip with a scalable architecture for learning in networks of spiking neurons *2011 IEEE Custom Integrated Circuits Conf. (CICC)* (Piscataway, NJ: IEEE) pp 1–4

[21] Serrano-Gotarredona T *et al* 2013 STDP and STDP variations with memristors for spiking neuromorphic learning systems *Front. Neurosci.* **7** 2

[22] Maria Tovar G *et al* 2008 Analog cmos circuits implementing neural segmentation model based on symmetric stdp learning *Neural Information Processing: 14th Int. Conf., ICONIP 2007, Kitakyushu, Japan, November 13–16, 2007, Revised Selected Papers, Part II 14* (Berlin: Springer) pp 117–26

[23] Yue K 2020 Circuit design with nano electronic devices for biomimetic neuromorphic systems *PhD Thesis* University of Southern California

[24] Indiveri G *et al* 2011 Neuromorphic Silicon Neuron Circuits *Front. Neurosci.* **5** 73

[25] Tovar G, Fukuda E, Asai T, Hirose T and Amemiya Y 2008 Analog CMOS circuits implementing neural segmentation model based on symmetric STDP learning *Neural Information Processing* (Lecture Notes in Computer Science vol 4985) (Springer) pp 117–26

IOP Publishing

Neuromorphic Circuits
A constructive approach
Alice C Parker and Rick Cattell

Chapter 7

The passive dendritic arbor

Chih-Chieh Hsu and Alice C Parker

This chapter begins with Elias' classic implementation of passive dendritic computations [4, 5]. Circuits performing passive additions of voltage in the dendritic arbor are covered next. The remainder of the chapter covers passive dendritic circuits researched by Hsu [6], followed by a survey of other research involving neuromorphic circuits performing dendritic computations.

7.1 Elias' passive dendritic model

A compartmental model of Elias' passive dendrite is shown in figure 7.1.

Figure 7.2 shows a segment of a dendritic branch and a sketch of a dendritic arbor. The branch contains five excitatory and five inhibitory single-transistor synapses. V_{rest} is the resting potential and V_{top} is the maximum membrane potential. Note that the top transistors (pull up transistors) are PMOS transistors, creating excitatory synapses, and the bottom transistors are NMOS transistors, creating inhibitory synapses, with gate inputs being synaptic inputs. The gate inputs to the excitatory synapses are inverted, so that an excitatory input is a low voltage. The bottom connection is ground, and the circuit direction towards the soma is to the right.

7.2 Passive voltage addition in the dendritic arbor

Most models of the dendritic arbor are current mode (including Elias' model), and add dendritic branch currents, just joining branches at a single node to add currents. Voltage mode circuits, like the BioRC circuits, usually convert voltages to currents, and add currents, converting back to voltages at the output of the current adder. A basic voltage adder by Chaoui, introduced earlier in chapter 3 figure 3.4 [2], is used in most of the BioRC dendritic arbors, although Hsu uses an average-amplify circuit to add voltages that requires tuning and is somewhat nonlinear, as shown in

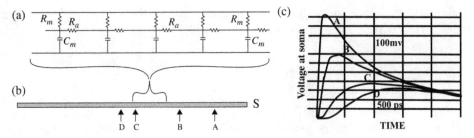

Figure 7.1. (a) Compartmental model of a passive dendrite. Each RC section, R_m, R_a, and C_m, is a compartment ; m indicates membrane, and a indicates cytoplasm. (b) Compartments abut to form silicon dendritic branches. (c) Measured impulse response of a single artificial dendritic branch due to transient transmembrane current at indicated locations on the branch. Reprinted from [5], copyright (1993), with permission from Springer Nature. (c) is redrawn for clarity.

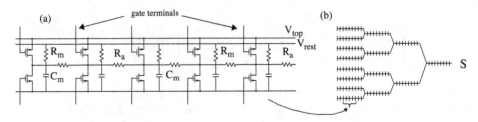

Figure 7.2. A section of dendrite (a) and a dendritic arbor (b). Reprinted from [5], copyright (1993), with permission from Springer Nature.

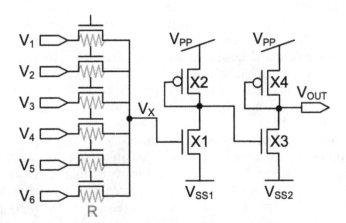

Figure 7.3. The *average-amplify* circuit [6]. The averaging resistor network implemented with N-type pass transistors is connected to an amplifier pair in common-source diode-connected configuration.

figure 7.3 and used in the dendritic spiking circuit in chapter 8. An advantage of the Chaoui adder is that it can add negative as well as positive voltages. A disadvantage of the Chaoui adder is that it is difficult to maintain zero output with zero inputs, and small errors accumulate. A dendritic arbor with 10 000 synapses could accumulate enough error to fire with all zero inputs to the synapses. A nonlinear adder was later developed in the BioRC group [9].

7.2.1 Hsu's average-amplify circuit

The summation of the postsynaptic potentials (PSPs) is computed by the *average-amplify* circuit shown in figure 7.3. The circuit first averages the voltage potentials at each input port through the resistive network that is modeled with pass transistors. By Kirchhoff's circuit laws, all current flowing into node V_X should sum to zero, hence according to equation (7.1), V_X is the average of the sum of input V_i. The gain, A_V, representing the overall amplification factor of the amplifier pair, can be derived from equation (7.2).

$$\frac{V_1 - V_X}{R} + \frac{V_2 - V_X}{R} + \frac{V_3 - V_X}{R} + \frac{V_4 - V_X}{R} + \frac{V_5 - V_X}{R} + \frac{V_6 - V_X}{R} = 0 \quad (7.1)$$

$$A_V = \left(-\frac{g_{m1}}{g_{m2}}\right) \cdot \left(-\frac{g_{m3}}{g_{m4}}\right) = \left(-\sqrt{\frac{(W/L)_1 \cdot \mu_n}{(W/L)_2 \cdot \mu_p}}\right) \cdot \left(-\sqrt{\frac{(W/L)_3 \cdot \mu_n}{(W/L)_4 \cdot \mu_p}}\right) \quad (7.2)$$

Since the geometric parameter (W/L) represents the strength (conductance) of the transistor, transistors X1 and X3 are stronger (wider) than X2 and X4.

7.3 Hsu's computations in the dendritic arbor

This section presents dendritic computations by modeling passive properties of the dendrites in cortical pyramidal neurons [6]. Hsu focuses on various types of PSP integrations in the dendrites and their impacts on a neuron's firing (spiking) state. She implements different dendritic mechanisms using neuromorphic circuits and demonstrates that the circuits mimic the passive biological response to the first order. In her thesis, Hsu models a temporal integration window as a function of the synaptic spatial distribution. Moreover, Hsu uses temporal summation as a means of sequence detection.

In addition, in the next chapter, chapter 8, Hsu's circuits implement nonlinear spatio-temporal dendritic computation (if spikes are close to each other and occur within a small time window), show that feedback from local dendritic branch and global neuronal output modulate dendritic excitability, and show that different dendritic spike mechanisms are used for learning (e.g. branch strength potentiation (BSP) and backward action potential (BAC)), as described in the next chapter, chapter 8. In these two chapters, Hsu validated her hypothesis that fine-grained dendritic modeling in neuromorphic circuits enhances:

- Spatio-temporal information processing in artificial auditory and visual neural networks;
- Dendritic spike-induced precise and reliable neuronal spike timing;
- Dendritic spike-induced coincidence detection and learning;

- Circuits for dendritic computation with an example border ownership network (see chapter 16, section 16.4);
- Excitation and inhibition: nonlinear/asymmetric integration;
- Synaptic distal and proximal spatio-temporal summation; and
- Active sodium and calcium dendritic spike-induced neural mechanisms.

Hsu's dissertation implemented circuit modules for dendritic plasticity, dendritic excitability up/down-regulation for BSP and branch reset mechanisms.

7.3.1 Shunting inhibition

Hsu conducted some experiments showing shunting synapse location matters in passive neural computation, described here.

An *up-stream* synapse means its location is farther away from the soma (cell body) than the reference synapse. On the other hand, a synapse *down-stream* means its location is closer to the soma than the reference synapse. For example, in figure 7.4(a), *Esyn1* is the *up-stream* synapse in reference to *Isyn* and *Esyn2* is the *down-stream* synapse.

A circuit with excitatory and inhibitory synapses is simulated to demonstrate the interactions between excitation and inhibition, as illustrated in figure 7.4(b). The input action potentials (AP_E) are applied to the excitatory synapses on all three branches and the input APs (AP_{I1}, AP_{I2}, AP_{I3}) are applied to the inhibitory synapses. The shunting inhibitory synapses are at different locations with respect to the excitatory synapses on the three branches. For example, on Branch1, the inhibitory

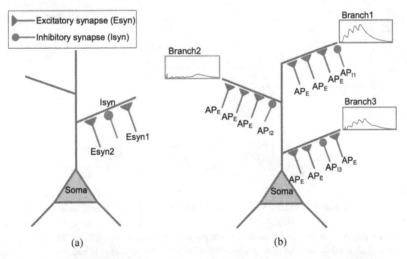

(a)   (b)

Figure 7.4. Shunting inhibitory synapse location variation [6]: (a) The red triangle represents an excitatory synapse and the blue circle represents an inhibitory synapse. *Esyn1* is the *up-stream* synapse in reference to the shunting inhibitory synapse *Isyn* and *Esyn2* is the *down-stream* synapse. (b) Neuron configuration to demonstrate shunting inhibition effect. The box next to each branch represents the dendritic potential of that branch when both *Esyn* and *Isyn* are activated.

synapse is located off the pathway to the soma while on Branch2, the inhibitory synapse is located on the pathway to the soma. Therefore, Branch1 has the largest potential and Branch2 has the lowest potential. The inhibitory synapse on Branch3 blocks the *up-stream* excitatory synapse but has no effect over the other two *down-stream* excitatory synapses.

The simulation result is shown in figure 7.5. The shunting inhibitory synapses on the three branches are activated in the following order: Branch1 at 200 ps, Branch2 at 400 ps (four input spikes) and 600 ps (one input spike), Branch3 at 800 ps. Branch1 has the largest dendritic potential because the inhibitory synapse is not on the pathway to the soma. Branch2 has the lowest dendritic potential because the inhibitory synapse is on the pathway to the soma. Therefore, the somatic potential (V_{SOMA}) has the largest potential when none of the inhibitory synapses are activated or only the one on Branch1 is activated. In contrast, V_{SOMA} has the smallest potential when the inhibitory synapse on Branch2 is activated and hence no output AP is initiated. The fourth trial shows spiking because the inhibition is weak. The fifth trial shows spiking because only one excitatory synapse is inhibited.

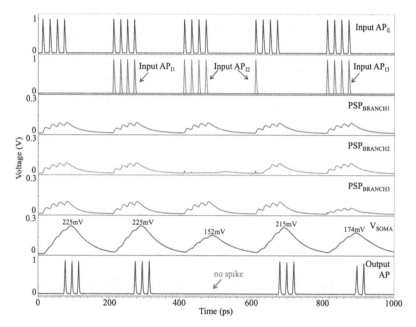

Figure 7.5. Nonlinear and asymmetric shunting inhibition effect [6]. Five scenarios are tested on the model neuron in figure 7.4(b). First, no inhibitory synapses are activated, the neuron fires three consecutive spikes. Second, when input AP_{I1} activates the shunting synapse on *Branch1*, no change on PSP$_{\text{BRANCH1}}$ is observed because the shunting inhibitory synapse is considered *off-path* to the soma. When strong input AP_{I2} (four spikes) activates the shunting synapse on Branch2, prominent change on PSP$_{\text{BRANCH2}}$ and no output AP spikes are observed because the shunting inhibitory synapse vetoes all other excitatory synapses on the same branch. However, if the input AP_{I2} is weak (one single spike), the inhibition is weaker resulting in the neuron firing. Lastly, when input AP_{I3} activates the shunting inhibitory synapse, only one excitatory synapse is vetoed resulting in a slight potential decrease on PSP$_{\text{BRANCH3}}$ and less output firing.

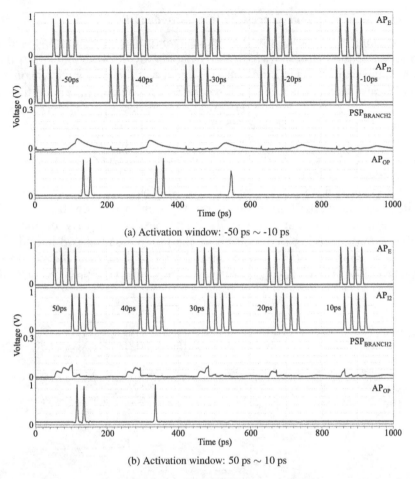

(a) Activation window: -50 ps ~ -10 ps

(b) Activation window: 50 ps ~ 10 ps

Figure 7.6. Time window for shunting inhibition effect. When the shunting inhibitory synapse is activated after the excitatory synapse within a certain time window (e.g., −20 ps ~30 ps), the inhibitory still can veto the rest of the excitatory synapses. However, when the delay exceeds 30 ps, the shunting inhibitory synapse can no longer veto the excitatory potential in time, hence the neuron starts firing spikes [6].

Next, using the same dendritic branch circuit containing inhibitory synapse AP_{12}, figure 7.6 shows simulation results for the neuron's firing state when the inhibitory synapse is activated early or late with respect to the excitatory synapse. The *effective inhibition time window* is defined as that time window during which the inhibition still has effect to veto the excitation even if they are not activated at the same time. This time window is defined as the difference between inhibitory input AP spike's arrival time and the excitatory input AP spike's arrival time, e.g., $t_{AP_I}-t_{AP_E}$. The waveform shown in figure 7.6(a) indicates that when the inhibitory synapse is activated more than 30 ps *before* the excitatory ones, the inhibition is no longer effective, hence the neuron starts firing. A similar result is observed when the inhibitory synapse is activated 40 ps or more *after* the excitatory synapses.

7.3.2 Spatiotemporal signal processing in passive dendrites

In this section, we discuss how the spatio-temporal information encoded in the synaptic activation patterns (*where* the synapses are located and *when* they are activated) can shape the dendritic potential and affect the final spike response of the neuron for passive dendrites, dendrites whose collective membrane potentials are the sum of the PSPs, but no greater. Active dendrites that produce superlinear membrane potentials will be presented later, in chapter 8. The mechanisms are different in active dendrites, with ion channels opening to introduce extra charges in active dendrites. We reference once again the excitatory synapses, and how the PSPs are modulated in figure 6.5.

Since signals can forward-propagate as well as backward-propagate in the dendrites, we model the bi-directional propagation using pass transistors in the diffuser network shown in figure 7.7(a). The passive property of the dendrite contributes to attenuation in amplitude of the PSP, spread in width, and delay in time of the membrane potential at different distances along the dendrite toward the soma. The half-width and rise time of the excitatory postsynaptic potential (EPSP) is

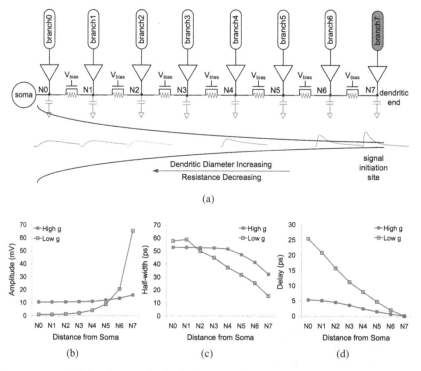

Figure 7.7. Characterized signal attenuation in the dendrite cable circuit simulation. (a) Dendrite model setup with Branch7 activated. Two sets of transistors are used to model high conductance (low impedance) and low conductance (high impedance). (b) Peak amplitude of V_{DEND} at each node along the dendrite. (c) Half-width of V_{DEND} increases as it travels towards the soma. (d) Delay at each node from the time Branch7 is activated until the signal reaches the specific node along the dendrite [6].

controlled by the voltage *DendDia* (modeling the dendritic diameter), as shown in figure 6.5. We increase *DendDia* to model the increasing dendritic diameter towards the soma. In biological pyramidal neurons, the unitary *EPSP* on the proximal site has less half-width and rise time than the one on the distal site [1]. The characterization of *EPSP* is shown in figure 6.5(b). By changing the control voltage at *DendDia* in the circuit, we plot the two parameters, half-width and rise time, of the *EPSP* with respect to the distance of the synapse from the soma. Figure 7.7(b), (c), and (d) demonstrate how the dendritic membrane potential signal, V_{DEND}, travels from the dendritic end of the neuron towards the soma in terms of the following parameters, *amplitude*, *half-width*, and *delay* under two conditions: high conductance and low conductance in dendrites. Figure 7.8(a) demonstrates how a signal

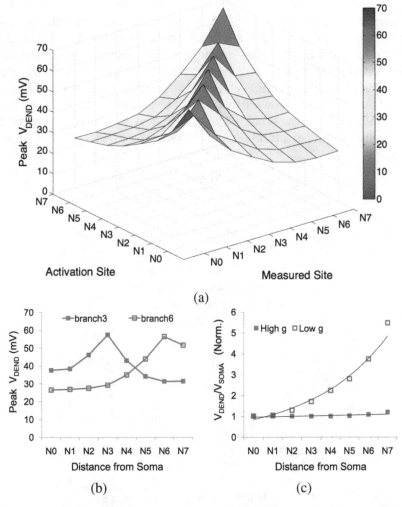

(a)

(b)   (c)

Figure 7.8. Potential attenuation in the dendritic cable circuit. (a) Peak of the dendritic potential (V_{DEND}) at different distances from the soma under different activation sites [6]. (b) Peak V_{DEND} under specific branch activation. (c) Ratio of the peak of V_{DEND} to the peak of V_{SOMA} as a function of the activation site and the conductance of the dendritic cable [6].

attenuates from its activation site as it moves in two opposite directions, since the cable we implemented is a two-directional diffuser circuit [6]. Figure 7.8(b) shows the peak dendritic potential (V_{DEND}) when either Branch3 or Branch6 is activated. Figure 7.8(c) represents the ratio of the peak dendritic potential (V_{DEND}) to the peak somatic potential (V_{SOMA}) as a function of the activation site under high and low conductive (g) dendritic cable configurations.

Next, we show how to include the passive nonlinear phenomenon that occurs when adjacent synapses are activated at once, causing the dendritic potential to saturate at a certain level and hence the actual potential becomes less than the ideal arithmetic summation. This is caused by the reduction in the driving force of synaptic current when multiple synapses are stimulated. In Hsu's circuit, this nonlinear saturation effect is embedded in her average-amplify summation circuit, in a way such that, when more synapses are activated, the current is reduced because of the increase of resistance. In biological neurons, thicker dendrites tend to have lower resistance and therefore smaller depolarization compared to thinner dendrites under the same amount of current injection. Therefore, we compare the nonlinear saturation effect in these two cases: one with a thick dendrite and another with a thin dendrite. The measured overall V_{DEND} of Hsu's circuit simulation compared to its linear arithmetic value is shown figure 7.9. The saturation factor (%) is calculated using equation (7.3) and is tabulated in table 7.1 as a function of the number of activated synapses. The saturation factor increases as the number of synapses increases.

$$\text{Saturation factor} = \frac{\text{Measured} - \text{Arithmetic}}{\text{Arithmetic}} \qquad (7.3)$$

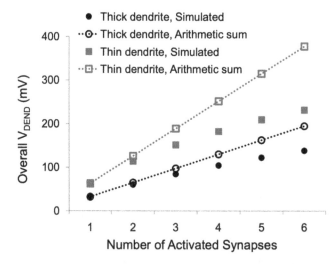

Figure 7.9. Saturation effect in passive dendrite. Black data-points represent thick dendrite (low resistance). Blue data-points represent thin dendrite (high resistance) [6].

Table 7.1. Nonlinear saturation factor for thick and thin dendrites. Reproduced from [6].

	Number of activated synapses				
	2	3	4	5	6
Thick dendrite	−7%	−13%	−20%	−25%	−29%
Thin dendrite	−9%	−20%	−28%	−33%	−39%

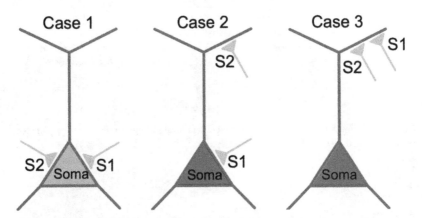

Figure 7.10. Synaptic spatial configuration for temporal integration experiment [6].

7.3.3 Temporal integration window effect

Next Hsu shows a passive dendrite model for different spatial and temporal configurations to demonstrate the temporal integration window effect. Figure 7.10 illustrates three synaptic spatial configurations: *Case 1*, two synapses are located at the soma, *Case 2*, one is located at the soma and the other at the distal dendrite, and *Case 3*, both are located at the distal dendrite. In these three cases, the two synapses are activated Δt time apart, ranging from 0 ps to 80 ps in a step size of 5 ps.

Case 1 simulation demonstrates that the peak somatic depolarization happens when both synapses are activated synchronously, $\Delta t = 0$, shown in figure 7.11. When the two synapses are activated more than 80 ps apart, there is no temporal summation observed. *Case 2* simulation demonstrates that the peak somatic depolarization happens when *S2* is activated 20 ps before *S1* (solid line: $t_{S2} - t_{S1} = -20$), shown in figure 7.12(a). However, when the sequence of activation is reversed, a smaller response is observed instead (dotted line: $t_{S2} - t_{S1} = 20$), since PSP_{S2} sums with attenuated PSP_{S1}. However, when we increase the activation time delay to 40 ps, the maximum somatic potential decreases, as shown in figure 7.12(b).

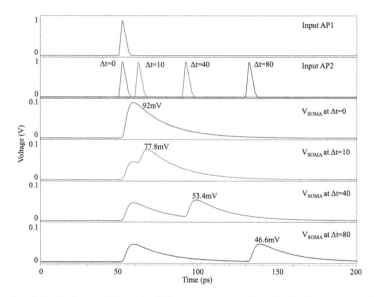

Figure 7.11. *Case 1* simulation result from the different temporal settings [6]. Both synapses are located at the soma and are activated Δ*t* = 0, 10, 40, and 80 ps apart.

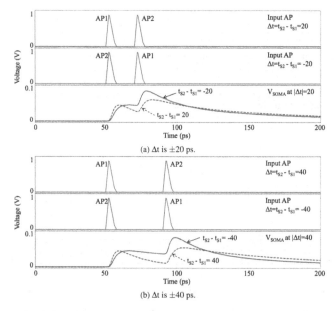

Figure 7.12. *Case 2* simulation result from the different temporal settings. Synapse S1 is located at the soma and synapse S2 is located at the distal dendrite. (a) The first two panels show that S2 is activated 20 ps *after* and *before* S1, respectively. The third panel shows the comparison between the two activation sequences given the two synapses are activated 20 ps apart. The solid trace (S2 *after* S1) and the dashed trace (S2 *before* S1) peak at different levels and times. (b) The same experiments are repeated when the activation time of S1 and S2 are 40 ps apart [6].

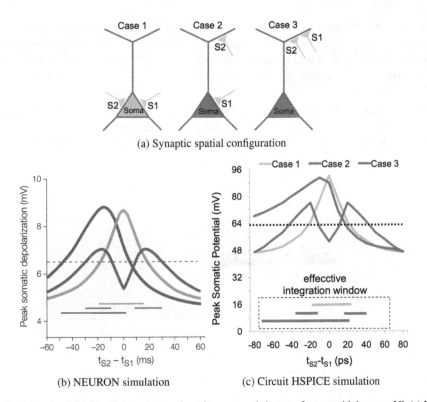

(a) Synaptic spatial configuration

(b) NEURON simulation

(c) Circuit HSPICE simulation

Figure 7.13. Passive dendritic effect on integration of two synaptic inputs of a pyramidal neuron [6]. (a) Model neuron setup for different synaptic activation sites. (b) NEURON simulation result from [8]. (c) Circuit simulation result. This experiment demonstrates a similar increasing temporal integration window for coincident inputs from distal and proximal synapses (red trace). Different color traces represent the three synaptic spatial configurations illustrated in (a). The color bars below the curves represent the integration time window for spike (AP) initiation.

Compared to the NEURON simulation of biological neurons from [8] shown in figure 7.13(b), the BioRC circuit simulation produces similar results in terms of the integration time window for spike initiation shown in figure 7.13(c). When the two synaptic activation sites vary, their effective temporal integration windows change accordingly. We observe that the temporal integration window is the largest when coincident inputs occur, i.e. synapses on soma and distal dendrite are activated (*Case 2*). In the scenario when both synapses are located in the distal dendrite, because small dendritic branch diameter results in large depolarization, when S1 and S2 are activated synchronously (less than 20 ps in the BioRC implementation) the saturation effect from co-activated inputs leads to a lower somatic potential (*Case 3*). The threshold to initiate an AP in Hsu's carbon nanotube circuit is approximately 163 mV (indicated by the dashed line in figure 7.13(c)).

7.3.4 Temporal summation for sequence detection

'Directional selectivity' is another phenomenon as a result of temporal summation observed in many neurons in the mammalian cortex. Direction-selective neurons found in many organisms from the fly's eyes to the mammalian cortex respond to stimuli motion in a preferred direction but not in the opposite direction (figure 7.14(a)) [7]. A directional-selective neuromorphic circuit for the retina based on reciprocal synapses in starburst amacrine cells has also been reported in the BioRC group [3].

This phenomenon can be explained with the RC filtering property in the dendrites. When the proximal synapse (closer to the soma) is activated first, the proximal PSP decays to a lower potential by the time the filtered distal PSP (further

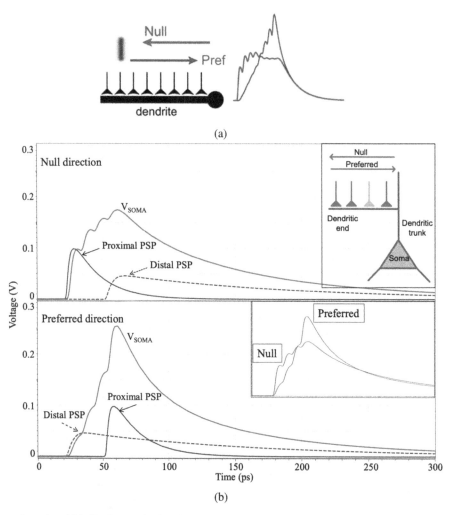

Figure 7.14. Dendritic filtering mechanism for directional selectivity. (a) When the visual stimulus moves in the preferred direction, from the left to the right, due to temporal summation, a larger voltage response is observed [6]. In contrast, when the stimulus is moving in the null direction, a smaller response is observed. Figure from London and Häusser [7]. (b) The simulation result of the activation on four synapses in different directions. The top inset represents the neuron setup used in this simulation. The bottom inset shows the comparison of the two V_{SOMA} at null and preferred directions, respectively.

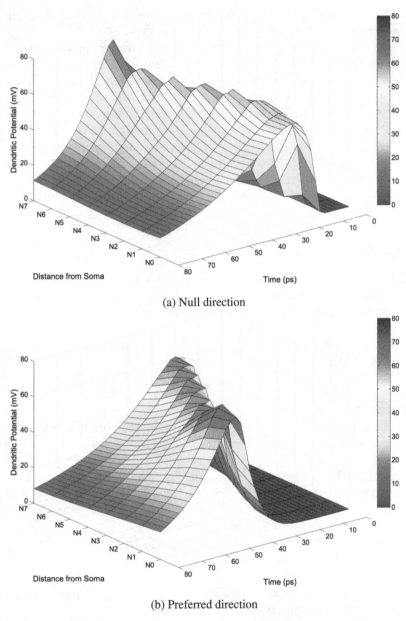

(a) Null direction

(b) Preferred direction

Figure 7.15. Temporal summation for direction selectivity. (a) Sequence Branch0 to Branch7 results in lower potential at the soma. (b) Sequence Branch7 to Branch0 results in higher potential because the lingering decayed distal PSP sums with proximal PSP [6].

away from the soma) arrives. Therefore, the overall somatic potential, V_{SOMA}, is smaller than the sum of the peak of proximal PSP and distal PSP. On the other hand, when the distal synapse is activated before the proximal one, the distal PSP is filtered (attenuated but widened) when it travels towards the soma. This delayed PSP gives time for the proximal inputs to sum temporally, thus the overall V_{SOMA} is larger compared to the null direction case mentioned earlier.

The simulation results of Hsu's implementation for these two directions are shown in figure 7.14(b) in which the top panel demonstrates synaptic activation in the null direction and the bottom panel demonstrates synaptic activation in the preferred direction. In the null direction, the proximal PSP (solid line) decays severely by the time the distal PSP (dotted line) is activated. In the preferred direction, the distal PSP is widened, which gives time for the proximal PSP to sum temporally. Therefore the overall V_{SOMA} results in a higher potential level.

We further demonstrate this directional selectivity effect with the dendrite RC model shown in figure 7.7(a). The seven branches are activated 5 ps apart in the null direction (figure 7.15(a)) and in the reverse direction (preferred direction, figure 7.15(b)).

7.4 Chapter summary

This chapter covered Elias' and Hsu's circuits performing passive dendritic computations. Elias' circuits are presented to give a historical perspective, and Hsu's circuits highlight the current BioRC approach to passive dendritic computations.

The next chapter focuses on active dendritic circuits, circuits that implement superlinear dendritic mechanisms.

7.5 Exercises

1. What circuit elements does Elias use to represent dendritic computations?
2. How does Elias create attenuation (lowering of voltage) in his dendritic arbor?
3. An inhibitory synapse on one dendritic branch can keep any of the excitatory synapses on that dendritic branch from having an effect on the neuron. Draw a picture of the branch and a small part of the dendritic trunk, with labels to show the location of the inhibitory synapse.
4. Elias' dendritic model (mark all correct answers):
   (a) Contains dendritic spiking;
   (b) Models dendritic plasticity;
   (c) Is a basic model of signal attenuation and spreading using resistance and capacitance;
   (d) Provides different membrane potentials at the soma depending on where the active synapses are placed on the dendrites

References

[1] Behabadi B F *et al* 2012 Location-dependent excitatory synaptic interactions in pyramidal neuron dendrites *PLoS Comput. Biol.* **8** e1002599
[2] Chaoui H 1995 CMOS analogue adder *Electron. Lett.* **31** 180–1

[3] Parker A C, Tseng K-C and Joshi J 2011 A directionally-selective neuromorphic circuit based on reciprocal synapses in Starburst Amacrine Cells *Engineering in Medicine and Biology Society, EMBC, 2011 Annual Int. Conf. IEEE* 5674–7

[4] Elias J, Chu H and Meshreki S 1992 Silicon implementation of an artificial dendritic tree *Proc. Int. Joint Conf. Neural Networks IEEE* 1 (Baltimore, MD: IEEE) 154–9

[5] Elias J G 1993 Silicon dendritic trees *Neural Comput.* **5** 648–64

[6] Hsu C-C 2014 Dendritic computation and plasticity in neuromorphic circuits *PhD Thesis* University of Southern California

[7] London M and Häusser M 2005 Dendritic computation *Annu. Rev. Neurosci.* **28** 503–32

[8] Migliore M and Shepherd G M 2002 Emerging rules for the distributions of active dendritic conductances *Nat. Rev. Neurosci.* **3** 362–70

[9] Zhou X *et al* 2013 Biomimetic non-linear CMOS adder for neuromorphic circuits *2013 6th Int. IEMBS Conf. on Neural Engineering (NER) IEEE* (Piscataway, NJ: IEEE) 876–9

IOP Publishing

Neuromorphic Circuits
A constructive approach
Alice C Parker and Rick Cattell

Chapter 8

Dendritic spiking and dendritic plasticity

Chih-Chieh Hsu and Alice C Parker

Chapter 8 covers dendritic plasticity, with an emphasis on dendritic spiking involving active dendrites. The focus of the chapter is on Hsu's dendritic spiking research, including spatio-temporal processing, precise action potential (AP) spike timing, and regulation of dendritic excitability (plasticity). A short section covers others' contributions. A section on border ownership neurons that uses dendritic computations is covered in chapter 16.

8.1 Introduction

As the text discussed before in chapter 1, biological neurons perform nonlinear computations in their dendritic arbors, and the dendritic computations vary depending on the situation, called *dendritic plasticity*. The *active* nonlinear computations are sometimes referred to as *dendritic spikes*. The bulk of this chapter covers dendritic spiking and dendritic plasticity as found in [8]. This chapter also covers several active dendrite circuits by other researchers.

In many neuroscience studies, the pyramidal neuron has been modeled using two-stage integration [16] with dendritic branch computations as the first state, and summation of dendritic branches as the second state; hence the text adopts this method and implements the dendritic arbor with a similar strategy. Figure 8.1 shows a pyramidal neuron cartoon (left), and its counterpart in circuit block diagram abstraction (right). The first stage, STAGE I (red Σ circle), carries out a 'within-branch' nonlinear active computation that has the capability to create a dendritic spike, as described more in section 8.2. Not shown in this figure are the positions of individual synapses that affect how the computation is performed, particularly for shunting inhibitory synapses. The second stage, STAGE II (blue Σ circle), performs 'among-branches' nonlinear integration based on their individual distances to the soma, because the locality of the branch influences its impact at the summation, again not shown in this cartoon. In this section, we focus on the STAGE II nonlinear

doi:10.1088/978-0-7503-5097-6ch8

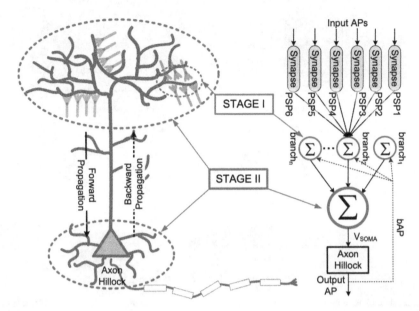

Figure 8.1. A pyramidal neuron cartoon (left) and its circuit implementation abstract (right) in two-stage representation [8].

location-dependent integration and we will discuss the STAGE I nonlinear regenerative spiking mechanism in the following section. The directions of forward propagation and backward propagation are shown in the figure.

A template of a dendrite is shown in figure 8.2 (a). In this template, the dendrite contains n segments with each equivalent to a 20 μm long dendrite. The resistance of each dendritic segment depends on the diameter of the dendrite; the thinner the dendrite, the higher the resistance. A hypothetical neuron shown in figure 8.2 (b), is configured to have two basal dendrites and two main apical dendrites each of which has branching nodes. Table 8.1 summarizes the parameters of the neural signals, AP and EPSP (excitatory postsynaptic potential), the dendritic cable we use in Hsu's carbon nanotube (CNT) circuit simulation and their biological counterparts. For voltage-related parameters, the scaling factor is approximately 8 compared to biological counterparts, with circuit voltages 8 times larger than biological voltages. For time-related parameters, the scaling factor is on the order of magnitude of 10^8, where biological signals are 10^8 times slower. Note that when the number of synapses per neuron and fan out of axons is scaled up to biological size, timing of electronic circuits will decrease significantly due to loading.

8.1.1 Excitation and inhibition integration

In the cortex, there are about 80% excitatory synapses and 20% inhibitory synapses. Inhibitory synapses play an important role in neuronal behavior. For example, the local inhibitory interneuron circuit controls the development of columnar architecture during a critical period in the primary visual cortex [7]. As in biological neurons,

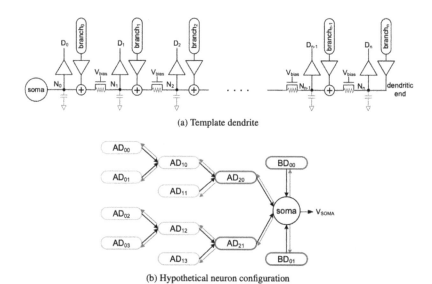

(a) Template dendrite

(b) Hypothetical neuron configuration

Figure 8.2. Template dendrite and neuron configuration [8]. (a) Template dendrite implementation for STAGE II integration. Each branch, e.g., Branch0, Branch1, ..., Branch$n$ represents STAGE I integration. (b) A hypothetical neuron configuration with two main apical dendrites and two main basal dendrites. AD refers to apical dendrites and BD to basal dendrites. Dark blue represents a strong branch and light blue represents a weak branch. Forward propagation is shown with black arrows and backward propagation with red arrows.

Table 8.1. Biological and CNT circuit parameters of neural signals and dendritic cable. Reproduced from [8].

Neural signals	Biological	CNT circuit
AP amplitude	110 mV	900 mV
AP half-width	0.5 ms	5 ps
EPSP amplitude	2.2–6.6 mV	18–24 mV
EPSP tail duration	6–10 ms	60–100 ps
Dendritic cable	Biological	CNT circuit
Dendrite length	20 μm	1 segment (node)
Space constant (λ)	1 mm	50 nodes
Time constant (τ_m)	10 ms	100 ps

there are two types of inhibition: hyperpolarizing inhibition and shunting inhibition. Hyperpolarizing inhibition generates a hyperpolarizing (opposite to depolarizing) potential, or in other words, a relatively negative potential to the resting potential. Shunting inhibition vetoes any *up-stream* excitatory synapses, however, has no effect on *downstream* excitatory synapses. Further demonstration of these two types of inhibition in Hsu's neurons are discussed in the following sections.

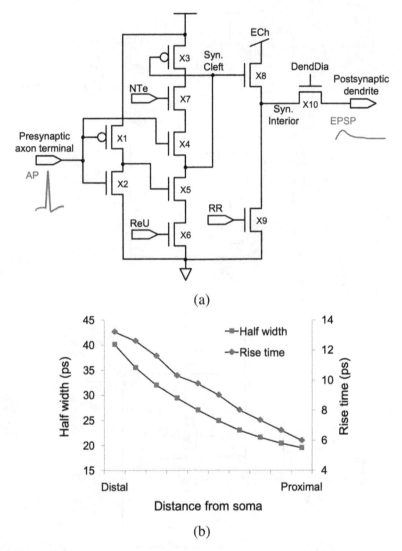

(a)

(b)

Figure 8.3. (a) A biomimetic excitatory synapse can be modulated by different neural mechanisms such as neurotransmitter concentration, reuptake, and ion pump. (b) EPSP half-width and rise time characterization. Distance from soma: Distal to proximal is modeled by *DendDia* control voltage [8].

The biomimetic synapses used in Hsu's dendritic arbor for various simulation experiments are shown in figures 8.3 and 8.4. They are modified versions from previous BioRC research [6] and [11]. In the synapse, when input AP comes in, the voltage at *Syn. Cleft* (synaptic cleft) increases, limited by the transistors X3 and *NTe* which model the release level of the excitatory neurotransmitters. The neurotransmitters then will be cleared from the synaptic cleft by the reuptake mechanism controlled by another input *ReU*. The voltage increase at *Syn. Cleft* will temporarily pull up the voltage at *Syn. Interior* close to the potential at *ECh*

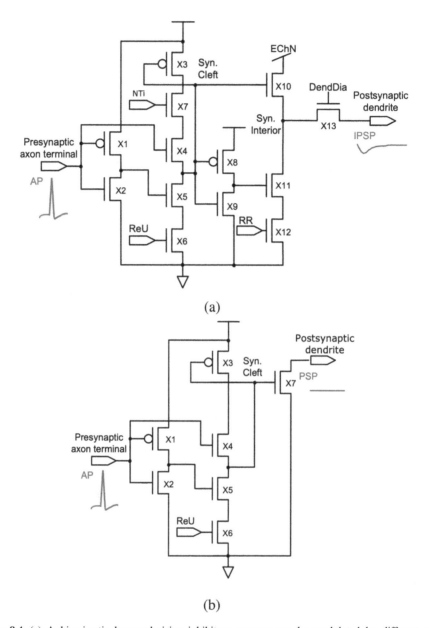

(a)

(b)

Figure 8.4. (a) A biomimetic hyperpolarizing inhibitory synapse can be modulated by different neural mechanisms such as neurotransmitter concentration, reuptake, and ion pump. (b) A biomimetic shunting inhibitory synapse is active when *AP* is asserted and pulls down the potential at postsynaptic dendrite to ground (circuit resting potential) [8].

which models the electromotive force. *Syn. Interior* is then pulled down to resting potential by the transistor X10. The timing of the falling waveform is controlled by *RR* (modeling the resting return); that is when *RR* increases, the EPSP falls to resting potential faster. Voltage at *Syn. Interior* is transferred to the postsynaptic dendrite by the transistor X11. The half-width and rise time of the EPSP is controlled by the voltage *DendDia* (modeling the dendritic diameter). We increase *DendDia* to model the increasing dendritic diameter towards the soma. In biological pyramidal neurons, the unitary EPSP on the *proximal* site has smaller half-width and rise time than the one on the *distal* site [3]. The characterization of EPSP is shown in figure 8.3(b). By changing the control voltage at *DendDia* in the circuit, we plot the two parameters, half-width and rise time, of the EPSP with respect to the distance from the soma. The hyperpolarizing inhibitory synapse (shown in figure 8.4(a)) works in a similar way except the electromotive force is now a negative potential (figure 8.5). The circuit representation of the shunting inhibitory synapse is shown in figure 8.4(b).

8.2 Active dendrites: dendritic spiking

First, this section discusses the neuromorphic circuits to implement a dendritic branch incorporating the local dendritic spiking mechanism with modifiable excitability. Spatio-temporal synaptic information processing in active dendrites follows. This section then shows results of an experiment to demonstrate the significance of incorporating dendritic spikes in the neuromorphic implementation for precise and reliable axonal spike timing enhancement.

After the discussion of local dendritic spiking effect on neuronal precise spike timing, an example demonstrates that the excitability of a dendritic branch is activity-dependent, and hence can be modulated by the spatio-temporal synaptic activation pattern. Two plasticity mechanisms are modeled in Hsu's neuromorphic circuit: short-term *local and global reset* on dendritic spikes and long-term *branch strength potentiation*.

The majority of cortical neurons (i.e., layer V pyramidal neurons) have long and broad dendritic structures that extend into all layers in neocortex. Distal inputs would attenuate greatly when they arrive at the soma if the dendrite were purely passive. Many studies have shown that when the distal inputs accumulate enough potential, the active conductances in the dendrites can amplify PSP and evoke a local dendritic spike that propagates more effectively than PSP alone [1, 12, 15]. In this section, we present a hypothetical neuron with a dendritic arbor that incorporates spiking behavior (primarily Na^+ spikes and Ca^{2+} spikes) along with the other mechanisms (e.g., synaptic integration in dendrites) mentioned in the previous chapter. Furthermore, the excitability of the dendrite can be up-regulated or down-regulated by different combinations of the neuron's spiking activities globally (from AP spike) or locally (from dendritic spike).

8.2.1 Neuromorphic circuit implementation

As discussed in chapter 4 (and shown later in this chapter in figure 8.28), we implement Hsu's neuron in a two-stage fashion, where *STAGE I* represents the local regenerative spiking mechanism within a dendritic branch and *STAGE II* represents the location-dependent integration among multiple branches. Therefore, each

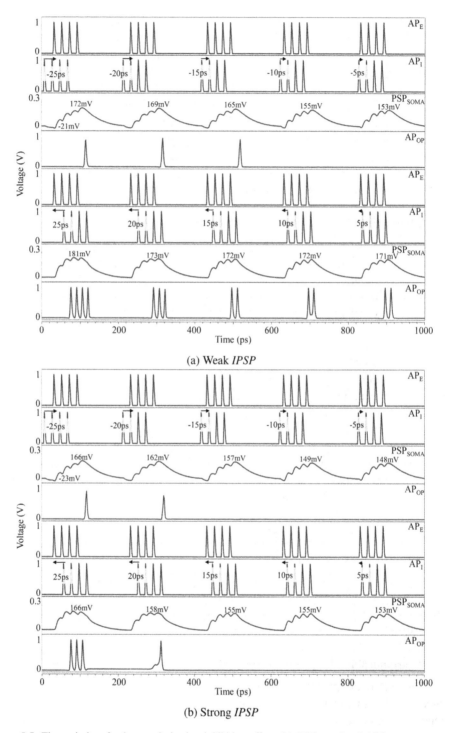

(a) Weak *IPSP*

(b) Strong *IPSP*

Figure 8.5. Time window for hyperpolarization inhibition effect. (a) With weaker Inhibitory postsynaptic potential (IPSP) the effective inhibition window is smaller, −10 ps ∼ 0 ps. (b) With stronger *IPSP* the effective inhibition window is larger, −15 ps ∼ 15 ps [8].

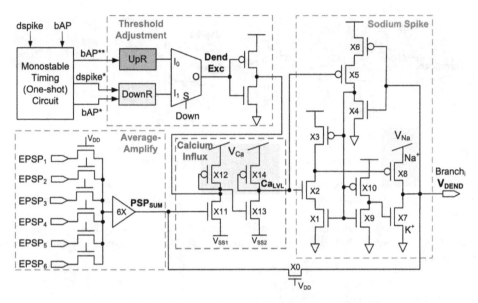

Figure 8.6. Dendritic branch module circuit implementation [8].

dendritic branch serves as an individual computational unit in Hsu's hypothetical pyramidal neuron implementation shown in figure 8.6. The active dendritic module is composed of several circuit blocks: *Average-Amplify*, *Threshold Adjustment*, *Calcium Influx*, and *Sodium Spike*.

The **Average-Amplify** section integrates six spatially-clustered PSPs that can arrive at different times on the same dendritic branch to produce an overall PSP, PSP_{SUM}. The **Threshold Adjustment** section modulates the dendritic excitability, i.e., to increase or decrease the threshold of spike initiation. The **Calcium Influx** section emulates the large inward current through the voltage-gated calcium channel (VGCC) when enough depolarization is reached at the dendritic membrane (as PSP_{SUM}). When sufficient potential is accumulated at Ca_{LVL}, a sodium spike is triggered. The **Sodium Spike** section undergoes a series of activation and inactivation of Na^+ and K^+ channels that is similar to the generation of an AP. However, since the Na^+ channel concentration in the dendrite is lower than that in the axon hillock, V_{Na} instead of V_{DD} is used to limit the overall Na^+ conductance. Transistor X0 is used to pass PSP_{SUM} if this potential is below the threshold to initiate a dendritic spike. Further discussion of each section follows.

8.2.1.1 The monostable timing circuit
Using a one-shot (monostable multivibrator) circuit (as described in section 3.2.2) in the dendritic branch module, changing the spiking threshold, we can generate different timings of control signals that either up-regulate or down-regulate dendritic excitability such as bAP^{**}, bAP^*, and $dspike^*$ used in the **Threshold Adjustment** circuit.

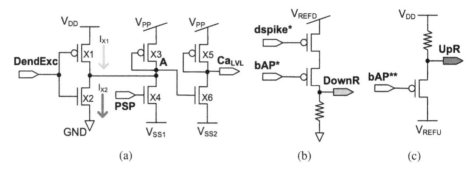

Figure 8.7. Modifiable dendritic spike threshold (a) This transistor-level circuit changes the threshold for dendritic spike initiation. Input *DendExc* modulates whether Ca_{LVL} is above or below the threshold of the spiking circuit. (b) Circuit implementation down-regulates the dendritic excitability. When both *dspike** and *bAP** are zero (no activity), *DendExc* is biased at $\frac{V_{DD}}{2}$ (no modulation on the excitability). (c) Up-regulation circuit implementation. *bAP* ** is a longer time constant than *bAP** to model the long-term branch potentiation [8].

8.2.1.2 Threshold Adjustment

The *Threshold Adjustment* circuit used to modulate the excitability (or threshold to spike) of a dendritic branch is shown in figure 8.7(a). The signal *DendExc* represents the dendritic excitability and is controlled by circuitry that modulates the threshold to spike in a dendrite. It can cause the output Ca_{LVL} to increase or decrease. The voltage at *DendExc* determines the amount of current drawn into node *A* from V_{DD} through X1 and the amount of current drawn out of node *A* to *GND* through X2. When the current injected into node *A* through X1 is greater than the current drawn from node *A* through X2, the current flowing through X3 decreases, hence the voltage at node *A* increases and voltage at Ca_{LVL} decreases. This will inactivate the spiking circuit and require a larger voltage on PSP to compensate for the elevated threshold. In contrast, when the current injected into node *A* through X1 is less than the current drawn from node *A* through X2, the current flowing through X3 increases, the resulting voltage at node *A* drops and voltage at Ca_{LVL} rises. This will activate the spiking circuit even if the voltage on *PSP* does not exceed the original threshold. By plugging in other circuits shown in figure 8.7(b) and (c) before this module to control the voltage at *DendExc*, we can implement *down-regulation* and *up-regulation* of the dendritic excitability to induce dendritic plasticity.

8.2.1.3 Calcium Influx and Sodium Spike

The *Calcium Influx* circuit (shown in figure 8.6) models the opening of the voltage-gated calcium channel by a sufficient amount of depolarization on the dendritic membrane. The amount of calcium influx can be controlled by the voltage source, V_{Ca}, that can be set externally to this circuit. The voltage-gated calcium channel is modeled by the P-type transistors (X12, X14) to draw current from the voltage source. When enough potential is accumulated at Ca_{LVL}, it triggers the *Sodium Spike* circuit. When Ca_{LVL} reaches the spike threshold, it turns on Na^+-activation segment (modeled by X1, X2) that later activates Na^+ channels (modeled by X8) rapidly.

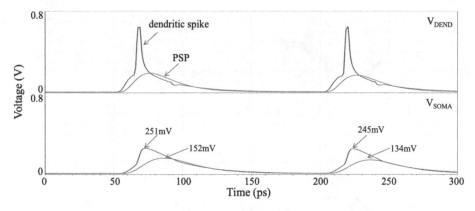

Figure 8.8. Comparison between dendritic spike and PSP at the distal dendrite and their attenuated potential at the soma. V_{DEND} represents dendritic potential and V_{SOMA} represents somatic potential. The attenuated dendritic spike has larger amplitude, 251 mV and 245 mV, compared to the attenuated PSP, 152 mV and 134 mV [8].

After some delay (X4) Na$^+$-inactivation (X3) then turns off Na$^+$ channels. This portrays the gradual inactivation of Na$^+$ channels when the membrane potential reaches a depolarizing state. K$^+$-activation (X10), after some more delay (X4), turns on K$^+$ channels (X7). Transistor X10 is designed to be more resistive than X3 by making the channel longer or narrower in order to mimic the biological behavior such that K$^+$-activation occurs a short period of time after Na$^+$-inactivation begins. K$^+$-inactivation (X9) turns off K$^+$ channels after a longer delay (X5, X6). Figure 8.8 shows that both dendritic spike and PSP dampen when traveling from the distal dendritic site (upper trace) to the soma (lower trace). However, the attenuated dendritic spike still has larger amplitude compared to the attenuated PSP at the soma. Therefore, the dendritic spikes forward propagate more effectively than PSP alone.

8.2.2 Spatio-temporal processing in active dendrites

In biological neurons, dendritic spikes are a result of coincident clustered synaptic activation on the same dendritic branch. Losonczy *et al* found that dendritic spikes occurred during co-activation of 20 synapses within 6 ms, within 20 μm of a dendrite [13]. Two parameters were used to measure the correlation between the spatio-temporal pattern and dendritic spike: (1) *ISI*, inter-stimuli interval, which represents the inputs' temporal synchronization, and (2) *n*, number of activated synapses, which represents the inputs' spatial clustering. Hsu simplified her dendritic arbor to have six synapses on each branch and adjusted the synaptic intensity to achieve the desired synaptic potential. For example, in order to initiate a dendritic spike, a threshold of approximately 18% of AP amplitude potential needs to be reached. Since she has designed six synapses per branch, each unitary EPSP should be greater than 3% of AP amplitude in order to produce a dendritic spike when all synapses are excited.

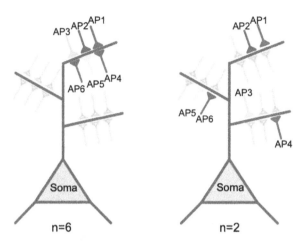

Figure 8.9. Spatial configuration. Spatially-clustered scenario: six excitatory synapses on one dendritic branch ($n = 6$, left). Spatially-distributed scenario: two excitatory synapses on each dendritic branch ($n = 2$, right) [8].

Hsu performed simulations to demonstrate that it is critical to have both temporally and spatially-clustered inputs to initiate a dendritic spike in her prototypical dendritic arbor. The spatial configurations of the neuron used for experimenting with the input pattern to a dendritic spike are illustrated in figure 8.9, where for simplicity only two cases ($n = 2$ and 6) are shown. A set of synaptic intensities that produce a unitary EPSP ranging from 3% to 6% of AP amplitude is applied to study the relationship between inputs' spatio-temporal patterns and the initiation of a local dendritic spike.

We summarize four spatio-temporal patterns of synaptic input activation: (a) spatio-temporal clustered, (b) spatially-clustered and temporally-distributed, (c) spatially-distributed and temporally-clustered, and (d) spatio-temporal distributed in figure 8.10. In the first two experiments, we activated six synapses ($n = 6$) on one dendritic branch and applied different inter-stimulus intervals to those synapses ($ISI = 2$ and 10). It is observed that if the synaptic activation is not in synchrony, clustered synapses would not generate the local dendritic spike shown in figure 8.10(a) and (b). In the other two experiments, we activated only two synapses ($n = 2$) on one dendritic branch and applied different inter-stimulus intervals to those synapses ($ISI = 2$ and 10). It is observed that even if synaptic activation is in synchrony, distributed synapses would not accumulate enough potential to generate a local dendritic spike, as shown in figure 8.10(c) and (d).

We further characterize the overall PSP on a single dendritic branch (shown in figure 8.11) and the initiation of a dendritic spike (shown in figure 8.12) based upon input spatio-temporal settings (n and ISI), synaptic intensity (controlled by the parameter NTe), and dendritic diameter (controlled by the parameter $DendDia$). Figure 8.13 demonstrates that as the synaptic intensity increases and dendritic diameter decreases, fewer number of synapses is required to initiate dendritic spikes. Figure 8.14 demonstrates that as the synaptic intensity decreases, higher input synchronization level is required to initiate dendritic spikes.

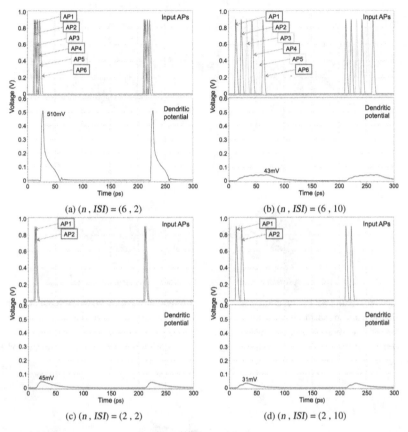

Figure 8.10. Synaptic spatio-temporal information encoded in active dendrite. The generation of dendritic spike requires both spatially-clustered and temporally-synchronized synaptic activation. (a) spatially-clustered, temporally-clustered. (b) spatially-clustered, temporally-distributed. (c) spatially-distributed, temporally-clustered. (d) spatially-distributed, temporally-distributed [8].

8.3 Dendritic spike-enhanced precise AP spike timing

In this section, we demonstrate that Hsu's neuron can detect coincident spatio-temporal input, and transform this neural information into a precisely-timed output spike, i.e., AP. The temporal structure of spike trains carries additional information beyond the mean firing rate in the cortical neurons. In artificial neurons the precision of these spikes is crucial, especially in large-scale neuromorphic networks, because the imprecision can accumulate between cascaded neurons and eventually can cause the neurons to fail to spike. We also demonstrate that dendritic spikes are key to enhancing precisely-timed input–output transformation within an individual neuron; without active dendritic modeling it would require more neurons to achieve the same level of precision. We also demonstrate that without active dendritic modeling, the neuron has a higher failure rate to produce output spike when there exists input jitter. Hsu's simulation results show reliable firing and improved precision of output

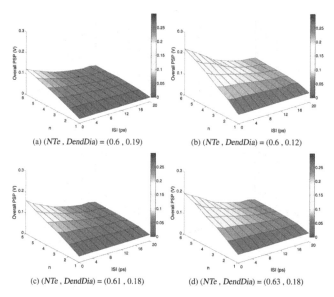

Figure 8.11. The overall PSP is a function of synaptic spatio-temporal setting under different configurations of synaptic intensity and dendritic morphology. Configurations (a) and (b) have the same synaptic intensity, however the dendritic branch in (a) is thicker. Hence, (a) has lower overall PSP. Configurations (c) and (d) have the same dendritic thickness, but synaptic intensity in (c) is lower than (d). Hence, (c) has lower overall PSP than (d) [8].

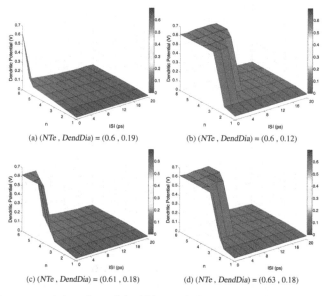

Figure 8.12. Different synaptic intensity and dendritic morphology on dendritic spike initiation. Based on the overall PSP in each configuration (shown in figure 8.11), the dendritic spike is generated once the threshold is reached [8].

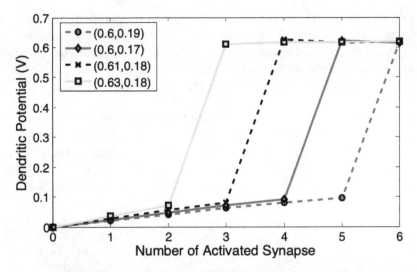

Figure 8.13. Dendritic potential as a function of synaptic spatial configuration (*n*), synaptic intensity (*NTe*), and dendritic morphology (*DendDia*). As the synaptic intensity increases and dendritic diameter decreases, the curve moves to the left indicating that a smaller number of synapses is required to generate dendritic spikes. The parameters shown in the legend are (*NTe*, *DendDia*) [8].)

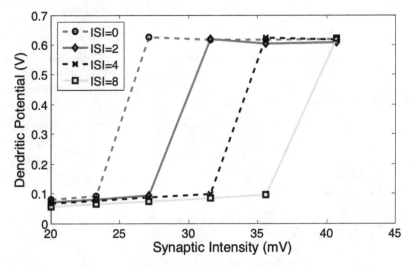

Figure 8.14. Dendritic potential as a function of synaptic temporal configuration (*ISI*), and synaptic intensity. Here the synaptic intensity is represented by the unitary EPSP given certain *NTe*. As the synaptic temporal configuration *ISI* increases, the curve moves to the right indicating that higher synaptic intensity is required to generate dendritic spike. (*n* = 4, *NTe* varies) [8].

spikes when a dendritic spike is initiated, and correlate well with biological experimental results.

Ariav *et al* have shown that synapses innervating onto the same dendritic segment, when activated synchronously, can initiate a dendritic spike which results in a precisely-timed AP at the neuronal output [1]. Figure 8.15 illustrates the experimental results from their study of 20 consecutive trials with the stimuli intensity set at a level such that an AP was generated at $80 \sim 90\%$ rate. The somatic responses were recorded under two different synaptic activation pairing protocols: apical activation with distributed basal EPSPs and apical activation with clustered basal EPSPs.

Hsu performed HSPICE simulations experimenting with different spatio-temporal input patterns to demonstrate her neuron's capability to generate precisely-timed APs, and to study the impact of dendritic spikes on precisely-timed AP. Three neuron configurations, N1, N2, and N3, are shown in figure 8.16. N1 and N2 emulate two neurons with the same dendritic property (active) but different spatial

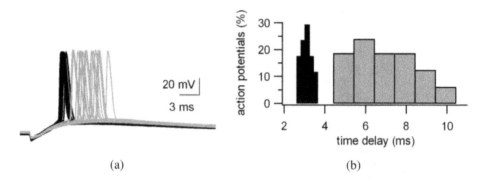

(a)   (b)

Figure 8.15. The temporal jitter and delay of axonal APs from CA1 pyramidal neurons. Cortical neuron response (a) temporally precise and imprecise firing. (b) delay histogram of APs. Black traces are somatic recording with fast Na^+ spikes initiated in the dendrites. Grey traces are somatic recording without Na^+ spikes (from [1], copyright 2003 Society for Neuroscience).

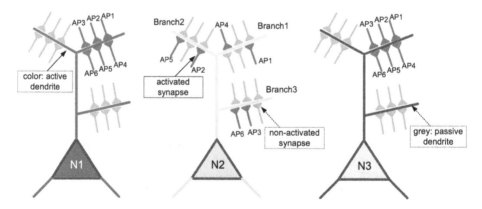

Figure 8.16. Neuron configurations for precisely-timed AP firing demonstration. Neuron configurations: N1 emulates a neuron with active dendrites and clustered activated synapses. N2 emulates a neuron with active dendrites and distributed activated synapses. N3 emulates a neuron with passive dendrites and clustered activated synapses. AP_i represents the input AP impinging on the synapse. Activated synapses are shown in red and non-activated synapses in pink [8].

synaptic distributions, N1 with clustered synapses and N2 with distributed synapses. N1 and N3 emulate two neurons with the same spatial synaptic distribution but different dendritic properties, N1 with active dendrites and N3 with passive dendrites.

The same input profile (temporal pattern and intensity) was applied to a pair of neurons in each of the following experiments. A consecutive 30 trials were carried out with a certain stimulus intensity such that the somatic PSP ranges from −5% to +20% of the threshold in order to initiate an AP. A range of synaptic intensity is chosen because of the stochastic nature of synaptic transmission, ion channel gating and background synaptic noise. We focus on two timing parameters: an output **AP jitter** (i.e., the timing variation among different trials' output APs) and **AP delay** (i.e., the peak-to-peak time between input stimulation and output response).

8.3.1 Effect of dendritic spike on AP spike timing

To investigate the effect of dendritic spikes on AP timing precision, we simulate two neurons with different spatial synaptic distributions: N1 with clustered synapses and N2 with distributed synapses, so that one neuron would generate a dendritic spike and the other would not. The synapses are all activated at the same time in this experiment. It is observed from figure 8.17 that a fast and large transient of dendritic spike (*dspike*) induces an invariant somatic potential in N1 while sub-threshold PSP in N2 induces a varying somatic potential.

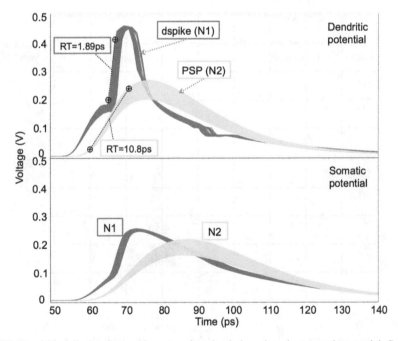

Figure 8.17. Dendritic spike has fast and large transient that induces invariant somatic potential. Comparison of dendritic potential (top) and somatic potential (bottom) measured in N1 and N2 [8].

Furthermore, we examine the relationship between the *dv/dt* (derivative of the rising phase, defined in equation (8.1)) of the somatic potential and the AP delay. It is noted that large *dv/dt* (AVG = 25.29 mV ps^{-1}) results in relatively invariant AP delay (SD = 0.31 ps) in N1 while small *dv/dt* (AVG = 9.57 mV ps^{-1}) causes a wider range of AP delay (SD = 1.27 ps) in N2 (figure 8.18).

$$\frac{dv}{dt} = \frac{80\% V_{\max} - 20\% V_{\max}}{\text{Rise time from 20\% to 80\%}} \tag{8.1}$$

The output response of N1 (with dendritic spike) and N2 (without dendritic spike) from 30 trials is shown in figure 8.19(a). Figure 8.19(b) shows the distributions of the output APs generated in N1 and N2, respectively. It is evident that the neuron with dendritic spikes (N1) can initiate APs more precisely (i.e., with smaller temporal

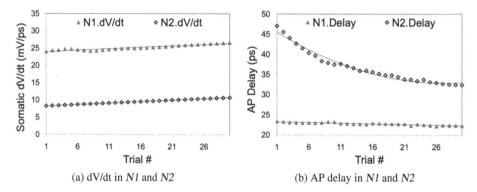

(a) dV/dt in *N1* and *N2*   (b) AP delay in *N1* and *N2*

Figure 8.18. Relationship between somatic *dV/dt* and AP delay in N1 and N2. Larger *dV/dt* leads to invariant and smaller AP delay N1. In contrast, smaller *dV/dt* leads to variant and larger AP delay in N2 [8].

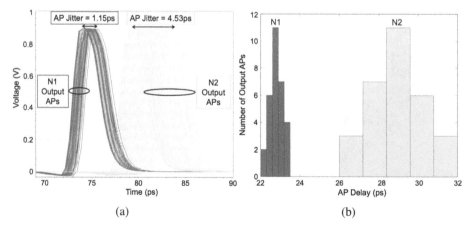

(a)   (b)

Figure 8.19. (a) AP temporal jitter of N1 and N2. (b) Histogram of AP delay of N1 and N2. For N1, the bin size is set to 0.3 ps where for N2, the bin size is set to 1.2 ps. Copyright 2014 IEEE. Reprinted, with permission, from [22].

jitter) than the neuron without dendritic spikes (N2). With a dendritic spike, AP jitter is improved by 74.6% reduction, and AP delay is improved by 21.5% reduction. It is worth mentioning that, in biological data, the temporal jitter for precisely-timed APs is about 30.9% of the AP spike width (810 μs), while in our simulation, it is about 28.75% of the AP spike width (4 ps). The neuron circuits at the transistor level were simulated using HSPICE and the data points (timing of each spike peak) were recorded. These data points then were extrapolated into repetitive trials stimulated at 20 GHz using MATLAB to demonstrate the spiking patterns in raster plots shown in figure 8.20. The data points were selected by a pseudorandom number generator.

Table 8.2 shows the AP temporal jitter and time delay between input and output from the biological recording [1] and from our simulation result. The time delay in biological recording was measured between the stimulation artifact and the peak of the axonal AP. The time delay in circuit simulation was measured from the peak of external input AP to the peak of output AP. The delay between peak of input AP to the peak of resultant EPSP is about 7 ~ 8 ps.

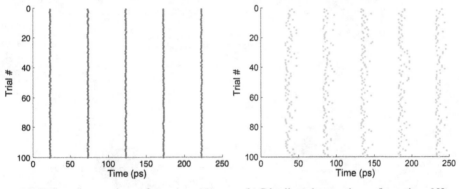

(a) Clustered synaptic configuration: *N1*   (b) Distributed synaptic configuration: *N2*

Figure 8.20. Raster plots for neurons with clustered and distributed spatial configuration. Temporal raster plots for neurons with (a) clustered and (b) distributed synaptic spatial configuration. The initiation of local dendritic spikes in scenario (a) induces more precise and reliable axonal spiking. Copyright 2014 IEEE. Reprinted, with permission, from [22].

Table 8.2. AP spike jitter and delay timing of biological recording and circuit simulation. Reproduced from [8].

	Biological recording		Circuit emulation	
	With *dspike*	No *dspike*	With *dspike*	No *dspike*
AP Jitter	0.25 ms	1.65 ms	1.15 ps	4.53 ps
Normalized (AP width)	0.25	1.65	0.23	0.91
AP Delay	4.39 ms	7.73 ms	22.76 ps	28.98 ps
Normalized (AP width)	4.39	7.73	4.55	5.79

8.3.2 Effect of synaptic activation level on AP spike timing

In this section, we study the scenario when the dendrites are passive (i.e., dendritic spike is absent even with coincident input) in our neuron. The synaptic activation level is represented by the number of the activated synapses which increases from 6 to 12 in N1 (active dendrites) and N3 (passive dendrites). Figure 8.21 illustrates the relative output AP jitter and delay between the two configurations. Table 8.3 summarizes the AP timing parameters used to evaluate the effect of synaptic activation level on AP spike timing. As observed in figure 8.22 these two timing parameters decrease more prominently in N3 (−73.26% in AP jitter and −23.68% in AP delay) compared to those in N1 (−16.38% in AP jitter and −11.64% in AP delay) when the number of activated synapses doubles. From this observation, we conclude that the AP jitter and AP delay become highly dependent on the synaptic activation

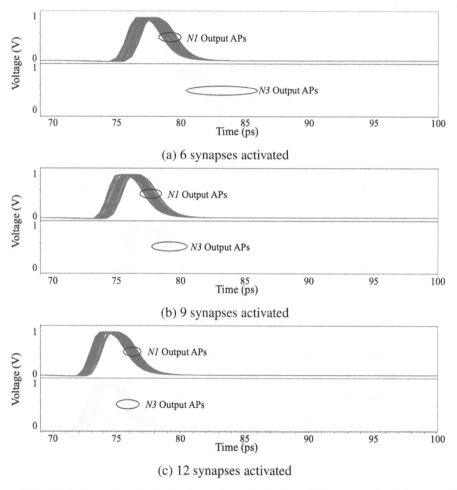

(a) 6 synapses activated

(b) 9 synapses activated

(c) 12 synapses activated

Figure 8.21. Effect of synaptic activation level on spike timing in N1 and N3, respectively. Only output APs are displayed here. Synaptic activation level refers to number of activated synapses in total: (a) six synapses, (b) nine synapses, and (c) 12 synapses. Copyright 2014 IEEE. Reprinted, with permission, from [22].

Table 8.3. Comparison between neurons N1 and N3 among different number of activated synapses. Reproduced from [8].

	6 synapses		9 synapses		12 synapses	
	N1	N3	N1	N3	N1	N3
AP jitter	1.16	4.45	1.16	2.09	0.97	1.19
AP jitter (norm.)	1	1	1	0.47	0.84	0.28
AP delay	25.43	29.09	24.03	25.43	22.47	22.20
AP delay (SD)	0.40	1.25	0.33	0.59	0.31	0.35
AP delay (norm.)	1	1	0.94	0.87	0.88	0.76

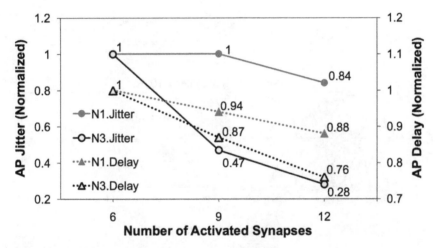

Figure 8.22. AP timing comparison between N1 and N3 under different synaptic activation level. Solid lines represent the normalized AP jitter (y-axis on the left) and dotted lines represent the normalized AP delay (y-axis on the right). Copyright 2014 IEEE. Reprinted, with permission, from [22].

level in the absence of active dendritic spiking. In other words, it would require more synapses activated by more neurons to achieve the same degree of precise firing.

8.3.3 Effect of input synchronization on AP spike timing

In biological neural networks, signals may not be perfectly synchronized, hence we introduce some input jitter to the experiment and evaluate the impact of the level of input synchronization on output AP timing in N1 and N2. We apply the ISI, the temporal interval between inputs AP_i and AP_{i+1}, to input APs and observed the output response caused by various ISI. Figure 8.23 shows the relative output AP jitter and delay among different input profiles, i.e., ISI = 0, 2, 4 ps. Table 8.4 summarizes the AP timing parameters used to evaluate the effect of input synchronization on AP spike timing. It is observed that when the ISI (input jitter) increases, both the output AP jitter and the AP delay increase. However, the rates of

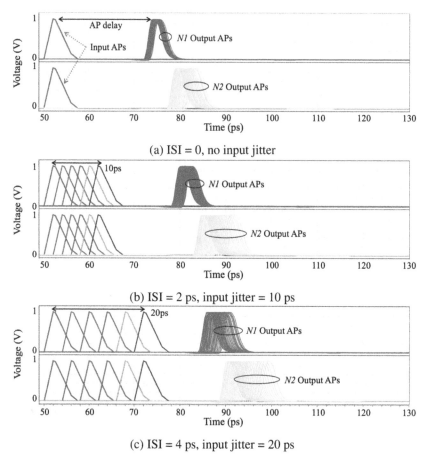

(a) ISI = 0, no input jitter

(b) ISI = 2 ps, input jitter = 10 ps

(c) ISI = 4 ps, input jitter = 20 ps

Figure 8.23. Effect of input synchronization on spike timing in N1 and N2, respectively. Input AP and output AP are displayed in the same panel. (a) ISI = 0 (no input jitter). All six input APs arrive at the same time. (b) ISI = 2 ps (input jitter = 10 ps). (c) ISI = 4 ps (input jitter = 20 ps). Copyright 2014 IEEE. Reprinted, with permission, from [22].

Table 8.4. Comparison between N1 and N2 among different ISI profiles. Reproduced from [8].

	ISI = 0		ISI = 2		ISI = 4	
	N1	N2	N1	N2	N1	N2
AP jitter	1.15	4.53	2.85	6.87	5.10	8.48
AP jitter (norm.)	1	1	2.48	1.52	4.43	1.87
AP delay	22.76	28.98	29.29	35.60	36.14	41.85
AP delay (SD)	0.31	1.27	0.75	1.93	1.42	2.36
AP delay (norm.)	1	1	1.29	1.23	1.59	1.44

increase are higher in N1 (+343.48% in AP jitter and +58.79% in AP delay) compared to those in N2 (+87.20% in AP jitter and +44.41% in AP delay) in the case when ISI is 4 ps. This phenomenon arises because the dendritic spike is more sensitive to the degree of input synchrony. Further increasing ISI beyond 4 ps makes N1 fail to initiate a dendritic spike. The comparison between N1 and N2 under different ISI is shown in figure 8.24.

Next, we examine the effect of input synchronization level along with the dendritic property on the output spike timing using the slope-sensitive *axon hillock* module described in chapter 3. Two neurons with the same synaptic spatial configurations are constructed and simulated, one with active dendrites and the other without active dendrites (can be considered as a point neuron). From the AP delay histogram in figure 8.25, it is observed that the neuron with active dendrites

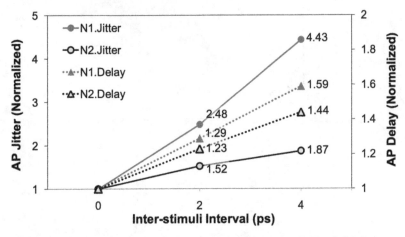

Figure 8.24. AP timing comparison between N1 and N2 under different ISI. Solid lines represent the normalized AP jitter (*y*-axis on the left) and dotted lines represent the normalized AP delay (*y*-axis on the right). Copyright 2014 IEEE. Reprinted, with permission, from [22].

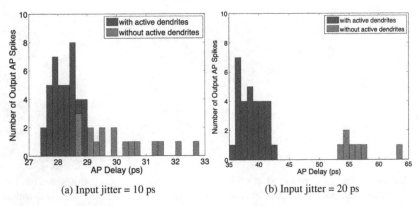

(a) Input jitter = 10 ps   (b) Input jitter = 20 ps

Figure 8.25. AP delay histograms for comparison of neurons with and without active dendrites. Neuron with active dendrites (blue bars) produces more reliable output spikes compared to neuron without active dendrites (grey bars) [8].

can tolerate input jitter and still produce reliable output spikes. In contrast, the neuron without active dendrites does not successfully produce reliable output spikes at a certain failure rate. As the input jitter increases from 10 ps to 20 ps, the failure rate increases from 57.5% to 76.7%.

The neuron circuit at the transistor level is simulated using HSPICE and then extrapolated into repetitive trials simulated at 20 GHz using MATLAB to demonstrate the spiking pattern in raster plots shown in figure 8.26. The input synchronization level can be interpreted as input jitter, i.e., lower input jitter refers to higher input synchronization. It is observed from the raster plots that the neuron

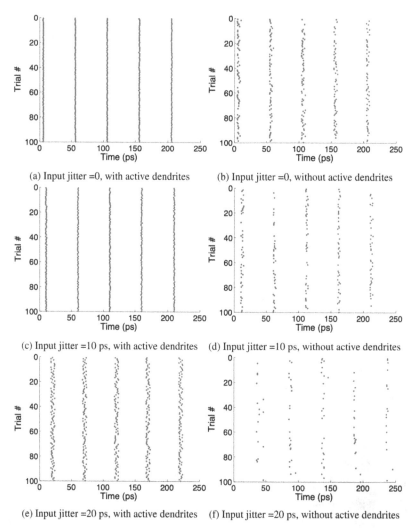

(a) Input jitter =0, with active dendrites   (b) Input jitter =0, without active dendrites

(c) Input jitter =10 ps, with active dendrites   (d) Input jitter =10 ps, without active dendrites

(e) Input jitter =20 ps, with active dendrites   (f) Input jitter =20 ps, without active dendrites

Figure 8.26. Raster plots for comparison of neurons with and without active dendrites. Neuron with active dendrites produces more reliable and precisely-timed output spike (a, c, e) compared to neuron without active dendrites (b, d, f). Standard deviation of the output spikes for each configuration (a–f) is 0.25, 1.44, 0.41, 1.21, 1.88, and 3.45, respectively [8].

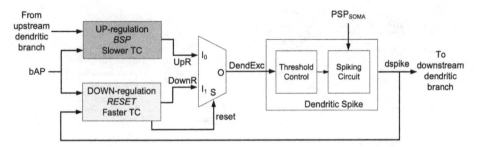

Figure 8.27. The control inputs to up-regulation of dendritic excitability are its up-stream branch *dspike* and *bAP*. The control inputs to down-regulation of dendritic excitability are its own *dspike* and *bAP* [8].

without active dendrites fails to produce reliable and precisely-timed spiking due to smaller somatic potential slope. The situation gets worse when the input AP jitter increases, e.g., the standard deviation of the output spikes increases from 1.21 to 3.45. In contrast, with active dendrites (capable of generating dendritic spike), the neuron seems to be more resilient to input AP jitter.

This chapter introduces circuits that change dendritic properties (dendritic plasticity) with different synaptic excitation patterns. The first section presents the *Reset* mechanism circuit that exhibits the property that the excitability of the dendrite is temporally reduced (down-regulated) by the previous local and global activities modeling a short-term depression in the dendritic spike. This mechanism imposes a limit on how fast the memory information can be retrieved. Second, the chapter presents the *branch strength potentiation* (BSP) mechanism, when the local synaptic activation coincides with bAP (back-propagating action potential), so that the local spike threshold on the weak dendritic branch decreases (up-regulation), implementing long-term potentiation.

Then the chapter demonstrates the coincidence detection mechanism induced by bAP activated calcium spike (BAC) firing that has been observed in layer V pyramidal neuron [12]. This is an example to demonstrate cortical neurons in different layers communicate through the apical and basal dendritic regions within a pyramidal neuron.

The block diagram of the proposed circuit implementation is shown in figure 8.27.

8.3.4 Down-regulated dendritic excitability

Down-regulation on dendritic excitability models the local and global *reset* mechanism (dendritic spike depression) observed in the pyramidal neuron which is described in chapter 2. In cortical pyramidal neurons, synaptic input activation less than 1 Hz would not trigger this *reset* mechanism, only when synapses activated at higher frequency, e.g., 5~10 Hz would set off dendritic spike depression. Since our CNT circuit runs at a much higher frequency, about 10^8 times faster than the biological neuron does, we scale the input activation frequency to 1 GHz in the circuit accordingly.

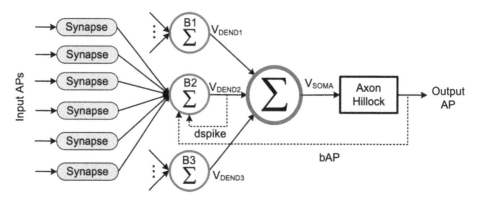

Figure 8.28. Two-stage neuron model for dendritic excitability simulation. The red circle represents the nonlinear integration within a single dendritic branch, and the big blue circle represents the integration at the soma. V_{DEND2} is the dendritic potential at Branch2. *dspike* represents the local control feedback and bAP represents the global control feedback. For simplicity only the detail of Branch2 is shown in this figure [8].

We perform simulation experiments to show different *reset* time effects and the local and global feedback mechanisms on the neuronal firing pattern. In these experiments, we configure a hypothetical neuron with three dendritic branches and as long as dendritic spikes are generated in two out of the three branches, the neuron fires. The circuit block diagram is shown in figure 8.28.

For the first set of simulations, a 1 GHz AP input is applied to the synapses clustered on each of the dendritic branches. We configure different *reset* time in our CNT neuron by adjusting the V_{CNTL} voltage in the *Oneshot* module (figure 3.15(a)). As a result, the comparison shows that with longer *reset* time, given the same input AP pattern, the output AP firing frequency reduces 500 MHz and 333 MHz in figure 8.29.

Next, we apply different input patterns on the three dendritic branches to demonstrate the effect of local and global control feedback on the neuronal output spiking. We investigate how the local and global *reset* mechanisms would impact each dendritic branch and the neuronal output. In this experiment setup, AP_1 is assigned to the synapses on Branch1, AP_2 to Branch2, and AP_3 to Branch3. The overall dendritic potential at each branch is named as V_{DEND1}, V_{DEND2}, and V_{DEND3}. We first enable both of the local and global feedback pathways and then disable them in our hypothetical neuron circuit. Figure 8.30(a) illustrates that the dendritic excitability can be down-regulated by the local activities (initiation of *dspike*) and by the global activities (bAP). For example, on Branch2, global bAP-induced dendritic spike depression occurs at t_3. The dendritic spike initiated at t_4 activation is limited to its local branch, therefore, only Branch2 is affected and the subsequent dendritic spike is suppressed at t_5, and Branch1 and Branch3 are left unaffected. When the same pattern of inputs (AP_1, AP_3) appear again at t_2, t_6, and t_8, the neuron does not respond to the pattern due to the *reset* caused by their previous occurrence at t_1, t_5, and t_7. When the local and global feedback pathways are disabled, there is no suppression on the dendritic excitability by the previous activity. Therefore, without

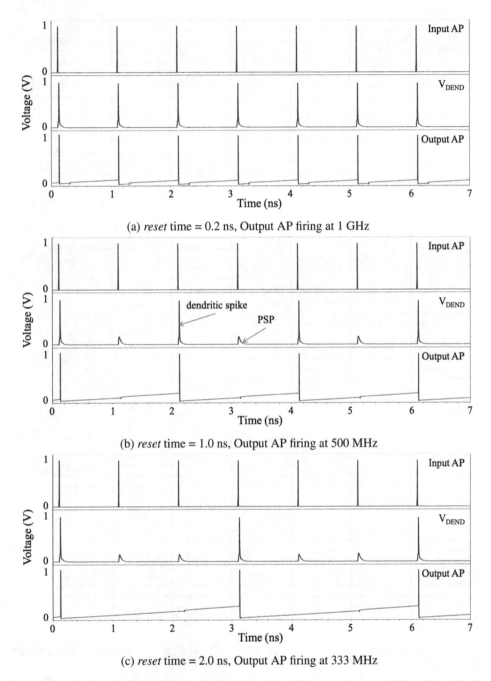

(a) *reset* time = 0.2 ns, Output AP firing at 1 GHz

(b) *reset* time = 1.0 ns, Output AP firing at 500 MHz

(c) *reset* time = 2.0 ns, Output AP firing at 333 MHz

Figure 8.29. Down-regulated dendritic excitability: dendritic spike *reset* time modulation. V_{DEND} is the potential at one dendritic branch [8].

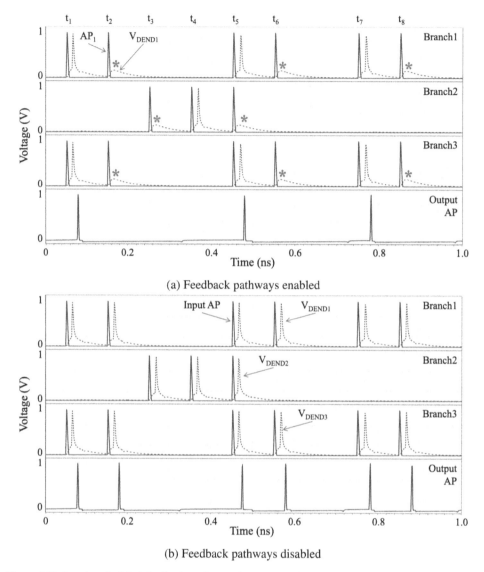

Figure 8.30. Local and global feedback pathways for *reset* mechanism. (a) With local and global *reset* mechanism, the dendritic spike depression occurs (marked with *) and hence the neuron fire less AP spikes. (b) Without local and global *reset* mechanism, the neuron fire more AP spikes [8].

the *reset* mechanism, the neuron fires more APs under the same pattern of inputs (figure 8.30(b)).

8.3.5 Up-regulated dendritic excitability

Up-regulation on the dendritic excitability is to model the BSPmechanism that enables dendritic spike to develop in the distal branch by coupling the local synaptic activation and the global feedback from bAP. This mechanism can enhance the neuron to generate more precise-timely AP spikes by propagating the strong dendritic spike more effectively from the distal dendritic branch towards the proximal dendritic branch.

As the dendrite bifurcates, it creates the parent–daughter dendritic structure shown in figure 8.31 where the parent branch is proximal to the center trunk, and the daughter branches are considered distal. When the repetitive stimuli alone are applied to the daughter branch, there is no recruitment of strong spikes in the downstream branch (parent branch). However, when the repetitive stimuli on a

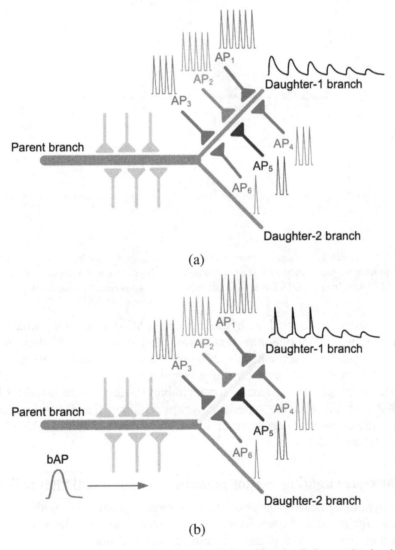

(a)

(b)

Figure 8.31. BSP formation in parent–daughter structure. (a) Repetitive stimuli alone on daughter branch, no potentiation occurs. (b) Repetitive stimuli on Daughter-1 branch coupled with bAP causes Daughter-1 branch to be potentiated (highlighted in yellow), capable of propagating strong spikes [8].

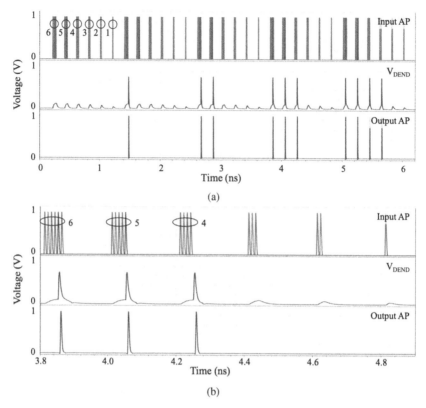

Figure 8.32. Up-regulated dendritic excitability simulation waveform. (a) The dendritic spike threshold decreases gradually from 0 spike generated to 4 spikes generated under the identical synaptic activation pattern. (b) Zoom-in during 3.8~4.9 ns. Inter-stimuli interval is set to 5 ps for synchronous synaptic activation [8].

daughter branch is coupled with acetycholine (ACh) activation, which usually happens during neuromodulatory exploratory behavior or bAP, there will be a slowly-developing enhancement of spiking on the weak dendritic branch.

In the following experiment, repetitive stimulation is applied on the six synapses on the daughter branch. Originally the excitability is low on the daughter branch, with bAP coupled with the repetitive synaptic inputs, the dendritic excitability increases, therefore, with less synaptic input, this branch is still capable of spiking shown in figure 8.32.

8.4 Back-propagating action potential activated calcium spike

Layer 5 pyramidal neuron has dendritic structures that extend into all layers in the neocortex, for instance, inputs from layer 2/3 innervate onto the apical dendrites while inputs from layer 5 innervate onto the basal dendrites. Larkum *et al* [12] discovered that when bAP coincides with distal dendritic depolarization within a few milliseconds time window, it facilitates the initiation of the dendritic calcium spikes. This mechanism is referred to as BAC. In addition, this BAC firing was found to

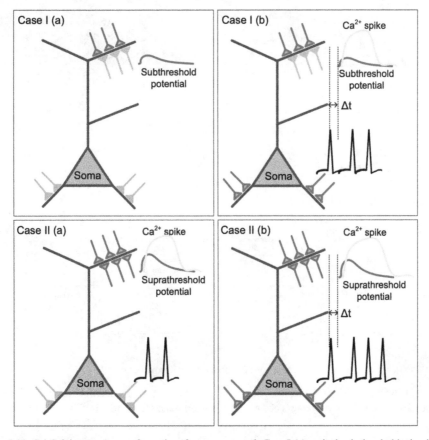

Figure 8.33. BAC firing neuron configuration: four cases tested. Case I (a): apical sub-threshold stimulation. Case I (b): apical sub-threshold stimulation coincides with basal stimulation. Case II (a): Apical supra-threshold stimulation. Case II (b): apical supra-threshold stimulation coincides with basal stimulation [8].

evoke a burst of axonal AP firing which was later interpreted as a coincidence detection mechanism to associate inputs arriving at different cortical layers.

To examine the effect of bAP on the Ca^{2+} spike threshold, we design four different synaptic activation scenarios, illustrated in figure 8.33. In Case I (a), only three synapses on the apical dendritic branch are activated which generates a sub-threshold depolarization, and therefore no Ca^{2+} spike is initiated. However, in Case I (b), when the apical sub-threshold depolarization paired with basal synaptic activation, the bAP lowers the Ca^{2+} spike threshold in the apical dendrite. As a result, the sub-threshold depolarization now can initiate Ca^{2+} spike. In Case II (a), all six synapses on the apical dendritic branch are activated which generates a supra-threshold depolarization, and subsequently a Ca^{2+} spike is initiated which later causes the neuron to fire AP spikes. In Case II (b), when the apical supra-threshold depolarization is paired with basal activation, the bAP further decreases the Ca^{2+} spike threshold in the apical dendrite. Hence a larger Ca^{2+} spike is generated in the apical dendrite, and as a result, the neuron fires more AP spikes. The CNT circuit simulation results are shown in figure 8.34.

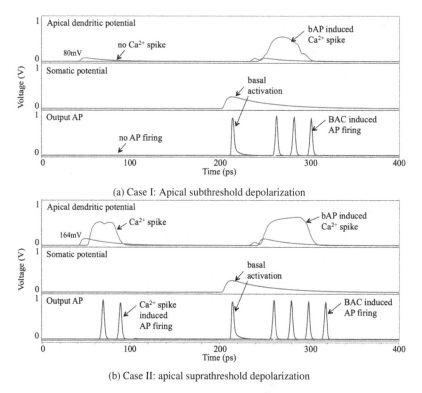

(a) Case I: Apical subthreshold depolarization

(b) Case II: apical suprathreshold depolarization

Figure 8.34. bAP activated calcium spike simulation waveform. Ca^{2+} spike induced AP firing is only observed in *Case I* and BAC induced AP firing is observed in both *Case I* and *Case II* with bAP-induced Ca^{2+} spike [8].

8.5 Back-propagating action potential characterization

Since bAP is crucial in many neural mechanisms especially when plasticity is involved, we characterize the bAP signal transmission in our artificial dendritic cable. Figure 8.35 shows the measurement of the three parameters: e.g., amplitude, half-width, and latency, of the bAP in the basal dendrite of the biological pyramidal neuron [15]. From this data, we observe that the amplitude of the bAP reduces to 36% from 100 mV, the half-width increases 3.5 times, and the latency increases to 0.45 ms (approximately 90% of AP half-width) at 150 μm from the soma. Figure 8.36(a) illustrates the dendritic cable configuration that allows back-propagation from the soma to the dendritic end. In Hsu's artificial dendritic cable, each segment, D_i, is equivalent to 20 μm of the dendrite. The CNT circuit simulation demonstrates a similar characterization of the bAP at the different distances from the soma, as shown in figure 8.36(b). The amplitude reduces to 35.6% from 0.9 V, the half-width increases 3.2 times, and the latency is 3.09 ps (approximately 88% of AP half-width) at the seventh dendritic segment, farthest from the soma.

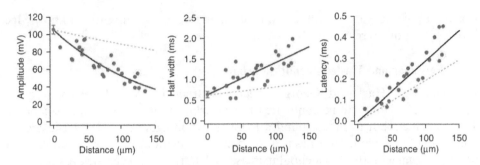

Figure 8.35. Measurements of bAP in basal dendrites of biological pyramidal neuron. Reprinted from [15], copyright (2007), with permission from Springer Nature.

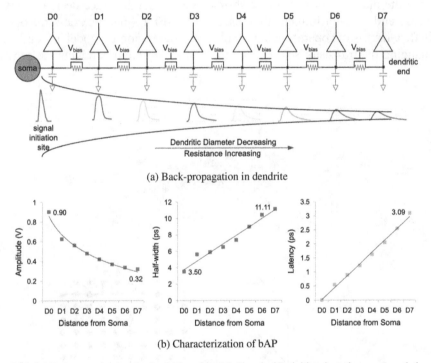

(a) Back-propagation in dendrite

(b) Characterization of bAP

Figure 8.36. bAP characterization in dendritic cable. (a) Signal, AP, initiated at the soma, and the signal attenuates when it back-propagates to the dendritic arbor. (b) Characterization, e.g., amplitude, half-width, and latency, of bAP in CNT neuron at different distance to the soma [8].

8.6 Other neuromorphic circuits for dendritic computations

Passive dendrite models were implemented with resistive switch-capacitor circuits in VLSI in early dendritic neuromorphic circuit designs [4, 17]. More recently, researchers in neuromorphic engineering have included active dendritic properties in their electronic neurons [2, 5, 9, 20]. Since the focus of this chapter is in modeling active dendritic arbors (dendrites with spikes) and dendritic plasticity with neuromorphic circuits, we will review three main research groups, to our knowledge, investigating this research problem.

8.6.1 Farquhar and Hasler's dendritic arbor

Farquhar and Hasler at Georgia Tech constructed a two-dimensional active dendritic arbor that can be configured to any arbitrary arbor pattern in silicon [5]. The dendritic arbor from that publication is shown in figure 8.37. The basic concept underlying Farquhar's dendrites is the exponential relationship between current and voltage, along with the exponential increase in dendritic diameter towards the soma. Charge moves as a result of diffusion current, and moves to reduce the difference between charge concentrations. A basic diffusor circuit used by Farquhar, is shown in figure 8.38.

Since the diameter of a dendrite shrinks and its conductance decreases towards the distal end of each branch, they used a MOSFET (metal-oxide-semiconductor field-effect transistor) operating in the sub-threshold region to model its conductance by changing the transistor's size. Each node has a different conductance controlled

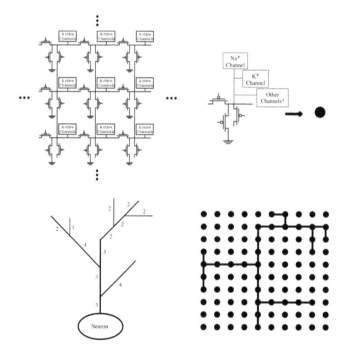

Figure 8.37. (a) A schematic for the 2D diffusor. Every node has a leak transistor to GND, and diffusive transistors to four other nodes. Active channels are at every node. The gate voltage on the diffusive/leak transistors varies the conductance through each transistor. High gate voltage can remove some nodes from the circuit. Upper right: a node of the 2D diffusor is shown as a dot. The lower left diagram shows how to make connections in the 2D array. The relative lengths of the dendritic arbor fit to the size of the array are shown in the lower right. In the upper left there is a schematic for the 2D diffusor. there is a leak transistor to GND, and diffusive transistors connecting it to four other nodes. Active channels are also present at every node. Caption and figure with permission from [5], copyright 2004 IEEE.

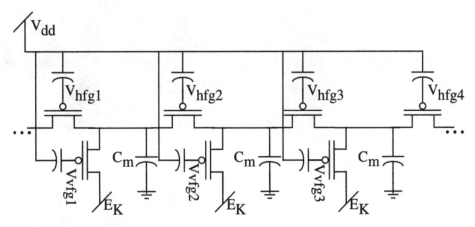

Figure 8.38. A basic diffusor circuit to model conductances of dendrites. Copyright 2004 IEEE, reprinted with permission from [5].

by the transistor gate voltage. To avoid the enormous amount of biasing control voltage, they proposed the idea of using floating gate transistors to program the diffusor array to overcome the pin limitations on-chip. To emulate the active property in dendrites, they inserted the circuits modeling the Na$^+$ and K$^+$ ion channels at every few nodes in the diffusor network. Their circuit demonstrates that the signal (they called it action potential, although it seems to be a dendritic spike) can travel robustly throughout the dendritic arbor, because it gets regenerated by the active channels in the diffusor network. A number of rapid inputs close to one point on the arbor structure could cause a potential like a dendritic spike to propagate down the dendrite, while a large number of simultaneous inputs at spread points on the structure might not. Figure 8.39 shows a large dendritic arbor as the 'AP' changes over time. In their implementation, previous neural activity would not affect the dendritic signal propagation.

8.6.2 Hynna, Arthur and Boahen's dendritic computations

Hynna and Boahen at Penn and Stanford University implemented a thalamic bursting silicon neuron by modeling the low threshold calcium current [9, 10]. They used a pair of current mirror integrators to mimic the activation and inactivation of the low threshold Ca^{2+} channel that is the trigger for bursting firing in a thalamic neuron. Different capacitors were used to provide fast integration for activation and slow integration for inactivation mechanisms for the Ca^{2+} channels in their circuits. Figure 8.40 shows the schematic for Hynna's T current. There is an activation and an inactivation current. The temporal dynamics of both of these currents are controlled using current mirror integrators. Each current mirror outputs a current equal in magnitude but opposite in sign to the input current. A capacitor on the gate of each input transistor provides an integration time constant while a source tilt on this transistor (V_{Sa} and V_{Sn} in figure 8.40) provides a constant gain to the output. The addition of a constant leak (V_h) to the inactivation mirror controls the rates of

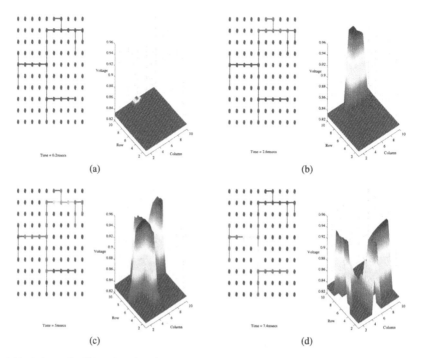

Figure 8.39. A large dendritic arbor showing change in the potential over the arbor over time. Each node is color coded as to its relative voltage, with red highest. (a) The array after stimulation at node [6,1] at 0.2 ms. Spiking occured at that point. (b) At 2.6 ms. a spike has occurred and has spread to the surrounding nodes. Unlike passive diffusion, the voltage is not decreasing as the voltage spreads. (c) At 5 ms. the original node voltage has returned almost to resting, but the potential has continued to spread. (d) The last node at time 7.4 ms. The remainder of the array begins to return to the resting potential. The potential is spreading to the final few nodes, but will die out very soon. Copyright 2004 IEEE, reprinted with permission from [5].

inactivation and deinactivation in the channel. Current into the activation and inactivation integrators (the latter we will call the deinactivation current) is controlled by the three transistors closest to ground in figure 8.40. The ratio of the output currents from the modified differential pair is controlled by the difference in the two gates voltages (V_{mem} and V_{thr}). V_{thr} is fixed to force a set voltage threshold for channel activation. The rising and falling T current is controlled by the fast and slow dynamics of the two current mirrors. More explanation of the timing of this circuit can be found in [10].

Arthur and Boahen then incorporated the Ca^{2+} spike as an active component in the dendrite to implement single-presentation learning in their silicon neuron [2]. The active basal dendrite provides a mechanism, calcium spikes, for reactivating patterns. Sufficient dendritic potential results in repeated calcium spikes at theta frequency (5~10 Hz) that then triggers bursting output at the soma. The learning process depends on two variables, the dendritic potential and synaptic input. The WTA (winner-take-all) circuits select the most active synapse (synaptic input) and the most active basal dendrite (dendritic potential). If the current flowing from this

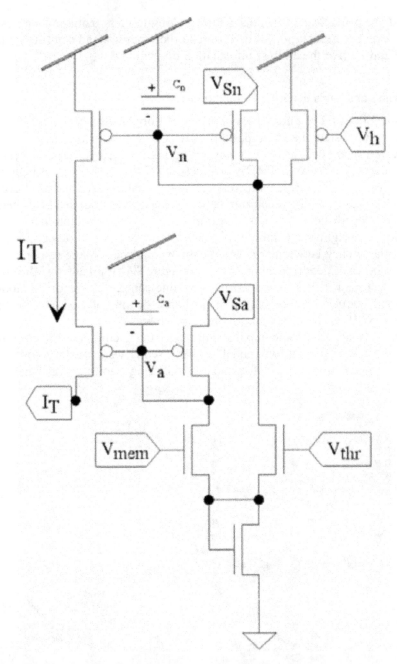

Figure 8.40. T channel electronic model. Copyright 2003 IEEE, reprinted with permission from [9].

synapse to the paired basal dendrite exceeds the learning threshold, this particular synapse is potentiated. By clustering strengthened synapses onto the same basal dendrite, the dendritic potential becomes sufficiently large which then initiates calcium spikes generating reactivation of the neuron. When the synapses are recruited from inactive pyramidal neurons, long-term potentiation occurs. AER (address-event representation) is used to send the synapse's and dendrite's addresses off-chip and receive the address information on-chip.

8.6.3 Wang and Liu's dendritic computations

Wang and Liu at ETH Zürich have modeled the nonlinearities in the dendrite as a function of input spatial and temporal patterns [19–21]. In their 2013 paper, there is a mathematical model showing spatial clustering and temporal coincidence. The circuit models AMPA and NMDA channels. NMDA channels have high calcium permeability. Their dendritic mathematical model is biomimetic and models calcium spikes. The dendritic spike generation depends only on the local dendritic membrane potential. A dendritic spike evoked within a subunit can facilitate dendritic spike generation in neighboring subunits. The active propagation of dendritic spikes shortens the latency between the synaptic inputs and the somatic response.

Wang and Liu's dendritic model, shown in figure 8.41 is an analog VLSI (aVLSI) model. Each neuron has nine dendrites and one soma. The dendritic model uses Mel's mathematical model [14] and includes details of spiking mechanisms (Including NMDA channels and inhibitory synapses).

There are nine dendritic compartments that can be configured to a number of morphologies in their neuron model. Cable circuits were used to configure the dendritic morphology and for spatial filtering among the neighboring

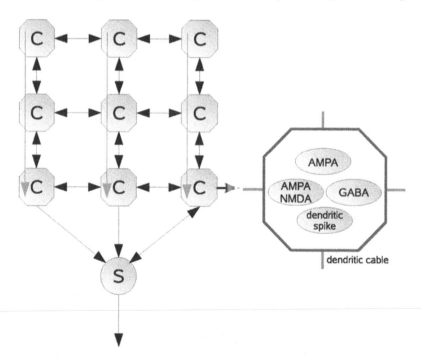

Figure 8.41. Neuron with active dendrites taken. Copyright 2013 IEEE. Reprinted, with permission, from [19].

compartments. The dendritic spike generation circuit employed two generally accepted dynamics of the ion channels: slow activation hyperpolarization current and fast activation depolarization current. They have a dendritic spike threshold bias voltage present in the circuit, however, it is not clear how this parameter can be controlled by other neural mechanisms. They used a sigmoidal curve to fit the dendritic and somatic membrane potentials as a mathematical function of the time interval between different synaptic activations. Therefore, their circuit does not have the ability to adapt to a specific biological scenario, for example, the down-regulation of the K^+ channel on the dendritic membrane that is caused by branch strength potentiation.

8.6.4 Comparison summary

All of these research groups being reviewed here have included an active dendritic property in their silicon neurons with CMOS technology. The transistors in their circuits operate in the sub-threshold regions which gives them three advantages, as follows. First, small changes in voltage (input) yield large changes in current (output), therefore a wide range of currents can be modeled. Second, many neuronal properties can be expressed in mathematical natural exponential equations, because transistors in the sub-threshold region also have voltage–current in an exponential relationship. Third, these circuits consume very low power because of the sub-threshold conduction current.

To our best knowledge, there are a few aspects missing or neglected in these groups' dendritic circuits that we think are important to capture in an artificial neuron implementation exhibiting plasticity: learning and memory formation. First, the excitability of the dendrite in this related research is not plastic due to the absence of feedback mechanisms from the local dendritic branch and from the global neuronal output. As discussed earlier in the neuroscience literature review, there are many neural mechanisms suggesting the excitability of dendrites can be modulated and can lead to coincidence detection enhancement and learning [13, 18]. Second, not all dendritic spikes have been incorporated in one single electronic neuron and the location e.g., basal or apical dendrites, where each type of dendritic spike, e.g., Ca^{2+} spike, Na^+ spike, or NMDA spikes initiated were not considered in their neuron implementation. In addition, an issue surfaces when the technology process scales down, the supply and threshold voltage could also scale down. The leakage current increases dramatically when the threshold and supply voltages decrease, therefore, their advantage over power consumption may not be prominent anymore. In addition, transistors operating in the sub-threshold region are susceptible to noise and process variations.

Another matter to point out is that they used mathematical equations to model the biological behavior and those biasing parameters were derived from curve-fitting. But it is not clear how a variation in a particular parameter can affect the simulation response in their circuits. However, using the design approach in the BioRC project, we gain direct control over certain transistors in the circuit, and use them as 'control knobs' to mimic the electrical and physiological properties in the synapse, dendrite, and axon hillock, for instance, the neurotransmitter concentration in synapse, dendritic diameter and channel density in dendrite, and activation/inactivation time of Na^+ channel in axon hillock. Another advantage of BioRC circuits is every computation is online and autonomous. There is no off-line communication overhead to our circuit, and there is no need for separate memory to store the synapse or dendritic compartment location.

8.7 Chapter summary

This chapter focused on Hsu's active dendritic arbor circuits. Other active dendritic arbor circuits included those by Farquhar and Hasler, Hynna and Boahen, and Wang and Liu.

The next chapter covers circuits implementing variable neural behavior, including noisy neurons and chaotic behavior.

8.8 Exercises

1. Farquhar's model of the dendritic arbor supports (mark all correct answers):
   (a) 3-D modeling of the dendritic arbor;
   (b) Dendritic spiking;
   (c) Two-directional spiking;
   (d) Dendritic plasticity.

References

[1] Ariav G, Polsky A and Schiller J 2003 Submillisecond precision of the input-output transformation function mediated by fast sodium dendritic spikes in basal dendrites of CA1 pyramidal neurons *J. Neurosci.* **23** 7750–8

[2] Arthur J V and Boahen K 2004 Recurrently connected silicon neurons with active dendrites for one-shot learning *Proc. IEEE Int. Joint Conf. Neural Networks* **3** 1699–704

[3] Behabadi B F *et al* 2012 Location-dependent excitatory synaptic interactions in pyramidal neuron dendrites *PLoS computational biology* **8** e1002599

[4] Elias J, Chu H and Meshreki S 1992 Silicon implementation of an artificial dendritic tree *Proc. Int. Joint Conf. Neural Networks IEEE* 1 (Baltimore, MD: IEEE) 154–9

[5] Farquhar E, Abramson D and Hasler P 2004 A reconfigurable bidirectional active 2 dimensional dendrite model *Proc. 2004 Int. Symp. Circuits and Systems (Vancouver)* 313–6

[6] Friesz A K *et al* 2007 A Biomimetic Carbon Nanotube Synapse Circuit *Biomedical Engineering Society Annual Fall Meeting*

[7] Hensch T K 2005 Critical period plasticity in local cortical circuits *Nat. Rev. Neurosci.* **6** 877–88

[8] Hsu C-C 2014 Dendritic computation and plasticity in neuromorphic circuits *PhD Thesis* University of Southern California

[9] Hynna K and Boahen K 2003 A silicon implementation of the thalamic low threshold calcium current *Engineering in Medicine and Biology Society, 2003. EMBS '03. 25th Annual Int. Conf. of the IEEE* 3 pp 2228–31

[10] Hynna K M and Boahen K 2007 Silicon neurons that burst when primed *Circuits and Systems, 2007. ISCAS 2007. IEEE Int. Symp.* 3363–6

[11] Joshi J *et al* 2009 A carbon nanotube cortical neuron with excitatory and inhibitory dendritic computations *2009 IEEE/NIH Life Science Systems and Applications Workshop* (Bethesda, MD: IEEE) 133–6

[12] Larkum M E, Julius Zhu J and Sakmann B 1999 A new cellular mechanism for coupling inputs arriving at different cortical layers *Nature* **398** 338–41

[13] Losonczy A, Makara J K and Magee J C 2008 Compartmentalized dendritic plasticity and input feature storage in neurons *Nature* **452** 436–41

[14] Mel B W 1993 Synaptic integration in an excitable dendritic tree *J. Neurophysiol.* **70** 1086–101

[15] Nevian T *et al* 2007 Properties of basal dendrites of layer 5 pyramidal neurons: a direct patch-clamp recording study *Nat. Neurosci.* **10** 206–14

[16] Poirazi P, Terrence B and Bartlett W M 2003 Pyramidal neuron as two-layer neural network *Neuron* **37** 989–99

[17] Rasche C and Douglas R J 2001 Forward- and backpropagation in a silicon dendrite *IEEE Trans. Neural Netw.* **12** 386–93

[18] Remy S, Csicsvari J and Beck H 2009 Activity-dependent control of neuronal output by local and global dendritic spike attenuation *Neuron* **61** 906–16

[19] Wang Y and Liu S-C 2013 Active processing of spatio-temporal input patterns in silicon dendrites *IEEE Trans. Biomed. Circuits Syst.* **7** 307–18

[20] Wang Y and Liu S-C 2009 Input evoked nonlinearities in silicon dendritic circuits *2009 IEEE Int. Symp. Circuits and Systems* (Taipei: IEEE) pp 2894–7

[21] Wang Y and Liu S-C 2010 Multilayer processing of spatiotemporal spike patterns in a neuron with active dendrites *Neural Comput.* **22** 2086–112

[22] Hsu C C and Parker A C 2014 A biomimetic nanoelectronic neuron with enhanced spike timing *2014 IEEE International Symposium on Circuits and Systems (ISCAS) (Melbourne)* 1560–3

IOP Publishing

Neuromorphic Circuits
A constructive approach
Alice C Parker and Rick Cattell

Chapter 9

Variable neural behavior

Jason Mahvash, Kun Yue and Alice C Parker

This chapter surveys circuits implementing neuromorphic neural behavior that is variable, either stochastic or algorithmic in nature, based primarily on the work by Mahvash, with a random pulse generator circuit designed by Yue included as well. The main goal of the research described in this chapter is modeling the intrinsic variability in neural networks at the circuit level and demonstrating the value of variability in behavior of neural networks. Variability in spiking thresholds and in synaptic strength is explored in the chapter.

9.1 Introduction

Our overarching goal for the BioRC (Biomimetic Real-Time Cortex) project is to demonstrate complex neural networks that possess memory and learning capability. Any artificial neural system designed to be brain-like, or biomimetic, might be enhanced by some variability in behavior. Artificial neurons that spontaneously fire without sufficient postsynaptic potential (PSP) could trigger brain activity that was unanticipated, but useful in triggering new or unexpected behavior downstream. To this end, we believe the behavior of such networks would be enhanced by the addition of variability. This chapter describes the design of a carbon nanotube neuromorphic cortical neuron with two main sources of intrinsic variability; neurotransmitter-release variability and ion-channel variability. Neurotransmitter-release variability and ion-channel variability are modeled at the circuit level using carbon nanotube circuit elements. We include a choice of two different types of signal variability in the transistor circuits in chapter 9, a signal with Gaussian noise and a chaotic signal. For neurotransmitter-release variability these signals are simulated as if they were generated internally in a synapse circuit to vary the neurotransmitter release in an unpredictable manner. Variation in neurotransmitter concentration in the synaptic cleft causes a change in the peak magnitude and duration of the PSP. For ion-channel variability, these signals are simulated as if they were generated internally in an axon hillock circuit to change the firing mechanism. The variable signal could force the neuron to fire if the variability strength were sufficient or could prevent the neuron from firing even with adequate membrane potential. When there is no PSP at the axon hillock (the cell membrane is at resting potential), the variable signal forcing the neuron to fire in fact models spontaneous firing of the neuron. For Gaussian noise, we include a file in our SPICE simulation consisting of random voltage samples that control neurotransmitter release volume. In implemented electronic circuits, device variability due to thermal effects, when amplified, could be used as a source of variability.

In this text we include neurotransmitter-release variability and ion-channel variability in a neuromorphic neural circuit. One approach to include variability in a neuronal circuit is to implement a deterministic Hodgkin–Huxley (HH) model with added white noise at the circuit level [5]. The earliest solution of the integrate-and-fire (I&F) model that included stochastic activity modeled the incoming signal from the synapse (PSP) as a random walk [13]. In 1965, the I&F model was formulated with stochastic input to include the decay of the membrane potential [21]. Stein discussed whether the variability is because of neural noise or whether it is an important part of the signal. A number of authors did theoretical and numerical analysis of the HH equations with stochastic fluctuations of the ion channels [2, 7]. This fluctuation can cause spontaneous firing and places limits on the miniaturization of the brain's wiring [10]. Overall, ion-channel variability has been studied and analyzed theoretically by several neuroscience researchers using the I&F and the HH models. However, they did not have a circuit implementation of the ion-channel variability

We present circuits in this chapter built in Parker's BioRC group (e.g., [15], and [18]) because they are designed to expand for greater control over specific mechanisms and to incorporate additional future mechanisms. Also, our approach is to include variability in transistors in the circuit that correspond to biological functions affected by variability and therefore Mahvash' approach is more biomimetic than Chen's [5]. At the time Mahvash's dissertation [20] was published, we were not aware of biomimetic ion-channel circuits that had variable behavior apart from the work by Chen.

In order to model ion-channel variability at the circuit level, a variable control signal is applied to the axon hillock circuit. The variable signal could force the neuron to fire if the variability strength were sufficient or could prevent the neuron from firing. The variable signal is independent of the PSP. When there is no PSP applied to the axon hillock (the cell membrane is at resting potential), the variable signal forcing the neuron to fire in fact models spontaneous firing of the neuron. We will talk about the circuit in more detail in this chapter.

9.1.1 Ion-channel variability in the Hodgkin–Huxley model

Neuronal action potentials (APs), generated by the actions of populations of ion channels, can typically be modeled using some variant of the classic phenomenological model of Hodgkin and Huxley. The membrane equation of the HH model describing the squid giant axon is given by the following equation:

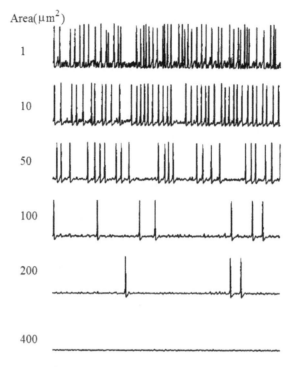

Figure 9.1. Spontaneous output from the simulation. Reprinted from [7], copyright 1996 The Biophysical Society. Published by Elsevier Inc. All rights reserved.

$$C\frac{dV}{dt} = \bar{g}_{Na}m^3h(V - E_{Na}) + \bar{g}_K n^4(V - E_K) + \bar{g}_L(V - E_L) \qquad (9.1)$$

where V is the membrane potential, E_{Na} and E_K are the sodium and potassium reversal or Nernst potentials, E_L is the resting leakage potential for a leakage conductance g_L, C is the capacitance and m, h and n are gating variables. If this equation is solved with discrete Markovian ion kinetics instead of the usual continuous rate equations, it could lead to spontaneous generation of APs. Figure 9.1 shows the output from the simulations for six values of membrane area. As we mentioned previously, the spontaneous rate is high for small membrane areas that correspond to small numbers of channels. As the membrane area is increased, the rate of spontaneous APs approaches zero, the expected rate from the deterministic model [7].

The probability density function (PDF) for the interspike intervals can also be estimated by solving the HH equation. The firing of an AP is governed approximately by a Poisson process and therefore the interspike interval has a negative exponential partial differential equation, shown in figure 9.2.

9.1.2 Ion-channel variability in the integrate-and-fire model

Ion-channel variability could be studied using the leaky I&F model, that assumes the neuron is a leaky capacitor driven by a current that simulates the actual synaptic

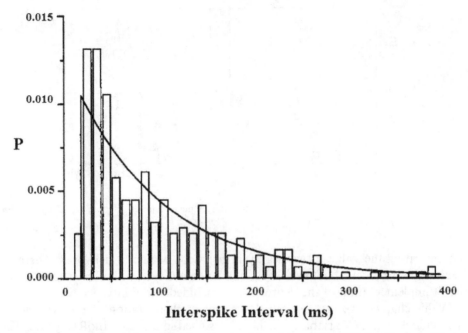

Interspike Interval (ms)

Figure 9.2. Interspike intervals from simulation. Reprinted from [7], copyright 1996 The Biophysical Society. Published by Elsevier Inc. All rights reserved.

inputs. A noise term is added to the equation to represent several internal sources of noise such as ion channel noise and synaptic noise to obtain a system described by the following Langevin equation:

$$C\frac{dV}{dt} = -gV + I(t) + \xi(t) \qquad (9.2)$$

where C is the cell membrane capacitance, V is the membrane potential, gV is the leakage term, g is a conductance, $I(t)$ is the input current and $\xi(t)$ is Gaussian noise. When the potential reaches the threshold V_0 an action potential is generated and the system returns to the equilibrium potential V_e [4].

Figure 9.3 shows the results of a numerical simulation of equation (9.2) in response to two different signals, in both cases in the presence of internal noise. Because of ion channel variability applied to the I&F model, there is a trial-to-trial variability in spike timing over 500 trials. When $I(t)$ contains high-frequency components (left portion of upper right signal), spikes are clustered more tightly to the upward strokes of the input and overall there is less trial–trial variability than in the constant input case. This is actually an advantage of having synaptic variability in the input.

9.2 Circuit implementation of intrinsic variability

As mentioned earlier, the main goal of the research described in this chapter is modeling the intrinsic variability in neural networks at the circuit level and

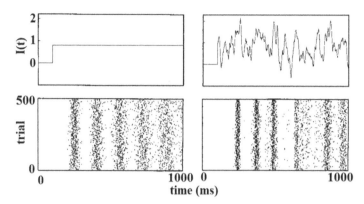

Figure 9.3. 500 responses to the constant and fluctuating inputs. Reproduced from [4]. Copyright 2000, National Academy of Sciences, USA.

demonstrating the value of variability in behavior of neural networks. There is a great deal of research about variability in the nervous system; however, there was no circuit implementation of the neurons with included variability.

In this chapter, we first explain the circuit implementation of the synapse and axon hillock with no variability included, designed in Parker's BioRC group. Then we discuss how we can include ion-channel variability and synaptic variability in the cortical neuron circuit. Finally, we conclude with a discussion of chaotic functions, and noise generated by photons. The use of noise in learning is discussed later in chapter 10. Figure 9.4 shows a simplified model for a cortical neuron, consisting of synapses, the dendritic arbor and the axon hillock. Excitatory and inhibitory synapses receive APs from presynaptic neurons and transfer a PSP to the dendritic arbor. The dendritic arbor consists of several adders that add all signals coming from synapses and generate one single signal. The arrangement of the adders and their linearity varies depending on the individual neuron and the synaptic location. The amplitude of the dendritic arbor potential signal is compared with the threshold voltage in the axon hillock. If the membrane potential is more than the threshold, a spike is generated at the output of the axon hillock. Otherwise there is no spike at the output.

Variability is not included in any part of this model. In order to include the intrinsic variability in the model, we will include neurotransmitter-release variability in the synapse circuit and ion-channel variability in the axon hillock circuit. Other aspects of neural activity could also exhibit variable behavior but the two aspects mentioned here are thought to be the most likely sources of variability.

9.3 Neurotransmitter-release variability in the synapse circuit

Figure 9.5 shows BioRC carbon nanotube excitatory and inhibitory synapse circuits [18]. This circuit models cell potentials and neurotransmitter concentrations with voltages, with a correspondence between circuit elements and biological mechanisms. In figure 9.5(a), the excitatory synapse circuit, the AP turns M5 ON. M7 and M6 are already ON. Therefore, the voltage at the source of M5 or gate of M7 increases until M7

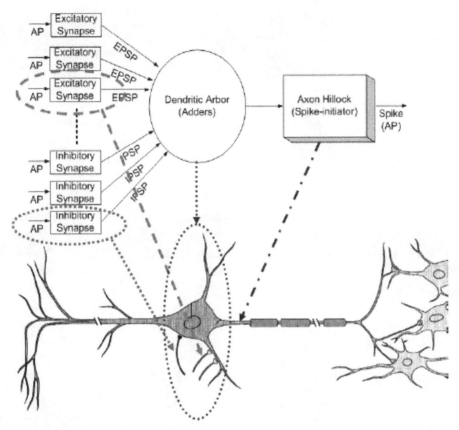

Figure 9.4. A system block diagram of the cortical neuron model with a pyramidal neuron cartoon. Copyright 2009 IEEE. Reprinted, with permission, from [17].

turns OFF, limiting the rise of voltage at the synaptic cleft. M6 controls the neurotransmitter concentration in the cleft. M3 models the reuptake process. The inverter containing M1 and M2 generates a delay between the AP and the neurotransmitter reuptake. The neurotransmitter release causes the ion channels to open. This depolarization is modeled by M13. The pull-up transistor in the neurotransmitter section (M6) modulates the neurotransmitter concentration in the synaptic cleft (the voltage at the synaptic cleft node). The voltage at the gate labeled *Neurotransmitter* controls the neurotransmitter release. This causes a change in the excitatory postsynaptic potential (EPSP) peak amplitude, directly altering the synapse strength.

In the circuit with no variability, the voltage applied to the gate labeled *Neurotransmitter* could be a fixed biasing voltage or the voltage could vary as the result of some *retrograde* process in the synapse arising in the postsynaptic neuron. In the case described in this chapter, the gate voltage is either an analog noise signal or a chaotic signal that makes the neurotransmitter release variable. This variable input causes the peak amplitude of the EPSP to be variable and varies the synapse strength stochastically or chaotically. Similarly, we produce variability in a BioRC

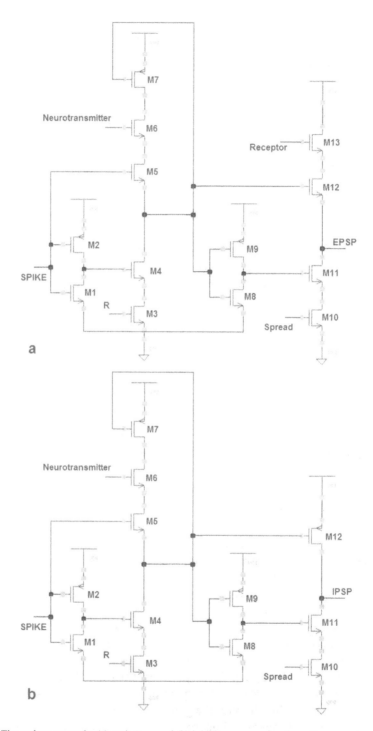

Figure 9.5. The carbon nanotube (a) excitatory and (b) inhibitory synapses where R represents reuptake [18].

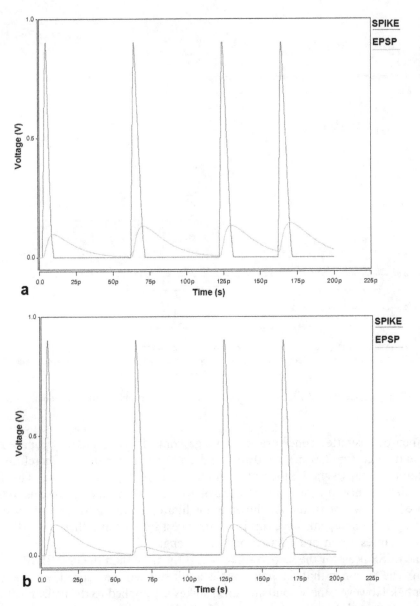

Figure 9.6. Input (pink) and output (green) of the excitatory synapse (a). No variability (b). With variability included [20].

inhibitory synapse. Figure 9.6 shows the result of the synapse circuit with and without variability.

Mahvash simulated the carbon nanotube cortical neuron consisting of three excitatory synapses with different strengths, one inhibitory synapse, a dendritic arbor and the axon hillock circuits in SPICE. He performed several experiments for neurotransmitter-release variability. First, he simulated the neuron with no variability. A spike was applied to the four synapses at the same time.

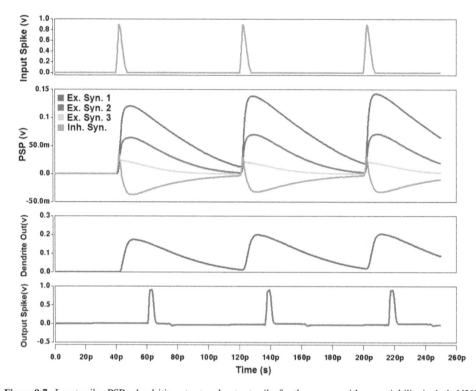

Figure 9.7. Input spike, PSPs, dendritic output and output spike for the neuron with no variability included [20].

The neurotransmitter concentration voltage controls for excitatory synapses one, two and three are 850 mV, 700 mV and 550 mV, respectively. Therefore, three excitatory synapses had different strengths (different peak EPSPs). The neuro-transmitter concentration voltage control for the inhibitory synapse is 700 mV. Figure 9.7 shows the result. As shown in the figure, the EPSP for excitatory synapse one has the highest peak since this is the strongest synapse and then the PSPs for the other synapses are in order based on their strengths.

The EPSP peak for the second spike is slightly more than the first EPSP peak and so on. The reason is that the first spike is applied when the neuron is at the resting potential. However, the second and third spikes are applied to the neuron before the neuron goes back to the resting potential, so there is temporal summation.

The output of the dendrite is a summation of all PSPs and when it crosses the threshold voltage (170 mV), the neuron fires. As shown in the figure, the neuron fires when all three excitatory PSPs peak. If we apply a spike to only one synapse instead of applying it to all synapses, the dendritic output is not sufficient to fire the neuron. We included neurotransmitter-release variability and calculated the probability of firing. For example, we applied a spike to the first synapse and instead of 850 mV fixed biasing voltage for neurotransmitter control voltage, we included a Gaussian voltage with mean $\mu = 850$ mV and standard deviation changing from $\sigma = 0$ mV to

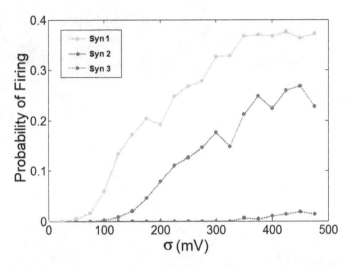

Figure 9.8. Probability of firing when a Gaussian voltage is included for neurotransmitter release control, resulting in synaptic variability; only one synapse has spike at the input [20].

$\sigma = 500$ mV and period of each sample 10 ps. We assume all other synapses have no spikes as inputs. The probability of firing is shown in figure 9.8. We changed the standard deviation from 0 mV to 500 mV with step size of 25 mV. For each standard deviation we ran the SPICE and MATLAB experiments 100 times with 100 different Gaussian samples. Among 100 experiments, we counted how many times the neuron fires. The probability is calculated by dividing the number of experiments that the neuron fires by 100.

When $\sigma = 0$ mV, meaning there is no synaptic variability, the PSP from one synapse is not strong enough to fire the neuron and then the probability is zero. When we allow synaptic variability and increase the standard deviation, the probability increases. Since synapse one is stronger, the PSP generated from synapse one can be closer to the threshold voltage and therefore the probability for variability in neurotransmitter release for synapse one causing the neuron to fire is higher. Synapse three generates a PSP that is much smaller than the threshold and even a strong synaptic variability cannot help the neuron to fire without spikes at other synapses in the dendritic arbor.

If we assume the PSP signal is Gaussian, we can calculate the probability of firing using acumulative distribution function of Gaussians and get similar results to do curve matching. This assumption might not be necessarily true. The following function shows the probability of firing for different PSP values. Each PSP value is a Gaussian random number. Figure 9.9 shows the result of plotting the following function versus σ in MATLAB.

$$p(V_{PSP} > V_{th}) = 0.5 - 0.5 \operatorname{erf}\left(\frac{V_{th} - \mu}{\sqrt{2\sigma^2}}\right) \tag{9.3}$$

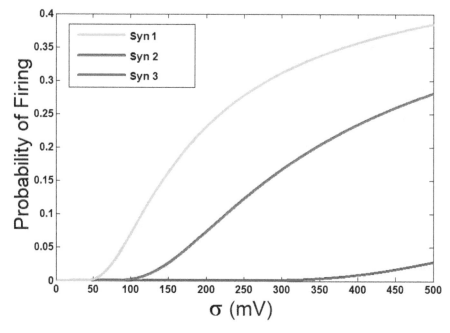

Figure 9.9. Probability of firing when a Gaussian voltage is included for neurotransmitter release control, resulting in synaptic variability, and only one synapse has spike at the input (**MATLAB** simulation) [20].

where μ is the mean of the PSP and σ is the standard deviation of the PSP signal, and substituting the non-variable PSP values for the three synapses as the means of the PSPs. Based on this function, we can conclude that the maximum probability is 0.5 if we include a strong Gaussian neurotransmitter release control (large mean). We did a similar experiment but, instead of Gaussian release control, we used a chaotic control mechanism. V_{pp} changes from 0 mV to 1000 mV. V_{mid} is the same as the fixed biasing voltage for neurotransmitter control voltage and V_{init} changes from $V_{mid} - V_{pp}/2$ to $V_{mid} + V_{pp}/2$. As shown in figure 9.10, traces with the same color are the results for one synapse with different initial conditions. When V_{pp} is low, the results for different initial conditions are almost the same, however, for higher V_{pp}, when the PSP is close to the threshold, the results are different, meaning that the effect of the initial condition on the probability of firing increases for PSPs close to the threshold voltage.

Mahvash applied a spike to all four synapses and included neurotransmitter-release variability in just one of them each time. He included a Gaussian neuro-transmitter-release variability with $\mu = 850$ mV and $\sigma = 0$ mV to $\sigma = 200$ mV in the first synapse and calculated the probability of firing. The mean of the Gaussian signal is the same as the fixed biasing voltage in the no-variability experiment because the Gaussian signal has a symmetric variation around this voltage, meaning that the probability of being more than 850 mV is the same as being less (50%). The dendritic output has a variable amplitude and therefore the neuron sometimes fires

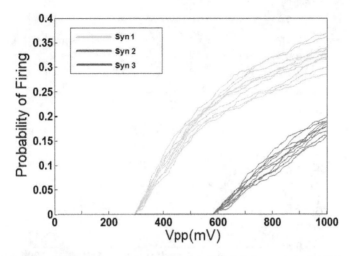

Figure 9.10. Probability of firing when a chaotic signal is included for neurotransmitter release control, resulting in synaptic variability [20].

and sometimes not depending on the dendritic output amplitude. He calculated the probability of firing. We did the same experiments for the variability in synapse two, three and the inhibitory synapse. Figure 9.11 shows the probability of firing when the synaptic variability is included in the excitatory and inhibitory synapses. All probabilities start from 1 because when there is no variability included, the peak of dendritic output (173.8 mV) is slightly more than the threshold voltage (170 mV) and the neuron fires as shown in figure 9.7. When the synaptic variability is included, the variability could push the output of the dendrite below the threshold. Therefore, the probability goes down from 1 to 0.5. The probability of firing when the variability in the inhibitory synapse is the lowest, meaning that the inhibitory synapse is more sensitive to neurotransmitter-release variability than the excitatory synapse. Also, by comparing the probability for three synapses, we can conclude that the neuron is more sensitive to neurotransmitter-release variability included in a weak synapse as compared to variability included in a strong synapse. He did another experiment similar to the previous one but he included the variability in two synapses; synapse one and synapse two. Gaussian signals included in two synapses have the same standard deviation and could be correlated. Figure 9.12 shows the probability of firing versus standard deviation in the MATLAB simulation. As shown in the figure, for higher correlation factor (ρ), the probability is lower, meaning when the variability of synapses is correlated, the variability is more effective and changes the firing probability more. He verified this statement by calculating the standard deviation of a Gaussian signal which is a summation of two Gaussian signals. The standard deviation is as follows:

$$\sigma_{PSP} = \sqrt{\sigma_{PSP1}^2 + \sigma_{PSP2}^2 + 2. \, \rho. \, \sigma_{PSP1}. \, \sigma_{PSP2}} \qquad (9.4)$$

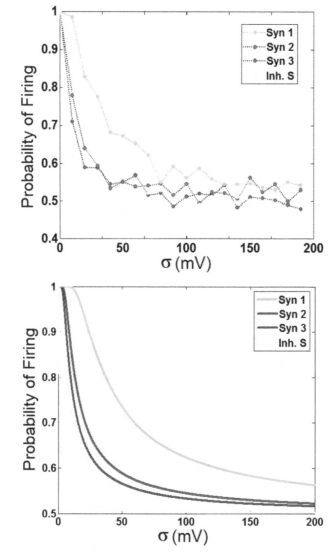

Figure 9.11. Probability of firing when neurotransmitter-release variability is included in one synapse. SPICE (top). MATLAB (bottom) [20].

As shown in the above equation, higher correlation factor means higher standard deviation and stronger Gaussian signal.

9.4 Ion-channel variability in the axon hillock circuit

Ion-channel variability is included into the axon hillock module that contains the input stage and the spike generation stage. The input stage consists of an amplifier and two inverters in cascade. It receives summation of EPSPs and IPSPs from the

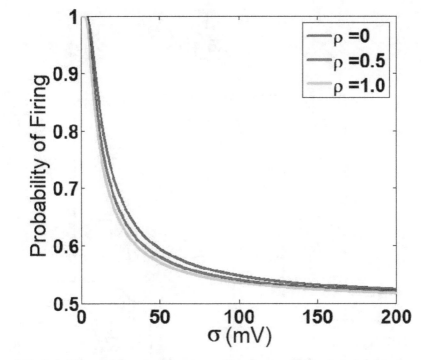

Figure 9.12. Probability of firing when neurotransmitter-release variability is included in two synapses. MATLAB [20].

dendrite arbor and after amplifying the signal and shaping the pulse, sends a rising edge to the spike generation stage circuit.

The spike generation circuit shown in figure 9.13 behaves like a self-resetting CMOS circuit. If the rising edge output from the input stage of the axon hillock crosses the threshold voltage, X2 turns ON. X1 is already ON in the resting state. Therefore, X1 and X2 pull the gate voltage of X8 low, opening the Na^+ ion channel. The output rises quickly to V_{dd}. As soon as the output goes high, the circuit resets itself; that means X4 turns ON, X1 turns OFF and finally X8 and X7 turn OFF and ON respectively. X7 is a model for K^+ ion channels. When X7 is ON that means K^+ ion channels open and the output returns to the low voltage (the resting potential). The width of the output spike is controlled by the delay of the inverter providing input to X7.

This spike-generation model can be used with no variability with ion-channel inputs controlled by the output of a simple amplifier (only necessary because the simplified experimental BioRC neurons used here have a small quantity of synapses) followed by an inverter pair that creates a fast rising edge required by the self-resetting circuit to generate a spike; i.e., opening and closing ion channels modeled by X8 and X7 is deterministic because the controls for these two channels have no variability. In order to include variability, we added X9 and X12 to the original input-stage circuit (figure 9.14) and applied a Gaussian noise or chaotic signal to the

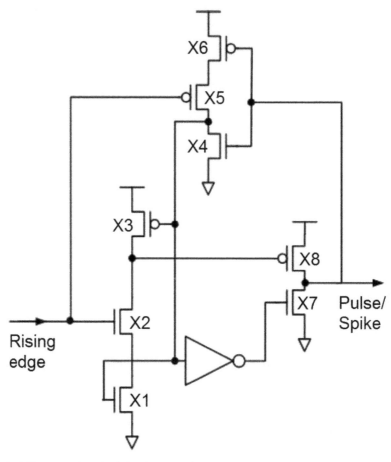

Figure 9.13. Spike generation circuit in the axon hillock module. Copyright 2009 IEEE. Reprinted, with permission, from [17].

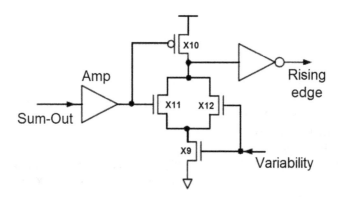

Figure 9.14. Axon hillock input stage with included variability [20].

gates of these transistors (labeled *variability*). The variable signal could prevent the neuron from firing or force the neuron to fire depending on the level of variability. When the variable signal is very small, X9 turns OFF; that signal could prevent the neuron from firing. When the *variability* signal rises to around 450 mV, X9 turns ON and the circuit behaves like the first inverter in the circuit with no variability. When the *variability* signal increases sufficiently, X12 turns ON and pulls down the output, sending a rising edge to the spike-generation circuit and the neuron fires. In this case, the variable signal forces the neuron to fire if the *variability* amplitude is sufficient. With a moderate change in input due to variability, the neuron fires reliably, depending on the membrane potential.

We also show how the variability changes the threshold voltage for firing. When the variable signal is low, it pushes the threshold voltage for firing close to V_{dd}. In this case, input to the axon that caused firing in the non-variable neuron is not able to cross the threshold and the variability prevents the neuron from firing. By increasing the variable signal, the threshold voltage is reduced and causes the neuron to fire even with low input, while the non-variable neuron would not fire. For a very high variability, the variable neuron fires with no input, that models spontaneous firing. Figure 9.15 shows the result for the experiments including ion-channel variability in the axon. We included a chaotic voltage signal with $V_{mid} = 450$ mV, $V_{pp} = 900$ mV and period of each sample 10 ps (green). At time 130 ps, PSP applied to the axon (purple) has an amplitude (200 mV) more than the threshold voltage (170 mV) and the neuron is expected to fire, however, because of the low chaotic signal at time 130 ps, the neuron does not fire (blue). In fact in this case, variability prevents the neuron from firing. At time 730 ps, the PSP is 150 mV less than the threshold voltage, but the chaotic signal at that time is strong enough to help the PSP to cross the threshold

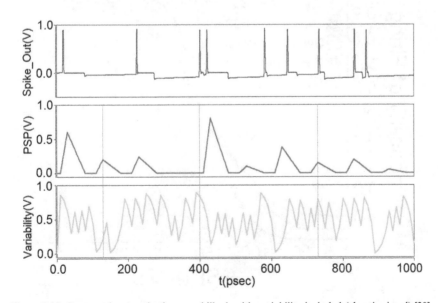

Figure 9.15. Input and output in the axon hillock with variability included (chaotic signal) [20].

and then the neuron fires. At time 400 ps, the PSP is 0 V, but variability forces the neuron to fire, modeling spontaneous firing.

We included Gaussian noise for the variability signal with $\mu = 450$ mV and $\sigma = 100$ mV in the axon. We applied several PSP samples with amplitude changing from 0 mV to 340 mV with 10 mV step size. For each PSP sample, we simulated the circuit 100 times with 100 Gaussian samples for ion-channel variability and summed the firing occurrences over 100 runs. We calculated the probability of firing for each PSP sample roughly by dividing the number of firing occurrences by 100. We repeated the experiment for Gaussian noise with different standard deviation ($\sigma = 200$ mV) and also for two types of chaotic signals, one with $V_{mid} = 450$ mV and $V_{pp} = 350$ mV, and another one with $V_{mid} = 450$ mV and $V_{pp} = 600$ mV. Figure 9.16 shows the result. The brown trace shows the result for the circuit with no variability. The threshold voltage is about 165 mV. When PSP changes from below the threshold to more than the threshold, the probability for the circuit with no variability jumps from zero to one. When small variability is included (green and blue traces), the probability changes less around the threshold voltage than the probability for the result with no variability. When variability is larger (purple and red traces), the probability changes are much smaller as PSP changes around the threshold voltage.

The results in figure 9.16 are approximately symmetric around the threshold because the mean of both the Gaussian signal and also the mid-point of the chaotic voltage are 450 mV. Therefore, the probability of variability forcing the neuron to fire is the same as the probability of preventing the neuron from firing. We ran the

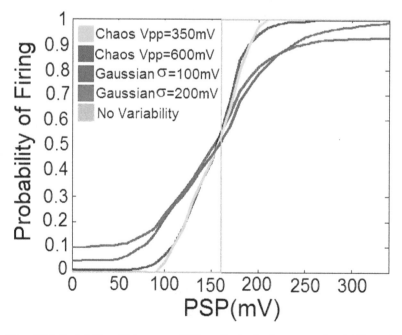

Figure 9.16. Probability of firing versus PSP amplitudes for four types of variability [20].

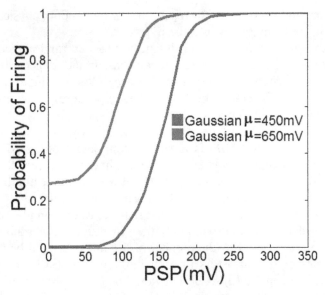

Figure 9.17. Probability of firing versus PSP amplitudes for Gaussian with two different mean values [20].

circuit for Gaussian noise with different mean (μ = 750 mV and σ = 100 mV). Figure 9.17 shows the result. When the mean of the Gaussian signal is higher, for the same PSP amplitude, the probability of firing is higher, meaning that the variability is more likely to force the neuron to fire rather than to prevent the neuron from firing. The probability of spontaneous firing (when PSP is zero) is higher when the mean of the Gaussian noise is higher.

9.5 Chaotic signal generation

9.5.1 Introduction

As we mentioned in the previous chapter, the source of synaptic variability or ion-channel variability could be either noise or chaos. In this chapter, both possible sources of variability are considered by embedding either Gaussian noise or a chaotic signal into the neuromorphic cortical neuron circuit. Therefore, we need to design two circuits, a noise generator circuit and a chaotic signal generator circuit.

Designing a good noise generator is not an easy task and is still a major research topic. The core of any kind of random number generator must be an intrinsically random physical process. So random generator designs range from tossing a coin, throwing a dice, drawing from an urn, drawing from a deck of cards and spinning a roulette to measuring thermal noise from a resistor and shot noise from a Zener diode or a vacuum tube, measuring radioactive decay from a radioactive source, integrating dark current from a metal insulator semiconductor capacitor, detecting locations of photo events and sampling a stable high-frequency oscillator with an unstable low frequency clock. The hard part of these designs is how to convert the noisiness of a physical process into a sequence of random numbers without suffering from the random and uncontrollable appearance of the random physical process and consequently introducing biases into the binary sequence.

Two well-known random generator designs are pseudo-random generators using LFSR (linear feedback shift register) and chaos-based random generators. Since the seventies, the use of chaotic dynamics for the generation of random sequences has raised a lot of interest. Several authors have already proposed to use chaotic systems as sources of physical randomness [24].

Beside the chaos-based random generator, LFSR is well known because of its simplicity. The output of LFSR is not a random signal but is pseudo random, because the output signal repeats after a certain time, and in fact the signal has a period. In LFSR, the period of sequence is $2^n - 1$ where n is the number of stages or number of flip-flops in the circuit. In order to get a signal closer to a random signal, the period needs to be a big number and that requires a large number of flip-flops in the design. In order to get approximately the same amount of randomness as the chaos-based random generator, the number of flip-flops needs to be more than 15. Assume the number of transistors in each flip-flop is at least 10, then the total number of transistors in the LFSR design would be 150. However, in a chaos-based random number generator, there are less than 40 transistors. Therefore, the chaos-based random generator has fewer transistors that make the size much smaller than the LFSR circuit and also the total power in the chaotic generator is lower.

For our cortical neuron circuit, we require a noise generator circuit and a chaotic signal generator circuit. For a noise generator circuit, we use the chaos-based random generator. Therefore, we only need to design a chaotic signal generator circuit. The output of that circuit could be applied directly to the cortical neuron circuit as a chaotic signal. Using the idea of chaos-based random number generators, we could generate random numbers after some data processing at the output of the chaotic signal generator.

In this chapter, we present a chaotic signal generator using carbon nanotube transistors. We first discuss different types of chaotic maps and choose one for this design, then we discuss the design at the transistor level and improve the design to get better performance.

9.5.2 Chaotic map

It is common to use a chaotic map for pseudo-random number generation. A chaotic map is in fact one or more nonlinear or piecewise linear functions and it is a nonlinear mapping, while most of the conventional random generators are linear (such as LFSR). Therefore, it is more complex and becomes a potential candidate to be a perfect random source. Some of the chaotic maps that are commonly used for the random number generator designs are a Logistic map, a Chebyshev map, a Skewed tent map, and a Sawtooth map. Among chaotic maps, we use a chaotic piecewise linear one-dimensional map because the implementation of this map can be done simply using switched capacitor or switch current circuits. We implement the design with switched current circuits that can operate at high frequencies [9].

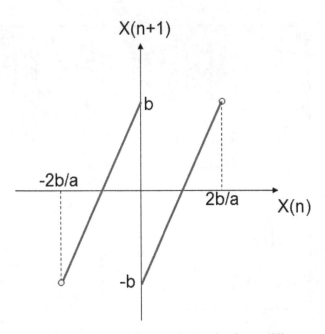

Figure 9.18. Transfer function for the chaotic map [20].

The chaotic map used in the design is described by the following recurrence relationship:

$$x_{n+1} = f(x_n) = \begin{cases} ax_n + b: x_n < 0 \\ ax_n - b: x_n \geqslant 0 \end{cases} \qquad (9.5)$$

where x_i is the ith sample of the generated sequence, and a and b are floating numbers. As shown in figure 9.18, the transfer function is mapping any $-2\frac{b}{a} < x_n < 2\frac{b}{a}$ to $-b < x_{n+1} < b$. Therefore, if $a < 1$, x_n converges and if $a > 2$, x_n diverges. Hence a must be in the range of $[1, 2]$ to ensure the output x_n, is in the range of $[-b, b]$. For a closer to 2, there is less redundancy and a better chaotic signal generator; however, when a gets closer to 2, there is a higher risk of appearance of periodic attractors and of breakdown of the chaotic signal generator [23].

In this map, x_n is a chaotic signal, however, if a random binary number is desired, based on the sign of x_n positive or negative, a binary one or zero is generated.

We analyzed this chaotic signal generator in MATLAB. Figure 9.19 shows a sequence of x_n for $a = 1.9$, $b = 1$, and $x_0 = 0.9$. In order to confirm the RNG designed here is an acceptable random generator, we did random property analysis (Bernoulli test) in MATLAB. We analyzed the number of ones and zeros and runs in the sequence of 100 000 bits of output.

9.6 Random pulse generation (RPG) noise generator

In modern digital systems, randomness is usually generated by a look-up table or linear feedback shift register and true random seeds [3], an approach that is actually

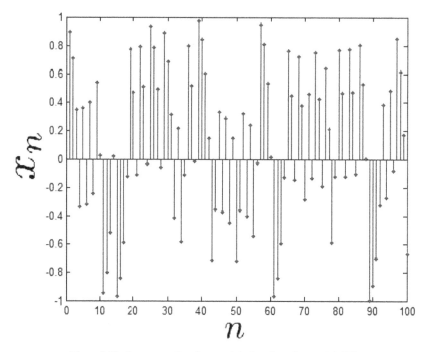

Figure 9.19. Sequence of x_n for $a = 1.9$, $b = 1$, and $x_0 = 0.9$ [20].

pseudo-random and may have problems with speed, power, and area cost. The digital nature of the signals may also cause accuracy issues when used with analog neurons. Analog devices are already prone to device mismatch or thermal noise, but the distribution of the noise is a mixture of multiple modes and stability is another issue of this kind of noise generation [14]. Moreover, the true randomness of the memristor, that shows a logarithmic distribution in resistance, is insufficient for modeling neural noise that has continuous variation in amplitude or frequency [12].

Here we present Kun Yue's CMOS-compatible true randomness generator using an opto-electronic device as a noise source for neuromorphic components in CMOS circuits. Photons generated by an LED, as a provably random quantum process, provide a way to realize a random pulse generator (RPG). Related work on noise generators has been widely reported but use in neuromorphic circuits has not been reported to date [22]. In neuromorphic circuits, independent randomness is important for noise to be a significant factor in neural information processing. Thus, in extensive neural networks containing noisy neurons, a large number of RPGs integrated in circuits can be expected, and, as a result, the RPGs must be power and area efficient.

The signals generated by an LED and single-photon avalanche diode are uniform distributed discrete pulses with Gaussian distributed amplitude. The photon intervals should be a Poisson distribution, but the constant quenching time of the single-photon avalanche diode device (SPAD) is much longer than the Poisson intervals [8]. To use the noise in this manner, Yue connects the RPG model followed

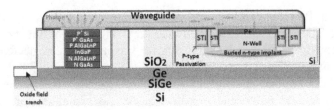

Figure 9.20. A cross-section view of the single-photon random pulse generator. Copyright 2017 IEEE. Reprinted, with permission, from [25].

by an amplifier to the neuromorphic circuit in our SPICE simulation. For continuous noise, Yue uses a current mirror circuit with certain leakage to convert the discrete signals to continuous signals, and then connect it in the SPICE simulation.

In order to model variability, the noise is applied as a neurotransmitter-availability control, noise is added to the PSP at the input of the dendritic arbor to model environmental noise, and noise is added to simulate threshold changes at the input of the threshold stage of the axon hillock that lies at the base of the axon. All three mechanisms model biological noisy behavior, bringing variability to the neuron in different ways and achieving more complex neural behaviors. These mechanisms have been developed in the past on the BioRC project by Mahvash and Parker [19], and more recently by Saeid and Parker [1].

9.6.1 Random pulse generator device

The RPG device consists of three parts: LED, SPAD, and waveguide. This structure has been experimentally verified by others [16]. Based on this structure, Yue assumes a red LED and SPAD device to implement an on-chip RPG. The cross-section of the device is shown in figure 9.20. using the platform SOLES reported by others [6]. The LED is compatible with CMOS technology.

The novel SPAD structure was emulated in SPICE using a CMOS 180 nm process [11]. A planar p–n junction is biased above breakdown in the core of SPAD, thus operating in Geiger mode. In this regime of operation, electron–hole pairs generated by photons can stimulate an avalanche breakdown by impact ionization. Because conventional avalanche photodiodes operate just below the breakdown voltage, the optical gain of the SPAD is high enough to enable single-photon sensing. Each photon absorbed in the active region can cause a large current to flow through the SPAD. In 180 nm CMOS circuits, both active and passive avalanche quenching schemes can be integrated, that enables this design to have a higher detection rate.

9.6.2 Discrete noise signals

LEDs are direct band gap devices that produce incoherent light by spontaneous emission, essentially a random process. If operated at sufficiently low power, an LED emits photons that are virtually independent of each other, this photon emission is a Poisson process, and the wavelength of photons is a Gaussian distribution. The exponentially-distributed time intervals of the Poisson process for photon emission and the photon loss in the waveguide are neglected, because the quenching time of *SPAD* is much longer.

In this RPG model, the output is uniform distributed discrete pulses with Gaussian distributed amplitude in µV. To use this signal in our neuromorphic circuits, we have to amplify it to a mV-scale pulse. The complete circuit of the discrete noise generator is shown in figure 9.21.

The photons are simulated as voltage responses in SPAD. The strength of photons depends on the wavelength, that is Gaussian. The photon detection efficiency of SPAD is also a Gaussian process related to wavelength. Thus Yue chose 615 nm peak wavelength and $\sigma = 30$ for both LED and SPAD as the simulation parameters. The simulation results of simulated photon voltage and noise signals are shown in figure 9.22.

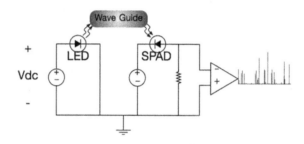

Figure 9.21. Circuit of the discrete noise generator. Copyright 2017 IEEE. Reprinted, with permission, from [25].

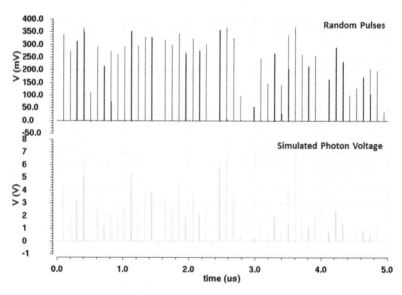

Figure 9.22. Discrete noise signals: random pulses (upper trace) and simulated photon voltage (lower trace). Copyright 2017 IEEE. Reprinted, with permission, from [25].

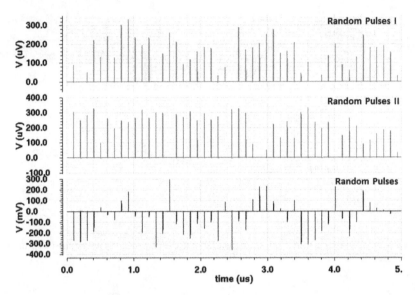

Figure 9.23. Corner situation of random pulses with positive and negative values. Copyright 2017 IEEE. Reprinted, with permission, from [25].

The above noise signals only include positive pulses. In neural systems, the noise can be both positive and negative. To accomplish this with our RPG, Yue uses two RPGs and connects them to one amplifier. The output can be calculated with the following equation:

$$V_{out} = -A(V_1 - V_2) + V_1$$

where V_1 and V_2 are the inputs to the amplifier and A is the gain of the amplifier. The corner situation is the two inputs having the exact same phase, so that the pulses could theoretically cancel each other. However, the amplitude of the two signals is usually different, and this allows the circuit to generate robust random positive and negative pulses (figure 9.23).

9.6.3 Continuous noise signals

To generate continuous noise signals, Hue connects the RPG to a current mirror (figure 9.24). The charge accumulates at the output, and gradually is discharged by the leakage signal. Thus Yue creates a continuous noise signal (figure 9.26(a)), but in this manner, the noise cannot be negative. The solution is the same as the method Yue used for discrete noise signals. Two continuous signals are connected to an amplifier (figure 9.25), one of the signals is inverted and the output is the summation of inputs. The result of the continuous noise generation is shown in figure 9.26(b).

9.6.4 Probability and distribution

The probability of the true randomness from a single-photon random pulse generator is determined by the quenching time of SPAD and single-photon

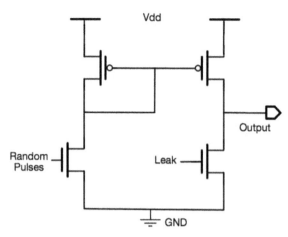

Figure 9.24. Current mirror circuit. Copyright 2017 IEEE. Reprinted, with permission, from [25].

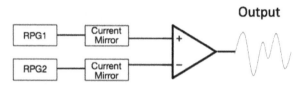

Figure 9.25. Circuit for continuous noise. Copyright 2017 IEEE. Reprinted, with permission, from [25].

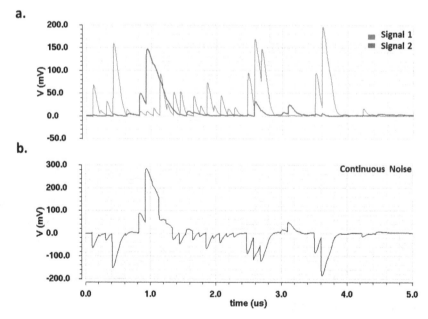

Figure 9.26. Continuous noise signal and summed positive and negative noise signals. Copyright 2017 IEEE. Reprinted, with permission, from [25].

generation. By varying the two parameters above, different probabilities can be achieved. Furthermore, combining more RPGs together also can change the probability significantly. The probability of the RPG is Poisson distributed, while the noise that comes from LED and SPAD is also Poisson distributed. The thermal noise from the amplifier could affect the probability distribution seriously, but with more advanced amplifier noise reduction technology and SPAD technology, the signal-to-noise ratio (SNR) can be controlled effectively. More future work has been scheduled to optimize the SNR. On the other hand, the thermal noise can be treated as another randomness source to be used in the neuromorphic system.

9.7 Chapter summary

This chapter focused on Mahvash's circuit implementations of neurotransmitter release variability and ion channel variability, using stochastic signals and chaotic signals. Chaotic signal and random signal generating circuits were discussed. The chapter concluded with Yue's circuits using random photons from LEDs to generate noise.

The next chapter focuses on learning and strengthening.

Certain sections of text in this chapter have been reproduced with permission from [19], [25] and [26]. Copyright IEEE.

References

[1] Barzegarjalali S and Parker A C 2015 A hybrid neuromorphic circuit demonstrating schizophrenic symptoms *2015 Biomedical Circuits and Systems Conf. (BioCAS) IEEE* (Piscataway, NJ: IEEE) 1–4

[2] BazsÛ F, Zal·nyi L and Cs·rdi G 2003 Channel noise in Hodgkin-Huxley model neurons *Phys. Lett.* A **311** 13–20

[3] Blum L, Blum M and Shub M 1986 A simple unpredictable pseudo-random number generator *SIAM J. Sci. Comput.* **15** 364–83

[4] Cecchi G A *et al* 2000 Noise in neurons is message dependent *Proc. Natl. Acad. Sci.* **97** 5557–61

[5] Chen H *et al* 2010 Real-time simulation of biologically realistic stochastic neurons in VLSI *IEEE Trans. Neural Netw.* **21** 1511–7

[6] Chilukuri K *et al* 2006 Monolithic CMOS-compatible AlGaInP visible LED arrays on silicon on lattice-engineered substrates (SOLES) *Semicond. Sci. Technol.* **22** 29

[7] Chow C C and White J A 1996 Spontaneous action potentials due to channel fluctuations *Biophys. J* **71** 3012–21

[8] Cova S *et al* 1996 Avalanche photodiodes and quenching circuits for single-photon detection *Appl. Opt.* **35** 1956–76

[9] Delgado-Restituto M, Medeiro F and Rodriguez-Vazquez A 1993 Nonlinear switched-current CMOS IC for random signal generation *Electron. Lett.* **29** 2190–1

[10] Faisal A A, White J A and Laughlin S B 2005 Ion-channel noise places limits on the miniaturization of the brain's wiring *Curr. Biol.* **5** 1143–9

[11] Faramarzpour N *et al* 2008 Fully integrated single photon avalanche diode detector in standard CMOS 0.18 μm Technology *IEEE Trans. Electron Devices* **55** 760–7

[12] Gaba S *et al* 2013 Stochastic memristive devices for computing and neuromorphic applications *Nanoscale* **5** 5872–8

[13] Gerstein G L and Mandelbrot B 1964 Random walk models for the spike activity of a single neuron *Biophys. J.* **4** 41–68

[14] Timothy Holman W, Alvin Connelly J and Dowlatabadi A B 1997 An integrated analog/digital random noise source *IEEE Trans. Circuits Syst.* I **44** 521–8

[15] Hsu C-C 2014 Dendritic computation and plasticity in neuromorphic circuits *PhD Thesis* University of Southern California

[16] Huang B *et al* 2011 CMOS monolithic optoelectronic integrated circuit for on-chip optical interconnection *Opt. Commun.* **284** 3924–7

[17] Joshi J *et al* 2009 *A carbon nanotube cortical neuron with excitatory and inhibitory dendritic computations IEEE/NIH 2009 LIfe Science Systems and Applications Workshop (LiSSA 2009)*

[18] Joshi J 2013 Plasticity in CMOS Neuromorphic Circuits *PhD Thesis* University of Southern California

[19] Mahvash M and Parker A C 2013 Synaptic variability in a cortical neuromorphic circuit *Neural Netw. Learn. Syst.* **24** 397–409

[20] Mahvash Mohammadi M 2012 Emulating variability in the behavior of artificial central neurons *PhD Thesis* University of Southern California

[21] Stein A R B 1965 Theoretical analysis of neuronal variability *Biophys. J.* **5** 173–94

[22] Stipčević M and Medved Rogina B 2007 Quantum random number generator based on photonic emission in semiconductors *Rev. Sci. Instrum.* **78** 045104

[23] Stojanovski T and Kocarev L 2001 Chaos based random number generators, part I: analysis *IEEE Trans. Circuits Syst.* I **48** 281–8

[24] Stojanovski T and Kocarev L 2001 Chaos based random number generators, part II: practical realization *IEEE Trans. Circuits Syst.* I **48** 382–5

[25] Yue K and Parker A C 2017 Noisy neuromorphic neurons with RPG on-chip noise source *2017 Int. Joint Conf. Neural Networks (IJCNN)* (Piscataway, NJ: IEEE) 1225–9

[26] Mahvash M and Parker A C 2011 Modeling intrinsic ion-channel and synaptic variability in a cortical neuromorphic circuit *2011 IEEE Biomedical Circuits and Systems Conf. (BioCAS) (San Diego, CA)* 69–72

IOP Publishing

Neuromorphic Circuits
A constructive approach
Alice C Parker and Rick Cattell

Chapter 10

Learning and strengthening

Jon Joshi, Kun Yue, Eric Evans, Dena Giovinazzo and Alice C Parker

This chapter provides a view of some advanced neural circuit structures that model biological mechanisms like learning and strengthening. The chapter begins by modeling structural plasticity, like that found in the barrel cortex of the rat, using neuromorphic circuits. The chapter then presents a neuromorphic blank slate neuronal network that models developmental learning. A developmental approach to learning is described in this section. Neurons are essentially blank slates, with no ability to respond differently to inputs. Training is done incrementally for each task, and only a few neurons are recruited for each task. As synapses are strengthened, their responses to presynaptic neurons become less noisy. Synapses are strengthened by synaptic timing-dependent plasticity (STDP) if training inputs and noise combined are sufficient to cause spiking in a postsynaptic neuron. Synapse strength is made persistent by dopamine when dopaminergic neurons fire to indicate successful learning. A programmable neuromorphic neuron architecture, PRONON, that supports learning, concludes the chapter.

10.1 Structural plasticity

An engineering solution to the rewiring of the cortex presents many challenges. The first challenge begins with silicon implementation of neural circuits, silicon being a substance that cannot change its structural properties over time. For a restructurable neuromimetic network we need new connections to be made with a hardwired approach in silicon; this proves virtually impossible without bulky, complicated reconfiguration circuitry. Changes in synapse numbers and usage call for new hardware to be created on the fly, a daunting task with our current technological capabilities in silicon. Hence, in this text, we must model structural changes in a silicon neural network behaviourally by anticipating such changes and designing in capabilities. Change in inter-neuron connection strength with increase or decrease in the number of synapses is a plausible contributor towards memory and change in sensory perception. The second challenge is to create a design methodology and a library of circuits representing neural compartments that can support the rapid design and implementation of neural circuits as additional significant neural mechanisms are understood, and can support the design of a wide variety of the cortical neurons without extensive redesign. A consequence of the second challenge is the need for the methodology to have circuits that are adaptable in a plug and play fashion, rather than with a black-box approach to designing complete neurons.

10.1.1 Approach to neuromorphic network restructuring using synapse claiming

Structural plasticity, in the form of network restructuring, is thought to be important to learning. To model structural plasticity, described in section 1.6, using a neuro-morphic circuit, Joshi introduced a method called *synapse claiming*, a circuit technique for network restructuring. Our first step towards structural plasticity is to claim inactive synapse structures autonomously and use them where activity warrants increased synapses in parallel with existing synapses. Our circuits monitor synapses for activity and when there is no activity for a long time (scaled down to order of nanoseconds for simulation) and the adjacent synapse is active, the inactive synapse is claimed to strengthen the active synapse[1]. All figures in this subsection were originally published in [3].

Figure 10.1 shows the detailed circuit schematic of a section of the network where a presynaptic neuron with increased activity can claim the synapse of a presynaptic neuron that has no neural activity. The switches shown are modeled using trans-mission gates. The switches emulate the creation and elimination of different synaptic connections. These switches are controlled using different time constants *ST* (slower time) constant and *FT* (fast time) constant. These time constants emulate different mechanisms behind the formation and elimination of a synapse. Some electrical connections (FT to ST and ST to FT) have been made to model their actions as system time constants without modeling the underlying mechanisms that are complex and not well understood. The synapses have been split into pre- and postsynaptic sections [3] to emulate synaptogenesis as discussed in section 1.6. The neuron circuits in synapse claiming include a spiking axon hillock, an excitatory synapse and an inhibitory synapse, as described in chapter 6.

The FT and ST circuits are basic four-transistor integrator circuits, as shown in figure 10.2, that are sized to provide required FT and ST constants. The input to each circuit is a train of spikes from a neuron and the output for control signals FT and ST is a rising (slow or fast) potential which falls at a rate controlled by *Vbias*.

Figure 10.3 shows the situation when both neurons N1 and N2 are active (black circle 1). N1 and N2 firing activate mechanisms FT1 and FT2, respectively (black circle 2). Active FT1 and FT2 control signals complete the neural connections to N3 (black circle 3) through synapses 1 and 2. FT1 and FT2 inactivate ST1 and ST2 (black circle 4) to prevent them from closing neural connections (black circle 5) by

---

[1] Note that reclaiming rarely-used synapses might be dangerous in that the rare firing might be the most important scenario, and should be investigated in the future.

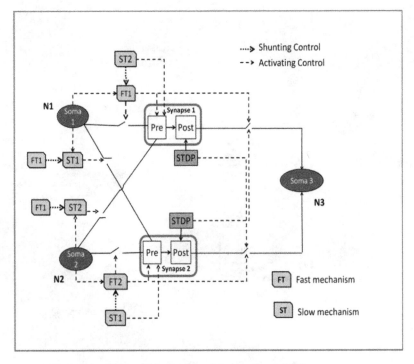

Figure 10.1. Synapse-claiming schematic [3].

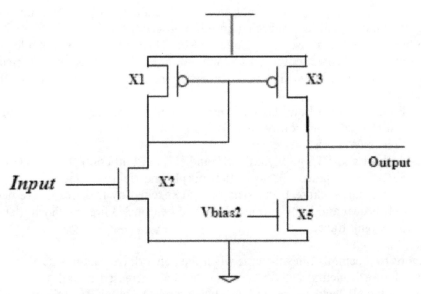

Figure 10.2. Circuit used to model the FT and ST time constants. Copyright 2013 IEEE. Reprinted, with permission, from [4].

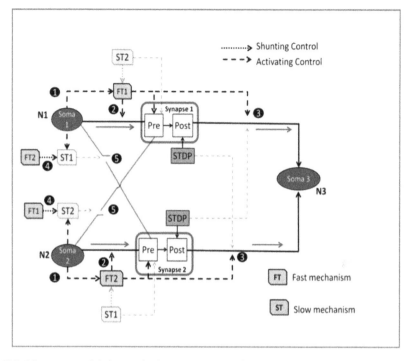

Figure 10.3. No synapse claiming as both neurons are active. Copyright 2013 IEEE. Reprinted, with permission, from [4].

grounding their outputs. This emulates the situation when neurons are actively firing; they have synapses connected and do not lose them.

Joshi simulated this case using Cadence SPECTRE (TSMC 18 technology) and the results are presented in figure 10.4. Simulation results for this case are presented in two halves, left and right. The results are explained with the following sequence of events:

1. Both neurons N1 and N2 (red and light pink traces), are active causing their fast time constant control signals (FT1 and FT2) to go high (left orange and right blue traces).

2. As FT1 and FT2 go high, the ST and FT constant control signals (ST1 and ST2) are grounded (disabled) (left purple and right red traces).

3. As a result synapse 1 and synapse 2 are excited by their respective neurons (left brown and right purple traces) and neuron N3 fires as shown (left/right dark pink trace).

Figure 10.5 demonstrates the case when the network restructures its connectivity due to change in neural activity. Neuron N2 has increased neural activity (black circle 1) while N1 lacks neural activity (black circle 2). N2 firing activates FT2 and ST2. FT2 deactivates ST1 so that N1 cannot form a new connection with synapse 2 (black circle 3). FT2 completes the connection with N3 via synapse 2 (black circle 4).

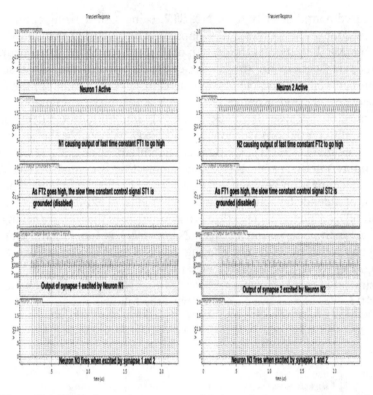

Figure 10.4. Simulation results: no synapse claiming as both neurons are active [3].

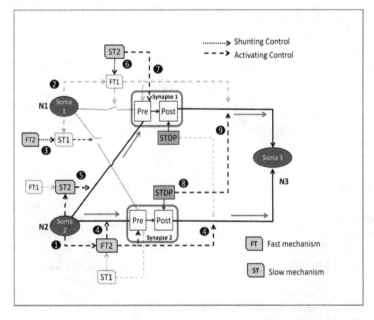

Figure 10.5. Synapse claiming as N2 is active and N1 lacks neural activity [4].

With increased neural activity from N2, ST2, being a slow rising control begins to make a new connection from N2 to synapse 1, which was left unclaimed by lack of activity from N1. This models the growth of an axon due to increased neural activity as described in section 1.6 (black circle 5). ST2 deactivates FT1 so that the connection between N1 and N3 is eliminated (black circle 6). With the connection formed between N2 and synapse 1, ST2 will activate the presynaptic side of the newly connected synapse 1 (black circle 7) emulating the effect of PRESD (presynaptic differentiation) (section 1.6). PRESD will enable the receptor side of synapse 1 to emulate POSD (postsynaptic differentiation) as described in section 1.6. With continuous activity the postsynaptic connection is completed (black circle 8) and so is the connection between synapse 1 and N3 (black circle 9). This emulates the growth of a dendritic spine with increase in local synaptic activity (section 1.6). As a result N2 is connected to N3 through two synapses thus strengthening its neural pathway. Also the connection between N1 and N3 is functionally eliminated by switching controlled by ST2, thus altering the connectivity of the network. Thus, by reusing hardware, we are able to change network properties.

Joshi simulated this case using Cadence SPECTRE and the results are presented in figure 10.6. The results are explained with the following sequence of events:

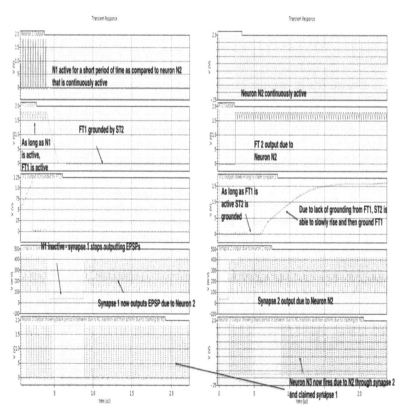

Figure 10.6. Simulation results: synapse claiming as N2 is active and N1 lacks neural activity. Copyright 2013 IEEE. Reprinted, with permission, from [4].

1. Joshi made N1 active for a short period of time (left red trace, 0–500 ns) as compared to N2 (right light pink trace) which is continuously active.
2. As observed in the figure, as long as N1 is active, FT1 is active (left orange trace) and ST2 is grounded (right red trace). This prevents N2 from claiming synapse 1.
3. When N1 is inactive (after 500 ns), synapse 1 stops outputting excitatory postsynaptic potentials (EPSPs) (500 ns to 900 ns).
4. During that interval as N2 is still active and due to lack of grounding from FT1, ST2 is able to slowly rise (right red trace) and then ground FT1. This indicates a loss of connection between synapse 1 and N1.
5. With ST2 rising, the switch between N2 and synapse 1 is closed thus indicating the formation of a new connection between N2 and synapse 1. This is demonstrated with synapse 1 outputting EPSPs after the interval (left brown trace, 900 ns) and neuron N3 firing (left/right dark pink trace, 900 ns).

Hence, synapse 1 is claimed by neuron N2. Joshi used this circuit in his thesis in an example that discusses the modeling of structural changes in the rat whisker receptive field.

10.2 The blank slate cortical column

10.2.1 Learning without forgetting

The research described in this section considers lifelong learning to be the ability of a system to retain skills and memory even when learning new skills or memorizing new information. The memory retained is not just facts but connections between them, and between steps involved in skill execution. The skills and memory are added during executions of behavior, and can be retrieved by triggering the neurons and neural connections with external inputs or situations related to their formation and utility. In order to exhibit lifelong learning without catastrophic forgetting, neuromorphic neural networks must possess the ability to learn on the fly, online, in real time, without forgetting previously acquired skills. Learning/training is continuous without distinct training and testing phases, and without supervision. The neuronal network continuously consolidates new information and ignores irrelevant information and noise. As skills and memories are retrieved, they could be edited with new situations or new inputs, and stored as variations to current skills and memory by adding additional inputs and neurons present in the cortical column but silent or weak. The system could learn new skills or carry out learned tasks with the same hardware, with inputs changing as tasks change. Old memories and skills are not forgotten as new skills and memory are added. In the research described in this section, these capabilities have only been tested at this point by adding one new skill, moving backward, triggered by fear, to the 'moving forward' skill triggered by desire.

10.2.2 Related research on dopamine

The neurotransmitter dopamine is used to create persistent synaptic strength in the synapses that cause movement. Dopamine is a complex neurotransmitter that falls into a class of transmitters called monoamine neurotransmitters. These transmitters contain a smaller group, the catecholamines, including norepinephrine and epinephrine. Dopamine regulates motor neurons, reward and pleasure, among other functions. Dopamine regulates neuronal behavior rather than acting as a data-processing transmitter. Dopamine can be transferred by being released near the presynaptic terminal by action potentials, called phasic transmission, or can be extracellular dopamine attached to receptors at the presynaptic terminal, called tonic transmission. Dopamine can excite or inhibit postsynaptic neurons, depending on the neural structure. It is worth noting here that dopamine is a neurotransmitter that has complex effects on neural circuitry, acting as a reward and also signals a reaction to surprise, for example. Here, dopamine is used as a reward to make synaptic strengths persistent, but there are many other meanings and reactions to dopamine in the human brain. The latest publications indicate that much is still missing in the understanding of dopamine in the human nervous system [5]. Other relevant dopamine publications are cited here [2, 7, 8].

10.2.3 Architecture of the blank slate cortical column

In the biological cortex, neurons are arranged in cortical columns. Neurons in sequence form chains. Each neuron in sequence in a chain belongs to a layer of neurons. Neurons in the chains, in the same layer or neighboring layers, connect with each other across the chains, usually in an inhibitory manner.

There are six layers in each biological cortical column, numbered I to VI, with the first layer being the outermost layer of the cortex and the sixth being connected to white matter. Signaling flow is columnar from layer VI to layer I and laminar between columns. Signaling between columns and between chains in the same column is often inhibitory. Figure 10.7 illustrates a biological cortical column. The blank slate cortical column is a neuromorphic structure designed to function somewhat like a biological cortical column, similar to the column shown in figure 10.7. The blank slate cortical column was designed to be used in a NeuRoBot cortex to support task learning without catastrophic forgetting when a new task is learned.

The NeuRoBot (robot with a nervous system) has been trained to walk forward and then backward using a cortical column of noisy neurons subject to STDP and made non-forgetting with synapses made persistent by dopamine. This section describes that cortical column.

Each cortical column of neurons contains dopaminergic neurons that respond if an input to them is detected that represents a different outcome from previous inputs, responding to novelty, or any outcome that stimulates the presynaptic dopaminergic neurons. The presynaptic dopaminergic signals can be from earlier neurons in the cortical column, another part of the robot's neural network, or from an external signal. In this NeuRoBot example, the signals come from the cortical column itself.

If a different outcome is detected from the network than previously, and the dopaminergic neurons fires, all synapse strengths that contributed to the outcome

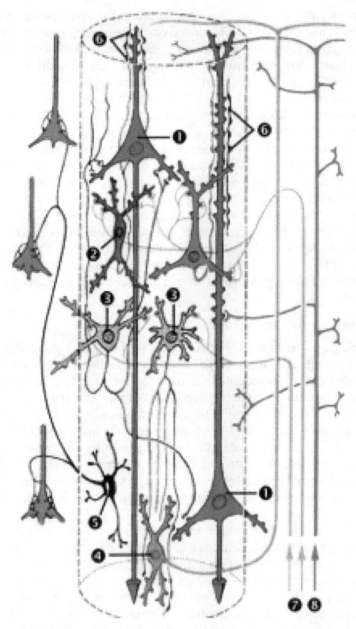

Figure 10.7. Cortical column in a biological neuron: simplified model of a cortical column. First hypothetical model of neuronal networks within a cortical column based on morphological data that included both principal, excitatory neurons and inhibitory GABAergic interneurons known at the time. Structures shown in black circles:1 pyramidal neurons in layers 2/3 and 5; 2 double bouquet cell; 3 spiny stellate neurons in layer 4; 4 Martinotti cells in layer 6; 5 basket cells in layer 5 establishing axo-somatic contacts with pyramidal neurons; 6 *en passant* axons of double bouquet cells establishing synaptic contacts on apical dendrites of pyramidal neurons. 7 Thalamic afferents; 8 asiational fibres from [6] (modified from *'Taschenatlas der Anatomie'* Thieme Verlag, Stuttgart/New York, copyright 2007, with permission from Springer Nature).

are made persistent (rewarded) by applying an input that represents an application of dopamine. Then the next task is trained on the remaining weak neurons (trained neurons essentially ignore the new inputs because the trained neurons become less noisy and hence less responsive). Mutual inhibition (inhibitory interneurons) separate neurons trained to different tasks that are organized in different rows of the blank slate network, as in biological cortical columns.

This approach has been applied to train a NeuRoBot's brain neurons to walk forwards or backwards depending on input signaling, using an electronic neural network. The neural network is designed and simulated using analog CMOS electronics. The input signals that trigger task learning and that the robot responds to are *desire* that causes forward motion and *fear* that causes backward motion.

Experimental circuits forcing the robot to freeze in the presence of sensed *pain* have also been developed and are covered in section 10.2.8.

The approach can also be used with software neural networks, or any neuromorphic computing network that has noisy neurons, control over synaptic strength persistence, STDP, and permanence caused by dopamine. A video can be accessed that shows the robot's legs moving forward and backward as training occurs[2].

10.2.4 Blank slate training approach

In the blank slate, neurons are essentially blank slates, with no ability to respond differently to inputs than other similar neurons. Training is done incrementally for each task, and only a few neurons are recruited for each task. In the blank slate, neurons are arranged in columns, input to output, and the chains of neurons mutually inhibit each other, similar to cortical columns in the biological cortex. All neurons begin with weak synapses. All synapses in the first layer of neurons receive all inputs. Neurons self-select for tasks depending on noisy synapses in those neurons that randomly respond to inputs. As synapses are strengthened, their responses to presynaptic neurons become less noisy. Synapses are strengthened by STDP if training inputs and noise combined are sufficient to cause spiking in a postsynaptic neuron.

This section presents an approach to lifelong learning without forgetting. Key to this learning approach is that neurons and their networks, including synapses, begin training with weak synapses that do not evoke spiking. A small group of neurons is randomly selected with sufficient noise and their synapses trained for a task, without activating large quantities of other neurons or synapses[3]. If the task is successful, trained neurons have their synaptic strengths made persistent. Using this approach, trained neurons must have persistent synaptic strength that cannot be erased when learning new tasks, inhibiting catastrophic forgetting. Once a neuronal network is trained, recruitment and activation of these neurons for further learning must be dampened. Neurons activated to implement a task must mutually inhibit neurons

---

[2] https://drive.google.com/file/d/1QVIZ7Ojyi_u4Dmx0Ib-xDCfxg79065qs/view?usp=sharing
[3] We associate strengthening synapses that connect to postsynaptic neurons with strengthening the neurons themselves.

that implement other tasks. While supervised training can achieve these goals, learning online, on the fly, is more practical when learning is autonomous. Although the implementation described here involves analog neuromorphic circuits, the basic principles support learning for any implementation framework.

The learning approach here shows that lifelong learning can be developmental, as in biological systems, with learning proceeding incrementally, and with neurons not involved in the learning weakly connected to other neurons. Neurons involved in learning exhibit synapse strengthening due to STDP that becomes persistent due to dopamine if those neurons contributed to success in carrying out a task. This results in a learning process that is more bottom-up than top-down, with a few neurons learning a task during that task's training.

In addition, the approach involves neurons that spike with several different spiking patterns (a neural code) that allows neurons to be reused for multiple, varying tasks, making networks more efficient. Frequency of spiking to subcortical neurons signals priority of movement as well as mode. Tonic spiking signals forward movement and fast spiking signals backward movement. The neural code allows neurons to selectively activate downstream neurons, supporting reuse of portions of neuronal networks to carry out different tasks, while avoiding modification of existing portions of neuronal networks that do not contribute to learning or carrying out the current task. One movement is triggered at a time, with all neurons on layer 1 of the blank slate network receiving all input 'emotions,' in the example cases of desire and fear.

Learning by training, whether autonomously or supervised, can occur top-down or bottom-up, whether one implements a neural network with software, digital hardware or analog hardware. Bottom-up training trains a neural network by training a neuron or small number of neurons at a time, then trains other neurons on a different task. If the tasks are stated to be mutually exclusive, the neurons are connected with inhibitory interneurons so that tasks are not confused, if the tasks are independent. Here, the approach is bottom-up, using analog hardware.

Synaptic noise (and threshold noise), as in biological neurons, support accidental firing so that neurons previously silent can begin training. Noise is the trigger for random selection of firing neurons that become trained to recognize the need for and carry out tasks. Noisy synapses isolate single neuron chains that lacked previous training coincident with 'emotions' like *desire* to find a target or *fear* that results in retreat. The manner in which these neuromorphic neuronal networks are trained involves several mechanisms. The approach involves weak synapses that are awakened randomly because they are inherently *noisy*. Noisy synapses are described in section 9.3. Conventional spiking neural networks can suffer from catastrophic forgetting, and have difficulties with generalizing, with learning competing tasks, and with few-shot learning. The noisy potential produced by a noisy synapse, if sufficiently large, could cause the postsynaptic neuron to spike, kick-starting the learning process. If the awakened synapses result in firing in the postsynaptic neuron, the synapses are strengthened using the *STDP* mechanism, as described in section 6.4. If the awakened synapses result in successful completion of a task, detected by a downstream neuron that signals with dopamine, as designed by

Yue [9], STDP-strengthened upstream synapses that contributed to the task completion will subsequently possess persistent strengths (long-term potentiation (LTP) in biological neurons) due to dopamine that cannot be easily weakened with subsequent training.

This approach assumes a pool of available synapses and neurons for learning. With bottom-up training, all neurons are not used in training like in top-down learning used in traditional spiking neural networks (SNNs). New synapses and neurons are recruited for new or generalized tasks while the remaining portions of the network are dormant.

Because any susceptible neuron could spike due to noise, and evoke a task further downstream, a method to signal specific tasks that are desired could (and perhaps should) include forcing the susceptible neuron to spike with a neural pattern or neural code that differed from codes used to invoke other tasks.

A neural code makes neural networks more efficient, since single neurons and their axons can convey different messages, using limited resources more efficiently. Learning without forgetting can be implemented overlaying new knowledge on the same neurons spiking differently, sharing limited resources. A specific spiking pattern by a neuron could indicate either new learning or previous learning. In the NeuRoBot described here, fast spiking signals a move backward, and normal spiking indicates a move forward.

10.2.5 Training the blank slate neuromorphic network

An initial example *blank slate* neuromorphic network is shown in figure 10.8. There are two inputs to the example blank slate network, *desire* and *fear*. After learning, desire should cause the robot to move forward and fear should cause it to move backward. All synapses in the blank slate network are weak. Two neuron chains are

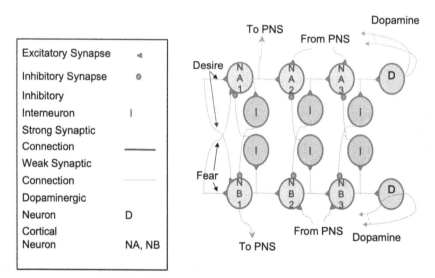

Figure 10.8. The initial blank slate network used to initiate the learning process.

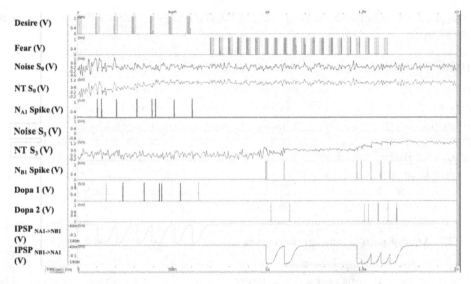

Figure 10.9. Simulation results for the blank slate network: results vary depending on the noise statistics.

shown, *NA* and *NB*. Interneurons that are inhibitory connect across the two chains. This helps one chain train for desire—forward movement, and the other train for fear—backward movement. Which chain performs which function is not predetermined.

The timing diagram (simulation results) are shown in figure 10.9. The simulation begins with neurons in a weak, resting state. The emotion spike *desire* is sent to both chains, but no spiking occurs until noise is added to the synapse of neuron A1, S0. A1 spikes, causing signals to be sent to the subcortical network. A signal is returned from the subcortical network. acknowledging the command sent, causing a second A neuron to fire. The third A neuron awaits a signal from the subcortical network that movement has occurred. When the movement signal is received, the third A neuron spikes. In the process of spiking, all neurons have their participating synapses strengthened due to STDP. The *NT* signal shows the neurotransmitter as noise is added/subtracted to the neurotransmitter produced by the *desire* signal. The next neuron in the chain, a D dopaminergic neuron, is triggered by the A neuron chain and sends dopamine to all A neurons that spiked previously, making their synapse strengths persistent. For the purposes of the experiment, noise is added to the NA1 and NB1 neurons, and the chain selected for movement due to desire is randomly selected depending on the different noise characteristics of the two neurons. Noise decreases in the trained A1 neuron, much like in the biological neuron.

In the video[4] the robot is seen to move forward. Random noise is now added to the B neuron chain along with the fear signal, but takes some time to be large enough to evoke spiking, so that the B chain is activated by fear only when there is

---

[4] https://drive.google.com/file/d/1QVIZ7Ojyi_u4Dmx0Ib-xDCfxg79065qs/view?usp=sharing

enough additive noise to evoke spiking in the B chain. The robot moves backward in the video.

10.2.6 The neural code in the blank slate

While the blank slate approach itself is developmental, signaling to the subcortical regions about intended motion is predetermined in this implementation. Signaling to subcortical regions has been reduced to a single *efferent* signal, with tonic spiking implying forward motion and fast spiking implying backward motion. Different *afferent* signals from the subcortical region imply that a motion signal has been received, or that motion has occurred. Once motion occurs, the dopaminergic neuron in the activated neuron chain releases dopamine, and nearby neurons have their synaptic strengths made persistent by the dopamine release.

10.2.7 Adding pain signals to the inputs

10.2.7.1 The chain architecture

There are two neurons and a dopaminergic neuron in the pain response chain. The first neuron receives a 10 ns continuous spike train as its input to the blank slate cortical column. The spike output of the first neuron is input to the subcortical system to signal it to stop moving, and is also input to the second neuron in the chain. The subcortical system sends its confirmation that it has stopped moving to the second neuron in the chain. When the second neuron receives inputs from both the subcortical system and the first neuron, it will also fire. Its output goes to the dopamine neuron, which releases dopamine to both neurons when the second neuron fires. Both neurons output high frequency spikes (higher than fear) that sit on a DC level. The chain architecture is shown in figure 10.10.

Currently, this neuron chain is missing an inhibitory neuron. That would be integrated when the pain circuit is integrated with desire and fear in the combined

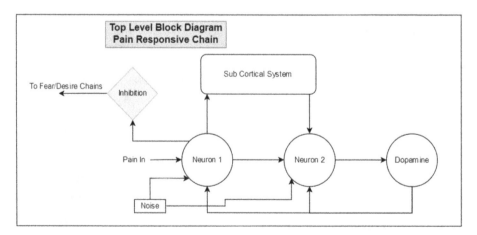

Figure 10.10. Top-level block diagram: pain-responsive chain.

cortical column. For this circuit, the subcortical and noise signals are digital signals that vary between supply and ground. A synapse can convert these digital signals to biological signals so that they more accurately mimic real life signals.

10.2.7.2 Results
The graph in figure 10.11 shows the full response of the pain-responsive chain. The first signal is the 10 nS pain input. The second signal is the noise present at the beginning of the simulation. The third signal is the subcortical response after going through a synapse. The third signal starts after the first neuron begins regularly firing. The fourth signal is the dopamine response. The first dopamine spike is a response to the first and second neurons randomly firing due to noise. The second dopamine spike is from the second neuron firing because it received inputs from both the first neuron and the subcortical system. The fifth signal is the action potential output of the first neuron, and the sixth and final signal is the action potential output of the second neuron.

10.2.7.3 Future work on the pain circuit
This neuron chain is capable of responding to pain, but it does not have the capability of learning from pain and avoiding it in the future. The article 'Rate and temporal coding mechanisms in the anterior cingulate cortex for pain anticipation' by Urien *et al* provides a hypothesis of how neurons can learn to avoid pain [10]. In short, there are neurons that specifically respond to pain once it has already occurred, and there are neurons that learn to avoid pain when they receive a 'trigger' input.

The memory neuron is only capable of firing when receiving the trigger signal and the output of N1. This is the neuron that learns to associate pain and the trigger

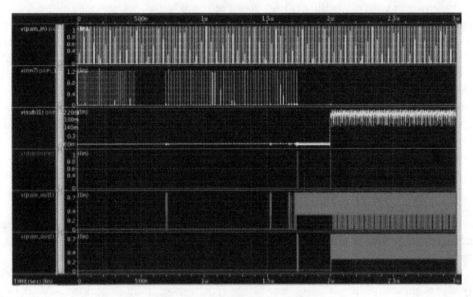

Figure 10.11. Simulation of the pain response circuit.

together. When it is successful, it causes a dopamine release to strengthen this bond. The pain avoidance neuron has two inputs: the trigger signal and the output of the memory neuron. Initially, the pain avoidance neuron only fires when the memory neuron fires, as well as receiving the trigger signal. After dopamine is released however, ideally this neuron is strong enough to fire from the trigger signal alone. This signal is sent to the subcortical system and tells the NeuRoBot to stop moving before any pain is felt or mirrored.

10.2.8 Future blank slate investigations

Many other biological mechanisms could be used to support learning without forgetting in neuromorphic neurons. Sleep cycles can sharpen neuronal network behavior, up-regulating strong synapses and down-regulating weak ones. Astrocytes can be used to synchronize neural firing, creating a focus of attention. Focus of attention when training new material avoids catastrophic forgetting. Astrocytes 1.7 can also be used to communicate between unattached neurons, assisting in generalization and providing fault tolerance, as described in [1]. Dendritic spiking isolates portions of the dendritic arbor, enhances coincidence detection, and can act as a gating mechanism for unrelated signals. Systems that can generalize (like biology) can also support categorization.

Silent synapses (found in biological systems) used in this approach could provide extra inputs to neurons for learning, generalization, and categorization. For future exploration, silent synapses could be activated when new learning occurs. Nearby activity could awaken silent synapses by opening N-methyl-D-aspartate channels as the cell membrane potential, as modeled by an internal voltage, rises. Silent synapses could be recruited to support learning without forgetting.

Future work involves illustrating how neuronal networks specialize or generalize on further training. If the second task is the specialization of the first task, the second neural network is joined with the first task whenever the tasks share common inputs. The two task outputs are distinct. The task that specializes includes the more general task as well as additional processing. For example, a network detecting four square corners (a rectangle) could be amplified with neurons detecting equal edges (a square). Generalization is more difficult than specialization (from squares to rectangles), because part of the square-detecting neuronal network that detects equal length edges is not part of the rectangle-detection network.

Bottom-up design hence could support generalization, and perhaps even categorization, while inhibiting catastrophic forgetting, since existing neural networks are not significantly modified, but incorporated into larger networks.

Another future line of investigation includes sleep cycles to sharpen neuronal network responses. Sleep can up-regulate strong synapses and down-regulate weak ones, analogous to a memory refresh cycle in dynamic electronic memories.

Further investigation should examine the role of astrocytes. Astrocytes strengthen synapses near recent activity and can synchronize neural spiking. Modeling astrocyte interaction is useful when synchronizing bursts to cause dendritic spiking, to communicate between unconnected neurons and to encourage structural plasticity.

Another avenue for future research involves dendritic spiking to enhance learning without forgetting. Dendritic spiking isolates portions of the dendritic arbor and enhances coincidence detection that sharpens the response of a neuron to stimulation of a few related synapses. Dendritic spiking supports neural spiking that indicates a cluster of synapses stimulated and supports STDP even if the neuron does not fire. Dendritic spiking contributes to burst spiking supporting LTP and the neural code, and causes LTP when, due to presynaptic bursts, makes neurons more noise-resistant, allows related portions of the dendritic arbor to generalize, and acts as a gating mechanism for unrelated signals.

Structural plasticity is also shown in long-term learning, although some structural plasticity investigations are controversial. More research should be performed on the role of structural plasticity in lifelong learning.

10.3 The PRONON programmable neuron

Chapters 1–9 have introduced neural structures that can be combined in different ways to create neuromorphic neural circuit structures. Considering CMOS layout approaches, Parker designed a neuron that has a physical layout that is arranged with rows of dendrites, called a *Programmable Neuron* (*PRONON*), as shown in figure 10.12. The arrangement of structures in the figure roughly corresponds to the intended physical layout structure. Each row represents a dendrite that has three excitatory synapses and one inhibitory synapse. The first two excitatory synapses, from the left, as combined with a nonlinear adder. The W inputs are weights that control synaptic strength. If both of the first two synapse inputs are high, and there is no inhibition, the output is enough to make the PRONON neuron fire. The inhibitory input keeps the dendrite from causing the neuron to fire. The third excitatory synapse adds to the nonlinear sum of the first two synapses, and the inhibitory synapse is shunting, blocking the excitatory synapses.

Synapses, dendritic structures and spiking circuits could be combined to produce a neuromorphic circuit containing PRONON neurons. To date, some experimental circuits and layouts were produced for the PRONON, and size estimates performed, but the PRONON neuron was not published.

10.4 Chapter summary

This chapter highlighted three BioRC projects, structural plasiticity implemented by Joshi, the blank slate cortical column implemented by Yue and Evans, and the PRONON programmable neuron. Giovinazzo researched adding pain to the blank slate neuronal network circuit.

The next chapter covers astrocytes, another brain cell. The astrocytes' roles in implementing neural communication, synchrony, retrograde signaling and self-repair circuits are covered.

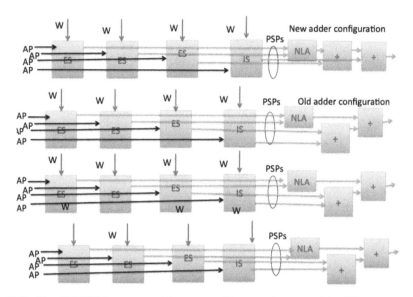

Figure 10.12. The PRONON programmable neuron. AP are action potentials, PSPs are postsynaptic potentials, W are synaptic weight controls (including STDP and dopamine controls), NLA are nonlinear adders, ES are excitatory synapses, and IS are inhibitory synapses. Two variations on adder configurations are shown in the figure.

References

[1] Delepine C *et al* 2022 Astrocyte glutamate transport is modulated by motor learning and regulates neuronal correlations and movement encoding by motor cortex neurons *bioRxiv* 2022–01

[2] Gadagkar V *et al* 2016 Dopamine neurons encode performance error in singing birds *Science* **354** 1278–82

[3] Joshi J 2013 Plasticity in CMOS neuromorphic circuits *PhD Thesis* University of Southern California

[4] Joshi J, Parker A C and Celikel T 2013 Neuromorphic network implementation of the somatosensory cortex *2013 6th Int. IEMBS Conf. Neural Engineering (NER) IEEE* (Piscataway, NJ: IEEE) 907–10

[5] Klein M O *et al* 2018 Dopamine: functions, signaling, and association with neurological diseases *Cell. Mol. Neurobiol.* **39** 31–59

[6] Lübke J and Feldmeyer D 2007 Excitatory signal flow and connectivity in a cortical column: focus on barrel cortex eng *Brain Struct. Funct.* **212** 3–17

[7] Meng X, Huguet G and Rinzel J 2012 Type III excitability, slope sensitivity and coincidence detection Discrete *Contin. Dyn. Syst. Ser.* A **32** 2729–57

[8] Wijekoon J H B and Dudek P 2011 Analogue CMOS circuit implementation of a dopamine modulated synapse *2011 IEEE Int. Symp. Circuits and Systems (ISCAS)* 877–80

[9] Yue K 2020 Circuit design with nano electronic devices for biomimetic neuromorphic systems *PhD Thesis* University of Southern California

[10] Urien L, Xiao Z, Dale J, Bauer E P, Chen Z and Wang J 2018 Rate and temporal coding mechanisms in the anterior cingulate cortex for pain anticipation *Sci. Rep.* **8** 8298

IOP Publishing

Neuromorphic Circuits
A constructive approach
Alice C Parker and Rick Cattell

Chapter 11

Astrocytes

Jon Joshi, Yilda Irizarry-Valle, Rebecca Lee and Alice C Parker

This chapter introduces neuronal-astrocyte communication, models the tripartite synapse, describes circuits that synchronize neurons with astrocytic control and repairs neurons with astrocytic intervention[1]. The BioRC group uses neuromorphic circuits to implement homeostatic mechanisms inspired by biological astrocytes to reorganize synaptic weights in electronic neuronal networks, compensating for damage or changing inputs. The BioRC neuromorphic circuits implement astrocyte circuits that can be used to control plasticity mechanisms when neural activity deviates from a set point. By varying the weights in the network, signals can be routed around areas where inputs are lost. Homeostatic plasticity mechanisms can also be useful for development and tuning of neural networks where synaptic weights start at zero or low values. The goal of this aspect of neuromorphic/gliamorphic networks is to demonstrate how astrocytic intervention can be advantageous to neuromorphic networks that model biological behavior.

11.1 Introduction

Biological astrocytes interact with neurons in a manner that enhances and changes neural behavior. This chapter describes a family of circuits that emulate this biological behavior. Biological astrocytes and their influence on neural computation have been studied for several decades, but little research has focused on models that emulate astrocytes and their communication with neurons. Mathematical models for neuronal-astrocyte interaction have been developed [1]. We believe that the earliest BioRC astrocyte circuits are the first attempt at this difficult modeling with neuromorphic circuits. The circuits build on Joshi's and Hsu's libraries of neurons that contain dendritic processing and dendritic plasticity [4], synaptic timing-dependent plasticity (STDP) [10], and other biomimetic features, many of which are introduced in earlier chapters.

---

[1] We suggest the reader review the material in section 1.7 before reading this chapter.

doi:10.1088/978-0-7503-5097-6ch11

Because of both the compartmentalized construction of BioRC neuromorphic circuits and also the ability to control neural parameters directly by means of specific control voltages, inserting additional mechanisms can be performed without extensive circuit redesign. This helped the BioRC group emulate astrocytic behavior in circuits in a compartmental approach, such that *intracellular* (within a cell) astrocytic calcium Ca^{2+} release causing glutamate release can be inserted easily into the neurotransmitter section of the BioRC synapses, and into the postsynaptic part of the neural synapse. Slow inward currents caused by astrocytes can also be inserted into neurons outside the synapses.

11.2 The tripartite synapse

One of the ways astrocytes and neurons interact is through the tripartite synapse, as described in Joshi's thesis [10]. Astrocytes are also known to exert modulatory properties on receptors located at the extrasynaptic side, while neurons, through the spillover of transmitters out of the synapse, can reach and modulate receptors in the outer membrane of the astrocyte. See figure 1.26 for a cartoon representation of a tripartite synapse, and the basis of the interaction between an astrocyte's process and a synapse. For the tripartite synapse, the BioRC group has chosen to model a single mechanism that captures signaling between astrocytes and neurons studied in the rat hypothalamus and cortex by means of the transmitter glutamate. In particular, BioRC circuits show a neural-glial neuromorphic system that demonstrates the role of astrocytes in facilitating neural firing when neighboring neurons share synapses in the same astrocytic *microdomain*, portions of a thin process of an astrocyte where calcium transients are active and can be observed [16]. Astrocytic microdomains are portions of astrocyte processes (arms) that interact with adjacent neurons. Each microdomain consists of several compartments, where each compartment is able to sense the modulatory effects of adjacent synapses.

The specific focus in this section is to show neuromorphic circuits that emulate the release of glutamate by astrocytes and show that it increases excitability in neurons located in the microdomain. The circuits also emulate the uptake of glutamate by astrocytes from nearby neurons that subsequently causes calcium concentrations to increase and spread, triggering the astrocyte's glutamate release and exciting nearby synapses. Although the effects shown in this section are first-order, they are a step towards demonstrating neuronal-astrocyte communication.

Figure 11.1 shows an excitatory synapse circuit modified from the current synapse circuit, as discussed in chapter 6 [10]. The circuit is divided into neurotransmitter (presynaptic) and receptor (postsynaptic) sections as shown. The voltage at the node labelled *synaptic cleft* represents the neurotransmitter concentration in the synaptic cleft. A modification has been made to the output of the neurotransmitter section, where an analog voltage adder [3] is connected, such that the cleft voltage is added to the neurotransmitter voltage contributed by the astrocyte circuit. AstroCa^{2+} is the control signal that causes the synaptic cleft to be offset by a voltage $V_{astro-glut}$. This models the amount of glutamate gliotransmitter that is injected into the cleft by the astrocyte. The operation of the synapse circuit was described in further detail in

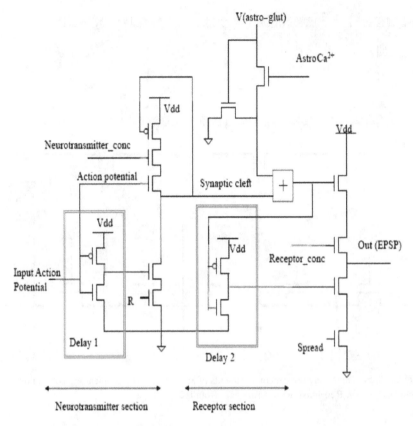

Figure 11.1. The BioRC excitatory synapse circuit with astrocyte compartment connections. Copyright 2011 IEEE. Reprinted, with permission, from [12].

chapter 6. Note that all transmitters and ions are emulated using charge, current and voltage in the neuromorphic circuits described here.

Figure 11.2 shows several compartments of a simplified astrocyte circuit. It is a distributed resistive (pass transistor) network that takes inputs from the voltages representing synaptic cleft neurotransmitter concentrations of different synapse circuits[2]. The neurotransmitter voltage from each synapse is fed into a non-inverting active delay circuit whose output voltage representing released neurotransmitters is summed [3] with delayed neurotransmitter voltages from other synapses. This models the time taken by the astrocyte to take up neurotransmitters and generate Ca^{2+}. The rise in potential at the resistive network ($AstroCa^{2+}$) models the propagation and spread in calcium across the astrocyte. Calcium wave mechanisms are not implemented here. The outputs of the astrocyte's compartments control transistors in each synapse. The synapse adds an offset voltage to the synaptic

---

[2] Actually the transistors form a distributed RC network that models the Ca^{2+} delays between portions of the astrocyte as well as attenuation.

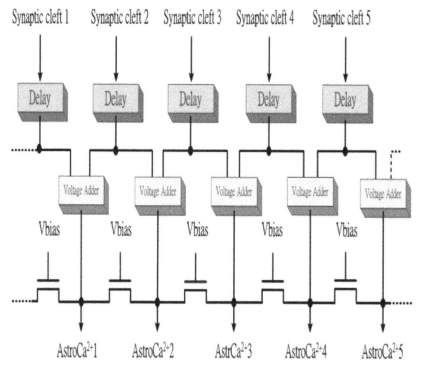

Figure 11.2. Circuit containing several compartments of an astrocyte communicating with multiple synapses. Copyright 2011 IEEE. Reprinted, with permission, from [12].

neurotransmitter concentration voltage to emulate the increase in neurotransmitters in the synapse due to the astrocyte's release of glutamate caused by astroytic intracellular calcium increase.

11.3 Experimental tripartite communication network

Figure 11.3 shows a network of silicon neurons [9, 10] along with an astrocyte spanning the neurons to create a microdomain. The goal is to test whether synaptic activity in one region of the network increases excitability at another. We set the firing thresholds for the neurons in such a way that the neurons fire when there is enough dendritic potential (about equal to the sum of the excitatory postsynaptic potential (EPSPs) of three synapses). Hence, as shown in figure 11.3, neuron 4 (N4) will fire as it is connected to three synapses whereas neuron 5 (N5) will not fire, as it has only two synaptic inputs. Neurons 1, 2 and 3 are input neurons to the network and will be given an action potential (AP) stimulus to fire. To demonstrate change in excitability we focus on the neurotransmitter (cleft) voltage and the EPSPs generated by synapse 5.

Circuit simulations were conducted using TSMC 180 nm CMOS technology in Cadence SPECTRE. We first show that without astrocytic communication provided to the network, synapses 4 and 5 do not produce sufficient neurotransmitter release

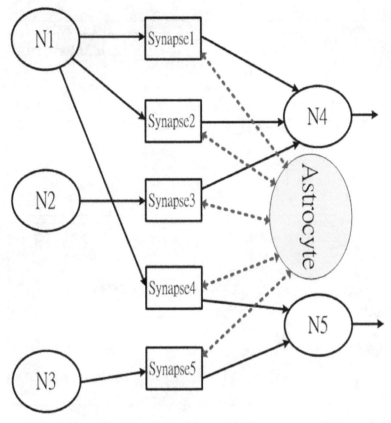

Figure 11.3. Neural network illustrating astrocyte microdomain. Copyright 2011 IEEE. Reprinted, with permission, from [12].

(represented by cleft voltages), resulting in inadequate EPSPs, so that N5 does not fire. As shown by the waveforms in figure 11.4, N1 and N2, when stimulated, generate APs (black trace). This causes N4 to fire due to sufficient dendritic potential (green trace). When Synapses 4 and 5 at N5 are excited by N1 and N3, their cleft voltages (pink trace) representing neurotransmitter concentrations are insufficient (comparison in figure 11.6) to generate sufficient EPSPs (figure 11.6) to make N5 fire (light blue trace, 0.0 V).

We then connect the astrocyte circuit and execute the same set of simulations. As shown by the waveforms in figure 11.5, when synapses 1, 2 and 3 are excited by N1 and N2 (black trace) the cleft voltage generated at the synapses (blue trace) causes the astrocyte circuit to generate a delayed voltage ($AstroCa^{2+}$ 1, red trace). As the Ca^{2+} signal propagates across the resistive network ($AstroCa^{2+}+5$, green trace) it causes the cleft voltage at synapse 5 to rise by an offset set by $V_{astro-glut}$, which in our experiments is 200 mV (pink trace) in figure 11.6. When N3 excites synapse 5 the cleft voltage (pink trace) rises high enough to generate a voltage greater than in case 1 (comparison shown in figure 11.6). This causes N5 to fire (light blue trace). Thus

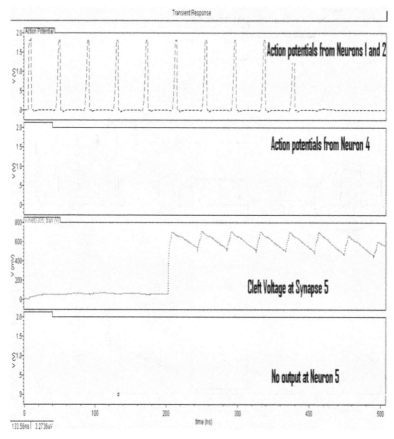

Figure 11.4. Case 1: simulation results for the network without astrocyte circuit. Copyright 2011 IEEE. Reprinted, with permission, from [12].

we implemented, in silicon, astrocytic monitoring of synaptic activity that can increase excitability of neurons close by, shown as a first-order effect.

11.4 Neural phase synchrony

There is no clock in the biological brain, and neurons can fire asynchronously. In the biological brain, synchronous firing of multiple neurons indicates importance of the signal connection in causing firing downstream. In neuromorphic circuits, signals that are synchronous contribute to increased spiking activity. In the biological brain, astrocytes play a role in neural phase synchrony. This section presents hybrid bio-inspired and biomimetic CMOS neuromorphic circuit designs and simulations as part of an initial effort to capture the role of astrocytes in phase synchronization of neuronal activity, found in Irizarry-Valle's thesis [6]. We present some gross first-order circuit designs and capture the main steps involved in the process of an astrocyte inducing synchronization in a small group of neurons. Biological exper-imental results have shown that a single astrocyte is capable of inducing

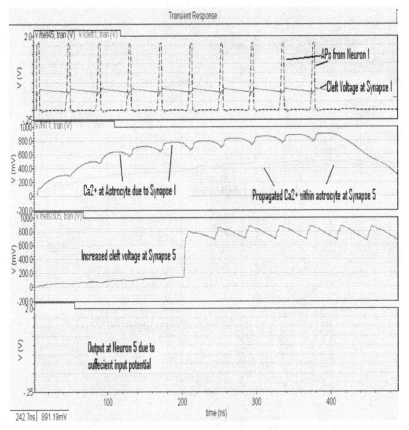

Figure 11.5. Case 2: simulation results for the network with the astrocyte circuit invoking excitability. Copyright 2011 IEEE. Reprinted, with permission, from [12].

simultaneous activation of neuronal *N*-methyl-D-aspartate (NMDA) channels located at the extrasynaptic side of neurons (away from the synapses). The activation of these channels elicits simultaneous slow inward currents (SICs) on adjacent neurons. The amplitude of SICs is several orders of magnitude larger compared to synaptic currents. A single SIC event drastically enhances the EPSP. Because the astrocyte induces SICs with a high degree of synchronicity, adjacent neurons experience a sudden rise in their membrane potential, firing synchronously in phase. Phase synchrony holds for a duration of time proportional to the time constant of the SIC decay. This decay is about sixty times slower compared to typical synaptic currents.

The amplitude of SICs is several orders of magnitude larger than synaptic currents. A single SIC event drastically increases an EPSP. Because the astrocyte induces SICs with a high degree of synchronicity, adjacent neurons experience a sudden rise in their membrane potential, firing synchronously in phase. Phase synchrony holds for a duration of time proportional to the time constant of the SIC

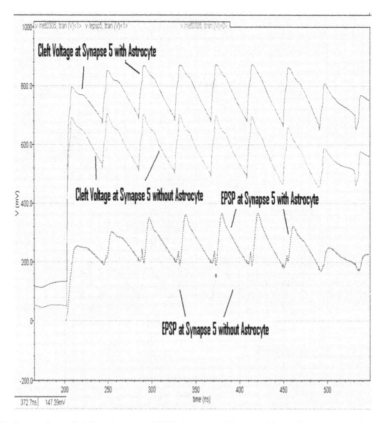

Figure 11.6. Comparison of cleft voltages and PSPs in cases with and without the astrocyte circuit. Copyright 2011 IEEE. Reprinted, with permission, from [12].

decay. Once the SIC decay has completed, the neurons go back to their natural phase difference, inducing desynchronization of their firing of spikes.

Using neuromorphic circuits, this section describes the ability of SICs evoked by the astrocyte, acting on extrasynaptic NMDA channels of adjacent neurons, to be a mechanism for phase synchronization. We describe important aspects of the process of communication between astrocytes and neurons. In this section we demonstrate, via circuit simulations, a model for the synchronization of adjacent neurons through astrocyte modulatory activity on extrasynaptic NMDA channels. In order to test the SIC mechanism, we perform simulations on circuits to emulate the indirect communication between two isolated small neuronal networks that are able to interact with each other, inducing SICs on adjacent synapses on each network by means of the activity in the astrocytic microdomains. This activity would be controlled by intracellular calcium waves evoked by neuronal stimulation. The compartments are designed using transistors as resistive and capacitive components forming a ladder network in the astrocyte. Irizarry-Valle used pass transistors for the interaction between microdomains.

11.4.1 Circuit implementation

This section describes each component used in our circuit demonstrating astrocyte-neuron signaling. We begin by describing the synapse circuit and the rule of firing in our neuron followed by a discussion of the extrasynaptic NMDAR circuit to be incorporated into the synapse circuit. We also discuss the astrocytic microdomain circuit and how the synapse and astrocytic microdomain blocks interact with each other. The circuits are simulated at accelerated time.

11.4.1.1 The excitatory synapse circuit

The tripartite synapse circuit used in this simulation test is shown in figure 11.7. Stages (1) and (2) show the pre- and postsynaptic sections separated by the synaptic cleft. The *cleft voltage* represents the neurotransmitter concentration in the synaptic cleft. The low-pass filtering characteristic of Stage (1) provides the cleft node with information about the average input spike rate. The pull-up transistors allow the cleft to be charged with a fast rise-time constant during the spike duration. The steady amplitude can be tuned by the input *NT Conc* (neurotransmitter concentration). The pull-down transistors allow the cleft to be discharged in the absence of a spike or some time after a spike has occurred. This mimics the drop of neurotransmitters in the cleft by the reuptake process which can be tuned by the input *Reuptake*. Stage (2) generates the *EPSP* voltage. The red arrow shows the extrasynaptic side used to emulate the NMDA channel contribution.

For the purpose of this work, since our interest is to show the influence of astrocytic evoked SICs on extrasynaptic receptors that leads to phase synchronization on postsynaptic neurons, we assumed no diffusion of gliotransmitters into the cleft; as in biological neurons, here we assume glutamate from an astrocyte mainly binds extrasynaptic receptors of postsynaptic neurons [2]. The extrasynaptic influence is shown by a red arrow on the top right-hand side that comes from the *extrasynaptic NMDA block* (see figure 11.10 and transistor X10 in figure 11.12). The release of neurotransmitters mimicked by the cleft voltage is of an excitatory type

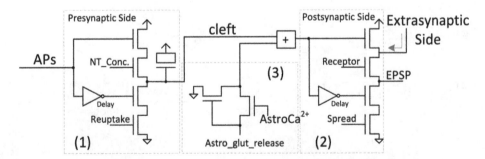

Figure 11.7. The BioRC synapse circuit. The presynaptic side is activated when an AP is received. The cleft node emulates the release of transmitters from the presynaptic side. Stage (1) behaves like a low-pass filter, where a high rate of input spikes increases the cleft node voltage accordingly. In Stage (2), an EPSP is produced when the cleft voltage is sufficiently strong. The red arrow shows the extrasynaptic side used to emulate the NMDA channel contribution [6].

and for the purpose of the discussion, by neurotransmitters, we mean glutamate transmitters. However, based on the application, a different interpretation may be given in the case of using a different type of excitatory transmitter. The synapse circuit is a first-order approximation and does not incorporate detailed receptor circuitry for the different types of transmitters as such receptor circuits would depend on the mechanisms being modeled.

11.4.1.2 Neuron block diagram and firing rule

In figure 11.8, we show a diagram of the different blocks of the neuron circuit, excluding astrocytic interaction. For simulation purposes, besides the astrocyte circuits, circuits used have been previously designed by the BioRC group [17]. The inputs AP1, AP2, ..., APn are action potentials or spikes that arrive at the presynaptic terminal of each synapse (the typical shape of an AP is shown in the simulation results in this section). The *Synapse* corresponds to the circuit shown in figure 11.7. The output of each synapse generates an EPSP voltage. The EPSP of the different synapses is then added at the *dendritic arbor* to produce the *total EPSP* voltage that is input to the *axon hillock*. We show a simplified arbor here. When the *total EPSP* voltage crosses the axon hillock threshold voltage from below, the neuron elicits an AP (AP$_{out}$).

A train of spikes at AP$_{out}$ is generated when the Total *EPSP* crosses the threshold from below on successive occasions. If presynaptic spikes (AP1, AP2, ..., APn) are in phase, such an output train of spikes would follow the input phase. When the arrival of presynaptic spikes is out of phase, then the neuron may enter an unreliable condition, since the amplitude of the total EPSP might not necessarily be enough to cross the axon hillock threshold to cause the firing of spikes. When the phase difference between input spikes is small enough to provide enough total EPSP for the neuron to fire, a phase shift may occur at AP$_{out}$. The neuron in the simulation test we perform is set to fire when the total *EPSP* is equivalent to the sum of the *EPSP* voltages corresponding to three synapses that are in phase. The BioRC group has also designed neurons that fire based on the rate of change of the membrane

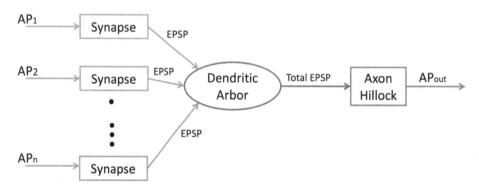

Figure 11.8. A system view of the neuron components. Copyright 2015 IEEE. Reprinted, with permission, from [7].

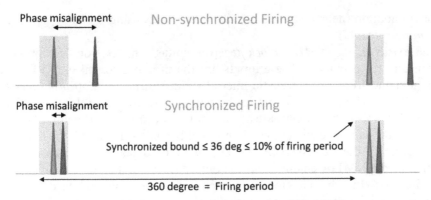

Figure 11.9. The concept of phase synchronization. Copyright 2015 IEEE. Reprinted, with permission, from [7].

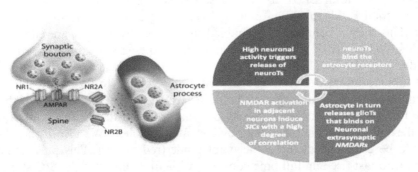

Figure 11.10. A system view: the extrasynaptic NMDA channel for the induction of SICs connected to the synapse and astrocyte. Left image reproduced from [20], copyright 2006 the American Physiological Society. Right image from [6].

potential, so that the threshold varies inversely with the rate of change [5], as discussed earlier in chapter 5.

Two neurons with the same firing rate are considered synchronized if their APs happen within 10% of phase difference. Considering 360 degrees of phase angle for each cycle starting with the rising edge of AP, we consider two series of APs phase synchronized if their phase misalignment is less than 36 degrees, i.e., maximum 10% misalignment (see figure 11.9).

11.4.1.3 Extrasynaptic NMDA block and the activation of SICs

SICs are initiated upon activation of NMDA channels. The block diagram depicted in figure 11.12 shows the connections between the *synapse*, the *extrasynaptic NMDA block*, and the *astrocyte microdomain*. The focus of the following description is on the *extrasynaptic NMDA block* (yellow-green-shaded box). This block has two outputs, in coordination, that enable the neuron to have a sudden rise of voltage in the neuron *total EPSP*. The *total EPSP* is a signal that represents the summation of each EPSP contributed by individual synapses, that is, the output of the dendritic arbor summation (neuroscientists usually refer to this using the more general term *membrane potential*).

The *extrasynaptic NMDA block* receives voltage inputs from the presynaptic neuron and the astrocyte. These inputs are the presynaptic spikes (AP1) and the calcium signal from the astrocytic microdomain (*astrocyte gliotransmitters GlioT* ($AstroCa^{2+}$)). The calcium signal in the figure represents the release of gliotransmitters. When these two signals are active, that is, the presynaptic neuron fires spikes (AP1) and the astrocyte elicits a calcium signal beyond a threshold, the first stage in the diagram of the *extrasynaptic NMDA block* becomes active. This models the opening of the NMDA channel and the output of the first stage is a pulse of short time duration. In the following paragraphs, the text provides the details of the generation and the changes in the neuron, in the assumption the channel is open, and SIC activity occurs, that is, the *SIC* and *control circuit* stages become active.

We focus on the two outputs of the *extrasynaptic NMDA block*. The output that connects to the total *EPSP* node only serves as a reset signal so that the neuron resets its total EPSP to resting potential according to the contribution of the SIC event. This output connection is enabled by two pathways that are controlled by switches SW1 and SW2. The dynamic activities of these switches will coordinate the time duration at which the neuron senses the SIC event. Switch SW1 is enabled for a short time duration, thus setting the total EPSP voltage to 0.0 V. Switch SW1 is disconnected after the duration of the pulse, which enables the voltage at the total EPSP to receive the incoming activity of synapses from the dendritic arbor, along with the SIC. The same pulse that enables and disables SW1 also forms the SIC event to be generated at the extrasynaptic side (red arrow). This pulse is characterized by a fast rise and fall time constant, while the output of the SIC stage has a fast rise time but very slow decay to approximate the biological response. When the total EPSP has fallen below 50% of the peak, the second pathway in the control circuit is enabled when switch SW2 closes, and becomes active for a short time duration. Switch SW2 is activated when the SIC event is reducing, and the EPSP voltage signal has decreased below 50% of its maximum amplitude. Activation of SW2 sends the total EPSP voltage to 0.0 V. Once SW2 becomes inactive, that is, the SIC event reaches its minimum voltage, the neuron output (AP_{out}) continues its normal nonsynchronized operation in the absence of an SIC event, receiving and integrating incoming information from its synapses.

The input block of the *extrasynaptic NMDA block* represents the NMDA activation section which includes the magnesium block removal (Mg^{2+} *BR*). The SIC stage is used for shaping the decay time constant of the SIC signal. While these blocks perform biomimetic functions, the *control circuit* is a bio-inspired circuit used as a reset mechanism that acts at the beginning and at the end of an SIC event, sensing the SIC activity and in the absence of an SIC event resetting the neuron to its natural firing phase of action potentials; its role will be discussed in detail in the next section. This reset mechanism is not biomimetic, and more modeling of the astrocyte physiology would be required to balance the SICs in the neurons so they are indeed synchronized in a biomimetic manner.

11.4.1.4 A system view of the network used for simulation experiments

Irizarry-Valle's simulation experiments are based on astrocyte compartments and neurons connected in a small network, with up to nine neurons and two astrocytic microdomains. We show a simplified system view in figure 11.11 of the circuit configuration Irizarry-Valle simulated. It combines the blocks in figures 11.8 and 11.12 along with the astrocytic microdomains in figure 11.13. She connected the *extrasynaptic NMDAR block* to only one postsynaptic neuron on each network. This block senses activity from the incoming presynaptic spikes and the astrocytic microdomain. The astrocytic microdomains individually sense information from their respective neurons and can interact with each other. The *extrasynaptic NMDAR block* is activated according to the strength of the signal (astrocyte gliotransmitters) and in the presence of presynaptic stimulation. The activation of the block induces a signal (red arrow) into the postsynaptic side that emulates the SIC event. Because of the interaction of the two microdomains, SICs will be induced simultaneously in both networks of neurons causing the neurons to be synchronized as they both cross the activation threshold simultaneously, which leads to the generation of APs (AP$_{out}$). The signal that is output from the *extrasynaptic NMDAR block* into the output of the *dendritic arbor* is used to reset the *total EPSP* (membrane potential of the neuron) initially, as it was already above the axon hillock threshold, and the neuron was spiking. This reset is the role of the *control circuit* block shown in figure 11.12.

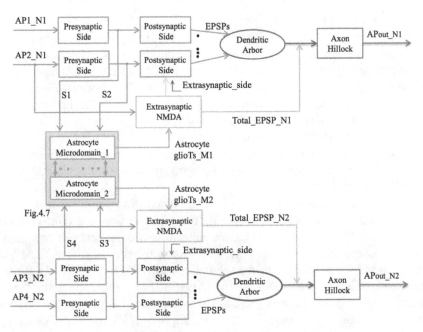

Figure 11.11. A system view diagram showing the main circuit blocks used for the neurons and astrocyte. Copyright 2015 IEEE. Reprinted, with permission, from [7].

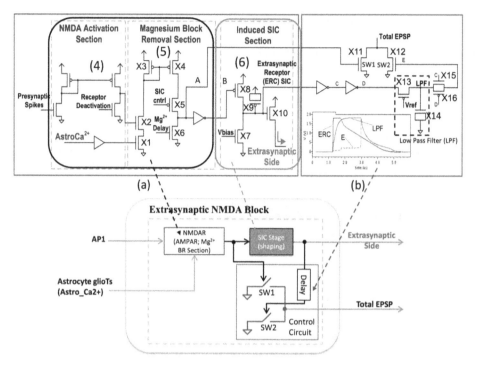

Figure 11.12. The circuit of extrasynaptic NMDA channel in (a), consists of sections (4), (5), and (6) with a compact control circuit shown in (b) [6].

11.4.1.5 Extrasynaptic NMDA channel circuit for SIC generation

This subsection presents and discusses the NMDA channel circuit used for extrasynaptic SIC generation in the neuron. Figure 11.12 shows the extrasynaptic NMDA channel (a) along with a control circuit (b) designed for the phase synchrony of adjacent neurons upon initiation of a SIC event. The bottom diagram corresponds to the *extrasynaptic NMDA Block* already discussed. Dashed lines are used to identify the circuit structure for each block. The *extrasynaptic NMDAR block* in figure 11.12(a) is divided into three main sections: the *NMDA activation* in subcircuit (4), the *magnesium block removal* in subcircuit (5), and the *induced SIC* in subcircuit (6). Subcircuits (4) and (5) are modified versions of previously published circuits to include the role of SICs [13].

The role of each subcircuit will now be discussed. Subcircuit (4) in figure 11.12 roughly plays the role of AMPA channels. The input section is activated to remove the magnesium block when coincidence detection occurs between the arrival of *presynaptic spikes* and the transmitters released by the astrocyte. The AMPA channel is usually needed to remove the magnesium NMDA block. As there is no clear evidence what triggers the AMPA activation, we follow the assumption that presynaptic spike stimulation is used as the coincidental stimulus that triggers the receptor activation. The basis for this assumption is Wade's model of neural-astrocytic interaction [19].

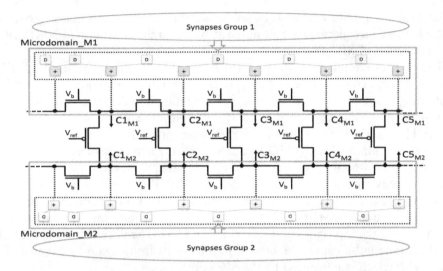

Figure 11.13. Two astrocytic microdomains (M1, M2) connected by pass transistors allowing interaction between synapses in group 1 and group 2. The nodes Ci_{MX} represent the astrocytic compartments. The voltages V_b and V_{ref} are bias voltages to control the resistive paths of the transistors. Copyright 2015 IEEE. Reprinted, with permission, from [7].

The voltage *receptor deactivation* in subcircuit (4) can be used to control the time duration at which the receptors remain active [13]. It is a fixed bias voltage of 350 mV that controls the resistance of its transistor. Subcircuit (5) is designed so that the removal of the magnesium block occurs only if there are three coincidental inputs (*AstroCa^{2+}*, *NMDA activation*, and *SIC cntrl*) for the activation of transistors X1, X2, and X5 simultaneously. This results in the production of a SIC event at the extrasynaptic side (in X10). The activation of X1 is controlled by the calcium level (*AstroCa^{2+}*) generated at the astrocyte compartment. The *AstroCa^{2+}* signal represents the astrocyte's contribution that triggers the SIC event. The activation of X2 depends on the AMPAR activation, that is, when there is presynaptic spike stimulation at subcircuit (4). Transistor X5 is controlled by the input SIC cntrl, a global periodic single pulse that emulates the time activity of SIC events. The pulse width of the SIC cntrl signal determines the minimum time window over which the SIC amplitude at the *extrasynaptic receptor (ERC)* remains at its maximum voltage. Astrocytes trigger SIC activity by a single glutamate release, correlated with calcium oscillations [13].

The control circuit presented here is bio-inspired, since it is not purely autonomous. The mechanism disables the current total EPSP to reinitiate EPSP at the exact time that the EPSP is reinitiated at other neurons, inducing synchronous firing. As future work, we plan to extend the astrocytic microdomain circuit (figure 2 in [22]) to generate different forms of calcium oscillations [23]. Thus, the SIC cntrl input is an artifice that will not be necessary once the calcium wave detection circuit is included and will be eventually produced from the astrocytic calcium oscillations. Subcircuits

(4) and (5) are modified versions of previously published circuits in our group [13], where here we incorporate the role of the astrocyte in the activation of NMDAR for the production of SIC events.

The control circuit in figure 11.12(b) is designed to discharge the total EPSP voltage at the axon hillock circuit [13] through either transistors X11 or X12, supporting the timing activity of the synchronization and desynchronization phases that happen at the beginning and at the end of SIC event occurrence (see figures 11.11 and 11.10 for the total EPSP node connection to the neuron).

Upon activation of the NMDA channel, when there is coincidental activity, a short time pulse impinges node A at section (5) that activates transistor X11. During this short activation of transistor X11, the total EPSP node resets the firing activity of action potentials. An SIC event is evoked at node ERC in section (6) to be further processed by the postsynaptic stage of the synapse through the extrasynaptic side (red arrow on the top right hand side in figure 11.7). The deactivation of X11 after the short time pulse causes the neuron to initiate its firing again by the rise of the total EPSP which is influenced by the SIC contribution.

Phase synchronization happens since neurons with adjacent synapses receive SIC events simultaneously, produced by their respective extrasynaptic receptors. Such events are strong enough to drastically increase the total EPSP of each neuron. Upon removing the SIC event, neurons are desynchronized through transistor X12 which is activated to reset the total EPSP node and so stops the firing of the corresponding postsynaptic neurons for a short time. Upon deactivation of X12, i.e. in the absence of SIC contribution to the total EPSP, the neurons return back to their initial conditions where they fire out of phase synchrony following the phase difference of their presynaptic neurons. We emphasize that phase synchrony happens only if the total EPSP of both neurons crosses the axon hillock threshold nearly simultaneously, i.e. when an SIC event is produced on adjacent synapses.

In figure 11.12(a), the SIC cntrl input contributes to the magnesium block removal by pulling down node B when coincidental input activity occurs. In other words, the current mirror in subcircuit (5) is properly biased if X1 and X2 are activated, thus enabling node A to rise when a single pulse SIC cntrl is applied. The voltage Mg^{2+} *delay* emulates the magnesium block removal delay, i.e. the time (at node B) that takes to deactivate X8 in subcircuit (6) after the SIC cntrl arrival. In our simulation it is a bias voltage of 450 mV. It contributes to increase the time width at which the ERC node remains at its maximum voltage. When X8 is deactivated, the ERC node decays with a slow time constant to 0.0 V, which emulates the SIC decay. This decay is controlled by the resistance of X7 and the capacitance of X9 along with the diffusion capacitances in the node. The small waveform diagram in figure 11.12(b) shows the ERC signal at the input of X10.

When node A is activated, the Total EPSP discharges down to 0.0 V through X11 at the control circuit in figure 11.12(b). Since node A sees a pulse of short duration, X11 is deactivated immediately after A returns to 0.0 V. That is when SICs are produced simultaneously into adjacent synapses of postsynaptic neurons through X10, causing the total EPSP of each neuron to rise simultaneously, and thus synchronizing the postsynaptic neurons in phase. Therefore, the total EPSP amplitude is increased by the increase of the EPSP for each synapse that receives the induced SIC event. After the ERC node drops to about 50% of its voltage, nodes C and D become high and low, respectively. This activates the transmission gate (X15, X16), transferring the low-pass filter (LPF) voltage to the gate of X12. Transistors X13 and X14, respectively, provide the resistance and capacitance of the LPF. Notice from the waveform diagram shown in figure 11.12(b) that the LPF voltage activates X12 for a short time. The activation of X12 indicates that the SIC event has passed and thus neurons are no longer synchronized in phase. The total EPSP is discharged, so that when X12 is deactivated the postsynaptic neurons return to the desynchronized state. Transistor X12 is deactivated through the pull-down path of the inverter connected at node D. The choice to use the ERC node when it drops to 50% of its voltage to desynchronize the neurons is not a biomimetic process and it is mainly inspired by the biological events reported by experiments. A more biomimetic design would require the desynchronization to wait until the signal ERC has reached its minimum voltage to emulate the absence of the SIC event. Whether neurons are desynchronized in the absence of an SIC event is not clear based on biological experiments.

Once X12 is deactivated, the total EPSP on each neuron is enabled to rise again. The phase difference between the neurons in the desyncronization state depends on the time at which each neuron crosses the axon hillock threshold. The maximum phase difference is proportional to the phase difference of the presynaptic spikes. When neurons are not synchronized in phase, the total EPSP is decreased, since it no longer receives the contribution of an SIC event. The circuit shown in figure 11.12 has a total active power of 148 μW. In the absence of an input stimulus, the circuit has no active path between V_{dd} and Gnd terminals. The inputs *receptor deactivation* and Mg^{2+} delay have bias voltages around the threshold of the transistor. Transistors X1 and X2 are enabled during the time their respective input signals are active. The SIC cntrl signal should be provided by a circuit that emulates the crossing of the astrocyte calcium wave threshold. A careful design should be done to capture calcium waves along with an activation threshold that is aimed to determine the activity of slow inward currents. Since SIC generation is expected to be active only under certain conditions, which depends on the intensity of glutamate release according to activity of calcium waves, we expect to have power savings.

11.4.1.6 The astrocytic microdomain circuit

As previously mentioned, the activation of the NMDAR extrasynaptic receptor requires sufficient calcium-level excitation ($AstroCa^{2+}$) at the astrocytic compartment associated with the synapse. In figure 11.13 we show two astrocytic microdomain circuits (orange boxes) able to interact with each other. Each microdomain consists of several compartments and is a distributed resistive (pass transistor) network that takes inputs from the voltages representing synaptic cleft neurotransmitter concentrations of different synapse circuits. The cleft voltage from each synapse (see figure 11.7) is fed into a non-inverting delay circuit (D) whose output voltage representing released neurotransmitters is summed with delayed cleft voltages from other synapses [12]. This emulates the time taken by the astrocyte to induce calcium waves at the astrocytic compartments due to the accumulation of neurotransmitters. In the next section we show a simulation test where M1 and M2 trigger SIC events on adjacent synapses according to the neuronal activity sensed by M1. We also show how the production of SIC events by the astrocytic calcium waves leads to phase synchronization on postsynaptic neurons. The rise of potential at the Ci_{MX} nodes in the resistive network emulates the increase and spread of calcium across the astrocyte [12]. In turn, these astrocytic outputs are able to influence the activation of the NMDA extrasynaptic receptor circuit when connected to the input $AstroCa^{2+}$ in figure 11.12.

A PMOS pass transistor between the outputs of each microdomain allows them to interact with each other, so that neuronal activity from both group of synapses can use the microdomains as a media to establish communication. For such communication to occur, any or both microdomain 1 (M1) and microdomain 2 (M2) need to sense a strong stimulation from the cleft nodes of their respective synapses. By tuning the widths and the lengths of transistor gates we can exploit the transistors' resistive and capacitive characteristics. Transistor size optimization was done in an ad hoc manner. Currently the sizes we have used in our design are in the range of 400 nm to 4 µm width and length. Transistors X9 and X14 behave as capacitances in figure 11.12, with sizes from 5 µm up to 8 µm.

The bias voltages V_b and V_{ref} at the microdomain circuit in figure 11.22 were set to 1 V and −1.8 V, respectively. These voltages have impact on the resistances of the transistors they control and also limit the interaction between any two nodes in the microdomain. The resistance between the microdomains controlled by transistors connected to V_{ref} is small so that both microdomains can have enough influence on each other. The nodes in the microdomains are influenced by their respective added synaptic clefts, their neighbor synapses added at the adjacent nodes from their own microdomain or the microdomains with which they interact.

11.4.1.7 Network configuration for our simulation experiments

Our simulation experiments illustrate the synchronization of unconnected neurons via astrocytic involvement, and the result of the simulation on a downstream neuron. The network depicted in figure 11.14 illustrates the configuration we used for this simulation test. It shows the neuro-astrocyte interactions of two small networks of silicon neurons, where synapses S1–S6 of Network 1 are spanned by the astrocytic microdomain M1, and synapses S7–S12 of Network 2 are spanned by M2. The astrocytic microdomains sense neurotransmitters released from their corresponding networks and feed back gliotransmitters, through the activity of calcium waves at each related compartment, to the extrasynaptic NMDA circuits corresponding to the synapses S3, S4, S9, and S10. Both microdomains are capable of interacting with each other, symbolized by the thick blue bidirectional arrow.

In this simulation test, Irizarry-Valle set the frequency of spikes of the presynaptic neurons in Network 2 lower than that in Network 1, so that we can show the capability of Network 1 to support the induction of SIC events in Network 2 by means of increasing the calcium waves in M2. In other words, M2 alone is not able to produce a substantial increase in the amplitude of calcium waves as it does not receive sufficient stimulation from its synapses.

Presynaptic neurons N1 and N2 at Network 1 have a higher frequency of spikes which increases the release of neurotransmitters at the synaptic clefts of S1–S6, sensed by microdomain M1, strengthening calcium waves at the compartments of M1 by means of increasing the amplitude at the Ci_{M1} nodes, as shown in figure 11.13. In the microdomain M2, calcium waves at compartments of M2, besides receiving the small influence from the weak release of transmitters from synapses S7–S12 of Network 2, also see the contribution of the calcium waves propagated from microdomain M1. we connected extrasynaptic NMDA circuits to each adjacent synapse S3–S4 and S9–S10 in Network 1 and Network 2, respectively. The induction of SIC events into these synapses is controlled by compartments $C3_{MX}$ and $C4_{MX}$ of their respective microdomain circuits. These compartment outputs act on the input *AstroCa^{2+}* of the extrasynaptic NMDA circuit, activating transistor X1 when the amplitude of the calcium wave signal is large enough (see figure 11.12). Calcium waves at nodes $C3_{M1}$ and $C4_{M1}$ are strong enough to soon propagate the signal to the compartments $C3_{M2}$ and $C4_{M2}$ of microdomain M2 through the related PMOS pass transistors (see figure 11.13). This causes the activation of the extrasynaptic NMDAR circuits of S9 and S10 in Network 2, inducing synchronized SIC events. In other words, each adjacent synapse (S3, S4, S9, and S10) receives SIC events triggered by the calcium wave induced at its respective astrocytic compartment.

As the simulations will show in the subsection below, the high degree of correlation of SIC events at the adjacent synapses of different postsynaptic neurons causes phase synchronization in the activity of neurons N3, N4, N7 and N8 on each network. We connected neuron N9 to postsynaptic neurons of Network 2 to show the role of neuronal excitability when postsynaptic neurons fire in phase synchrony. The latter is discussed in Irizarry-Valle's thesis [6].

11.4.1.8 Simulation results for Network 1 and Network 2
Results for the phase of the firing of postsynaptic neurons N3–N4 and N7–N8, corresponding to Network 1 and Network 2 are shown in figures 11.15 and 11.16. We set the firing threshold such that these neurons fire in the presence of enough dendritic potential (about equal to the sum of the EPSPs of three synapses). Postsynaptic neurons N3–N4 and N7–N8 can initially fire since they each receive the contribution of the coincident EPSPs of three synapses (see figure 11.14).

The top panels in figures 11.15 and 11.16 show the Total EPSPs for neurons N7–N8 and N3–N4. The middle panels show the Aps of each neuron. The bottom panels show a zoom-in of the APs for two different regions. This simulation was conducted for $V_{bias} = 700$ mV, $V_{ref} = 1.8$ V and $V_b = 1$ V.

The frequency of postsynaptic spikes is the same as that of the presynaptic neurons. Thus, in the absence of an SIC event, the asynchronous phase differences of APs on each pair of postsynaptic neurons, N3–N4 and N7–N8, are, respectively, proportional to the phase difference of their corresponding presynaptic neurons. The circuit simulations were conducted in TSMC 180 nm technology using a power supply of 1.8 V. The input frequencies were set at 8.3 MHz for Network 1 and the higher frequency is 33.3 MHz for Network 2, respectively.

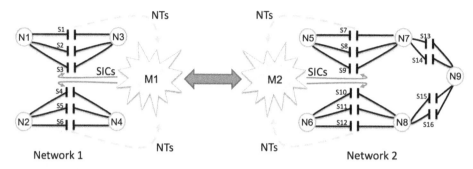

Figure 11.14. Two small neural networks interacting with astrocyte microdomains M1 and M2. The green (dashed) arrows represent the release of neurotransmitters (NTs) from synaptic clefts to the astrocyte microdomain. The blue (solid) arrows labeled SICs illustrate glutamate binding the extrasynaptic receptors to produce SICs on nearby synapses. Copyright 2015 IEEE. Reprinted, with permission, from [7].

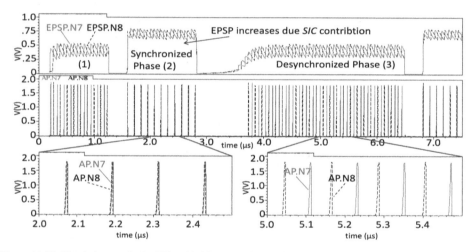

Figure 11.15. Simulation results for N7 and N8 in network 2, as shown in figure 11.14. Copyright 2015 IEEE. Reprinted, with permission, from[7].

In order to synchronize the firing of neurons in the presence of a SIC event, the NMDA block removal section of each adjacent synapse in both networks must be activated via meeting the necessary conditions discussed in subsection 4.1.5, leading to the activation of X11 of each synapse (refer to figure 4.6). Upon triggering X11, the total EPSP on each of the postsynaptic neurons, i.e. EPSP.N3, EPSP.N4, EPSP. N7 and EPSP.N8, is initially discharged to 0.0 V (at time 1.25 µs in figure 4.9; the end of section (1) of the simulation trace). This causes N3–N4 and N7–N8 to stop firing in the time interval corresponding to the pulse width at node A. SICs are simultaneously produced (at 1.6 µs in figure 4.9; the beginning of simulation trace section (2)) on the extrasynaptic side of synapses S3–S4 and S9–S10, i.e. when the NMDA block removal is activated. The simultaneous raise of the SIC event allows the neurons to cross their activation thresholds at the same time by the increase of the total EPSP, enabling N3–N4 and N7–N8 to begin firing synchronously with

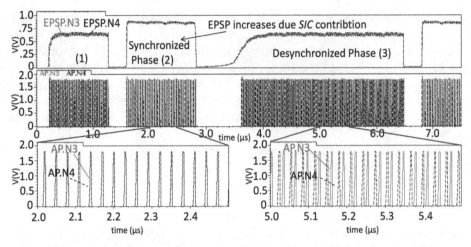

Figure 11.16. Simulation results for N3 and N4 in network 1, as shown in figure 11.14 [6].

each other. While the SIC event is active, neurons N3–N4 and N7–N8 remain synchronized in phase. Note that the increase of the EPSP amplitude in the synchronized phase (section (2) in figure 4.9) is due to the contribution of SIC amplitude (the top panels in figure 4.9(a) and 4.9(b)). Neurons N3–N4 and N7–N8 remain synchronized while the SIC amplitude is high enough not to trigger X12 by the E path in figure 4.6. After the SIC event has passed, X12 is activated and the neurons arrive at a desynchronization phase. Thus, X12 in each of these neurons simultaneously discharges the corresponding Total EPSPs to 0.0 V in a short time (at 2.8 μs in figure 4.9; the end of section (2)). Upon passing this time, i.e. when X12 is deactivated, the total EPSPs of N3–N4 and N7–N8 are charged to new states in which the firing of neurons is desynchronized in phase (at 3.6 μs in figure 4.9; the beginning of section (3)). The phase difference depends on the time at which the total EPSP of each neuron crosses its axon hillock threshold. In the desynchronized phase (section (3) in figure 4.9), the total EPSP receives only the contribution of synapses connected to each postsynaptic neuron and lacks the SIC event, so the phase difference between postsynaptic neurons on each network is dominated by the phase difference of their corresponding presynaptic neurons.

Besides synchronizing neurons not directly connected to each other, astrocytes also preserve homeostasis when synapses become inactive. This occurs when astrocytes participate in retrograde signaling, as described in the next section.

11.5 Retrograde signaling

Circuit designs that model retrograde messenger signaling[3], particularly involving astrocyte-neuron signaling (from Lee's thesis [15]), are presented in this section. The circuits include effects on synaptic plasticity in CMOS circuits modeling astrocytes and neurons. Furthermore, in this section we cover how the circuit models could be

---

[3] Signaling from postsynaptic to presynaptic neuron at the synapse.

used to repair networks with synaptic faults. Healthy synapses are strengthened in order to compensate for broken synapses that do not contribute to network behavior. Repair occurs autonomously in an activity-dependent manner. This type of self-repair would be good for highly active networks with low numbers of faults. If activity levels are insufficient, the necessary amount of potentiation at healthy synapses would not occur and self-repair might not occur.

A hardware model of retrograde signaling in astrocyte-neuromorphic circuits is presented in this section, including CMOS circuit models of neurons and astrocytes with retrograde signaling mechanisms. The CMOS circuits model a type of homeostatic mechanism where synaptic potentiation and depression caused by retrograde messengers balance each other out. The circuits are used to demonstrate a self-repairing neuromorphic hardware circuit inspired by [18]. Similar circuits and results were presented in [14] and will be covered in this section.

The block diagram of a neuron circuit with retrograde signaling mechanisms presented in this chapter is shown in figure 11.17. This type of neuron will be referred to as the neuron$_{RG}$ circuit. It is modified from the BioRC neuron circuit, and the pathways between synapses and astrocytes are also shown. Briefly, presynaptic APs (AP$_{pre}$) impinge on synapses. The synapses also respond to retrograde activity. EPSPs output from the synapses are summed by the dendritic arbor, and the total EPSP is sent to the axon hillock. When the total EPSP is above the firing threshold, the axon hillock emits an output spike (AP$_{post}$). The *retrograde messenger (RGM) generation* block raises voltage signals that mimic increases in the concentration of RGMs in the synaptic cleft in response to postsynaptic activity. The amplitude of RGM increases with more AP$_{post}$ spikes. Short-term synaptic plasticity mechanisms mediated by RGMs are included. The RGM signal is sent back to the excitatory synapses to suppress activity through RG depression. RGM is also sent to the astrocyte block where it increases intracellular Ca^{2+}. The astrocyte then releases glutamate (Glu$_{astro}$) in response to its Ca^{2+} level. Glu$_{astro}$ is sent back to the synapses and globally potentiates activity through the RG potentiation mechanism.

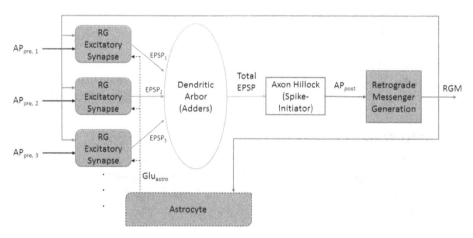

Figure 11.17. A block diagram of the neuron$_{RG}$ circuit [15].

The dendritic arbor and axon hillock components of the circuit are the same as previous designs from the BioRC group. Three new circuits were designed: (1) the RGM generation circuit block; (2) the astrocyte circuit; and (3) the retrograde (RG) excitatory synapse circuit. The RGM generation circuit converts postsynaptic activity of a neuron into a voltage that represents the concentration of RGM released back into the synaptic cleft. The astrocyte circuit detects neural activity and emulates the release of glutamate to presynaptic terminals. The circuit for the astrocyte is based on previous designs from the BioRC group but uses a different approach based on RGM concentrations instead of neurotransmitter concentrations. The RG excitatory synapse circuit is based on previous synapse designs from the BioRC group. However, the neurotransmitter concentration of the synapse can be modulated due to potentiating and depressing effects via astrocytes and retrograde signaling. CMOS designs for the new circuits will be presented in this section.

11.5.1 The retrograde messenger (RGM) generation circuit

In their biophysically-based computational model for astrocyte-neuron systems, Wade *et al* assumed that a postsynaptic neuron releases RGMs every time it fires. They described the dynamics of RGM generation and decay with the following equation [18]:

$$\frac{d(\text{RGM})}{dt} = \frac{-\text{RGM}}{\tau_{\text{RGM}}} + r_{\text{RGM}}\delta(t - t_{\text{sp}})$$

RGM represents the amount of retrograde messengers in the synaptic cleft. τ_{RGM} is the decay rate, and r_{RGM} is the production rate of RGMs. t_{sp} is the time when postsynaptic spikes are emitted.

A circuit model for RGM production and decay with a current mirror at its core is shown in figure 11.18. When a postsynaptic neuron fires, AP_{post} momentarily goes high, creating a current through transistors M1–M3. This current is mirrored to the

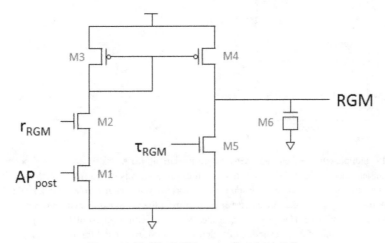

Figure 11.18. The RGM generation circuit [15].

pathway through transistors M4–5, and some charge gets stored on the capacitance formed by the gate of transistor M6. The output of this node (RGM) represents the amount of RGM in the synaptic cleft. The increase in RGM's amplitude every time a spike is fired is controlled by the signal r_{RGM} and the resistive properties of transistor M2. When r_{RGM} is high, more current is allowed to flow through the paths of the current mirror and RGM increases more. RGM decays through transistor M5. The rate of decay is controlled by the resistance through this path which is set by the bias voltage τ_{RGM}.

Sample outputs from the RGM generation circuit are shown in figure 11.19(a). The amplitude of RGM can be tuned by varying the voltage r_{RGM}. Higher r_{RGM} results in higher RGM amplitude. The time constant of RGM can also be tuned by varying τ_{RGM}. Higher τ_{RGM} voltages result in faster decay time constants. Using the resistive and capacitive properties of the RGM generation circuit, RGM can increase even further depending on the level of postsynaptic activity. Figure 11.19(b) shows the response when the postsynaptic neuron is very active. The postsynaptic neuron fires six action potentials with a period of 10 ns. Charge accumulates on transistor M6 in figure 11.18, and RGM increases with every spike. It increases to a final value of 0.92 V before decaying back to 0 V in the absence of firing activity. Figure 11.19(c) shows the case when activity in the postsynaptic neuron is low. The neuron fires with a period of 20 ns. RGM increases due to charge accumulation on transistor M6 after each spike, but it decays to 0 V during quiescent periods through transistor M5 and τ_{RGM} in figure 11.18. RGM never increases

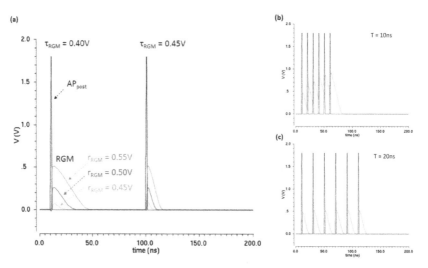

Figure 11.19. Sample outputs from the RGM generation circuit. (a) A postsynaptic action potential (AP$_{post}$) causes a transient increase in RGM. The rate of production r_{RGM} was varied from 0.45 V to 0.55 V and the RGM signals were plotted. The decay constant, τ_{RGM}, was 0.4 V for the first spike and 0.45 V for the second spike. (b) A train of AP$_{post}$ spikes (black curve) emitted from the postsynaptic neuron can cause *RGM* (blue curve) to increase even more. Here, six AP$_{post}$ spikes were fired with a period of 10 ns. (c) A train of AP$_{post}$ spikes fired with a period of 20 ns cannot cause increased RGM. In (b) and (c), τ_{RGM} was set to 0.45 V and r_{RGM} was 0.55 V [15].

above 0.53 V. This shows that sustained, intense levels of postsynaptic activity are required for RGM to increase significantly, similar to results found in biology.

11.5.2 The retrograde (RG) excitatory synapse circuit

Figure 11.20 shows the circuit for the RG excitatory synapse circuit from figure 11.17. It is a modified version of the BioRC excitatory synapse circuit that has been demonstrated previously. The BioRC excitatory synapse circuit converts a fast input action potential AP_{in} into a slow EPSP whose amplitude depends on the amount of neurotransmitter concentration (NT) in the synaptic cleft. Of course, rapid APs also increase the EPSP due to temporal summation. In the RG excitatory synapse circuit, We added presynaptic mechanisms that modulate the amount of NT. The mechanisms arise from the effects of RGMs on presynaptic neurotransmitter release. In the circuit, NT_{base} represents a baseline neurotransmitter concentration when effects of retrograde signaling are omitted, and NT represents the actual amount of neurotransmitter in the synaptic cleft. ΔNT represents the change in presynaptic neurotransmitter release due to RG depression and RG potentiation. When retrograde signaling and astrocytes are omitted, ΔNT is zero and NT is about equal to NT_{base}. When retrograde signaling and astrocyte mechanisms are included, ΔNT varies and is added to NT_{base} through an analog adder in order to modulate NT. ΔNT is the sum of two signals representing RG depression and RG potentiation mechanisms. The glu_{astro} signal represents glutamate released from an adjacent astrocyte, and the circuit generating this signal will be presented later in the next section.

In this model, it was assumed that the effects of RG depression on presynaptic neurotransmitter release are proportional to the amount of RGM released by the postsynaptic neuron, similar to the model presented by Wade *et al* [18]. The RG depression circuit module (also built around a current mirror) converts a positive RGM signal from figure 11.18 into a proportional negative signal *RG_dep*. *RG_dep* effectively decreases the value of *NT*, emulating the suppression of presynaptic neurotransmitter release by activation of RGM receptors. The value for VSS in the

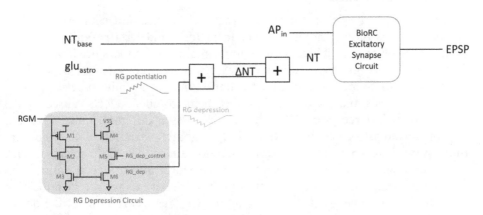

Figure 11.20. The RG excitatory synapse circuit [15].

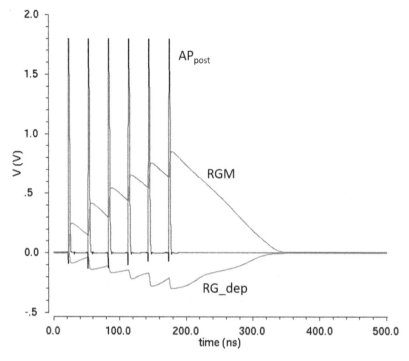

Figure 11.21. Sample results from the RG depression circuit block when *RGdepcontrol* = 0.4 V and *VSS* = −0.4 V[15].

experiments shown here was −0.4 V. The magnitude of RG depression is controlled by the signal *RG_dep_control*.

A demonstration of the RG depression circuit is shown in figure 11.21. Postsynaptic APs (AP$_{post}$) generate the RGM signal. The RGM signal is converted into a negative signal (*RG_dep*) whose value is proportional to RGM.

11.5.3 The astrocyte circuit

The circuit used to model interactions between astrocytes and neurons is loosely based on previous BioRC circuits designs from Joshi and Irizarry-Valle [7, 8, 11]. The circuit model presented here is different from previous works since it models the influence of RGMs on astrocytic Ca^{2+}. Previous designs consider astrocytic Ca^{2+} concentrations to be increased from activation by neurotransmitters released from presynaptic neurons, but the design described here considers effects caused by the activation of RGM receptors. This design also uses a different model for Ca^{2+} microdomains in astrocytes. In previous designs, spatial variation of Ca^{2+} concentrations were included in the astrocyte microdomain model. Ca^{2+} levels at each location of a microdomain were dependent on the neurotransmitter concentration in two adjacent synapses, and the amount of gliotransmitter released at each location was controlled in a fine-grained manner by the Ca^{2+} concentration. In the design described here, it is assumed that the Ca^{2+} concentration is the same at all locations within a microdomain. It is assumed that microdomains ensheath small groups of functionally-related synapses, and the microdomain concentration reflects the average Ca^{2+} level caused by the activity at all synapses connected to the micro-domain. When the Ca^{2+} in a microdomain is high enough, it can propagate and affect concentrations in adjacent microdomains.

A diagram illustrating the design methodology for the astrocyte circuit is shown in figure 11.22. It shows an astrocyte process that contains two microdomains. Each microdomain ensheathes three synapses in this example. Neural activity causes each synapse to release RGMs that are taken up by the microdomains. It is assumed that increases in RGMs cause a proportional increase in Ca^{2+}. The Ca^{2+} concentration in each microdomain can then be represented by averaging the RGM signals from each of its synapses. The amount of neurotransmitter (glutamate) that is released from each microdomain depends on the Ca^{2+} level, and it is the same at each synapse in the microdomain's territory. Ca^{2+} signaling also allows microdomains to commu-nicate with each other so that the synaptic activity in one microdomain can affect the activity in an adjacent microdomain. The astrocyte circuit is comprised of three subcomponents: (1) the microdomain Ca_{2+} circuit; (2) the microdomain coupling circuit; and (3) the astrocytic glutamate release circuit. The designs for these subcomponents are presented below.

The microdomain Ca^{2+} circuit is shown in figure 11.23. The RGM signals for each of the synapses connected belonging to the microdomain are connected to non-inverting, amplifying delay blocks (D). The outputs of the delay blocks are sent to a resistive averaging network, and $Ca_{microdomain}$ models the intracellular level of Ca^{2+} in the microdomain.

The microdomain coupling circuit is shown in figure 11.24. $Ca_{microdomain}$ signals from adjacent astrocytic microdomains are linked through NMOS pass transistors. When the $Ca_{microdomain_i}$ signal for a microdomain is above a threshold, the output (thr_i) of the coupling threshold circuit block goes high and turns on the pass transistor connecting it to an adjacent microdomain. Intracellular Ca^{2+} can propagate through an astrocyte when the concentration is high enough. The

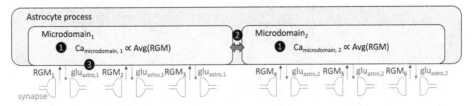

Figure 11.22. Design methodology for the astrocyte circuit. Astrocytes are divided into microdomains that ensheathe groups of synapses. Microdomain₁ and Microdomain₂ ensheathe three synapses each in this example. Each synapse releases an amount of retrograde messenger depending on its activity level. The RGM_i signals from each synapse get sent to their associated microdomains. The microdomain Ca^{2+} concentration ($Ca_{microdomain,i}$) is represented by the average of RGM signals (1). $Ca_{microdomain,i}$ signals from adjacent microdomains can influence each other (2). Microdomains release glutamate (glu_{astro}) in a $Ca_{microdomain}$-dependent manner. Glu_{astro} is the same for all synapses in the same microdomain. Synapses in Microdomain₁ receive $glu_{astro,1}$, and synapses in Microdomain₂ receive glu_2 [15].

1 Microdomain Ca^{2+} circuit:

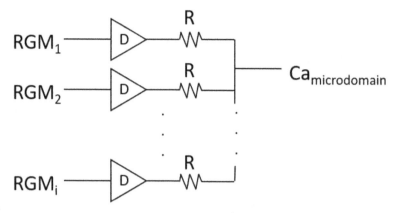

Figure 11.23. Microdomain Ca^{2+} circuit [15].

2 Microdomain coupling:

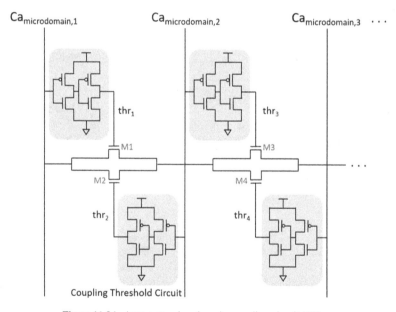

Figure 11.24. Astrocyte microdomain coupling circuit [15].

threshold for propagation can be controlled by precise sizing of transistors in the coupling threshold circuit blocks.

The astrocytic glutamate release circuit is shown in figure 11.25(a). It is a bio-inspired circuit based on the model proposed by Wade *et al* [18]. Their model included complex, biophysically-based dynamics that created Ca^{2+} waves in astrocytes. They assumed that astrocytes release a pulse of glutamate whenever the intracellular Ca^{2+} concentration rises above a threshold from below. The circuit model proposed in figure 11.25 is a simplified view of Wade's model that omits the complicated dynamics of Ca^{2+} waves and glutamate release. In the circuit models, the astrocyte Ca^{2+} signals represent time-averaged concentrations. It is assumed that an astrocyte periodically releases glutamate when its intracellular Ca^{2+} level is sufficiently high. In the circuit, the frequency of glutamate release is set by the control voltage f_{glu}, the amplitude is set by r_{glu}, and the decay rate is set by τ_{glu}. The Ca^{2+} for glutamate release is controlled by the sizing of transistors M1 and M2. Initially input $Ca_{microdomain}$ is below the threshold and glu_thr is high at V_{dd}. Transistor M3 is off and glu_pulse is held at ground through M5, so the output glu_{astro} is at ground. Once $Ca_{microdomain}$ exceeds the threshold, glu_thr falls to ground, turning on M3 and increasing glu_pulse to V_{dd}. M8 turns on and the left side of the capacitor (C) falls to 0 V. This causes the right side of the capacitor to also fall

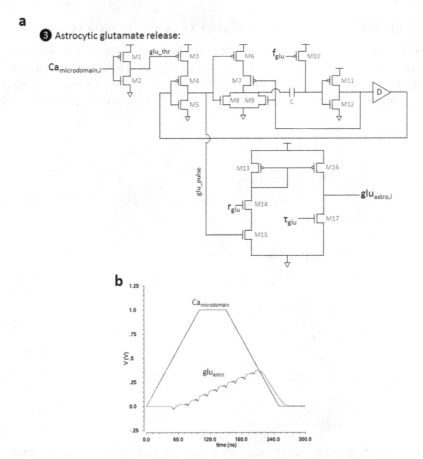

Figure 11.25. (a) The astrocytic glutamate release circuit. (b) Example output from the circuit when $f_{glu} = 1$ V, $r_{glu} = 0.32$ V, and $\tau_{glu} = 0.35$ V. The circuit output, glu_{astro}, starts to increase when $Ca_{microdomain}$ is over a threshold of 0.49 V [15].

to 0 V, and the output of the inverter formed by M11 and M12 rises to V_{dd}. This is sent through a non-inverting delay block (D) that turns on M5 and turns off M4 after a short period of time, and *glu_pulse* quickly falls back to 0 V. M6 then turns on and the capacitor slowly charges up to V_{dd} at a rate controlled by f_{glu}. Once the capacitor is sufficiently charged, the output of the M11–M12 inverter falls to 0 V, turning off M5 and turning on M4. If $Ca_{microdomain}$ is still high, this process can start over and another quick voltage pulse is generated at *glu_pulse*. *glu_pulse* is input to a current mirror formed by transistors M13–M17. Whenever *glu_pulse* goes high, a quick pulse of current flows through M16 and M17, and charge is stored on the transistor capacitances connected to glu_{astro}.

Sample results from the astrocytic glutamate release circuit are shown in figure 11.25(b). At 52 ns, $Ca_{microdomain}$ rises above the threshold of 0.49 V and glu_{astro} begins to increase. During the time that $Ca_{microdomain}$ is above the threshold, glu_{astro} increases every 20 ns. At 202 ns, $Ca_{microdomain}$ falls below 0.49 V. glu_{astro} is increased one last time before it decays back to 0 V.

11.6 Self-repair by RGM-mediated synaptic plasticity

The RGM signaling circuits were implemented in a feed-forward astrocyte-neuron network. The configuration is shown in figure 11.26(a). The network consists of five neurons (N_1–N_5), eight synapses (S_1–S_8), and an astrocyte with two microdomains (Microdomain$_1$ and Microdomain$_2$). Input APs, $AP_{in,1}$–$AP_{in,4}$, connect to N_1–N_4

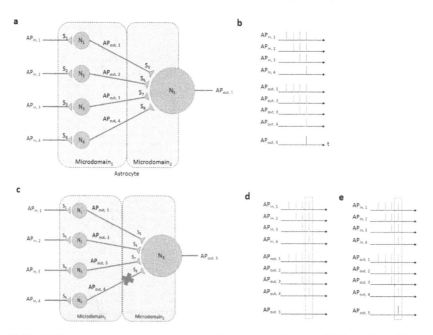

Figure 11.26. (a) The astrocyte-neuron network used to demonstrate self-repair. (b) Illustration of the expected results during normal operation. (c) The network with one synaptic fault at S_8. (d) Illustration of the results when no self-repair is used in the damaged network. (e) Illustration of the desired results when self-repair is used in the damaged network [15].

through synapses S_1–S_4. The strengths of these synapses are adjusted such that one input AP is sufficient to cause firing (AP_{out}) in the neuron. N5 receives inputs from synapses S_4–S_8. The strengths of the synapses are such that N5 should receive coincident action potentials $AP_{out,1}$–$AP_{ou,4}$ in order to fire. The expected behavior of the network when it is functioning normally is shown in figure 11.26(b). N5 emits $AP_{out,5}$ when all four inputs $AP_{in,1}$–$AP_{in,4}$ are given.

The situation when a synaptic fault occurs is shown in figure 11.26(c). Here, S8 is broken (red cross mark) so N5 does not receive input from N4. If no self-repairing mechanisms are used, N5 will not be able to fire regardless of the inputs as shown in figure 11.26(d). Using the circuit designs presented in the previous section, this would correspond to the case where RGM signaling mechanisms are disconnected. When self-repair by RGM signaling is implemented, we expect the network to regain function-ality similar to its normal state as shown in figure 11.26(e). When large activity is detected in astrocyte Microdomain$_1$, it should couple to Microdomain$_2$ through Ca^{2+} signaling and stimulate the release of glutamate that potentiates S_5–S_7. When S_5–S_7 are sufficiently strong, N5 regains functionality and is able to emit action potentials.

Circuit simulation results are shown in figure 11.27. In all simulations, $V_{dd} = 1.8$ V, $VSS = -0.4$ V, and input action potentials are triangular pulses with an amplitude of 1.8 V and width of 2 ns. The circuit was designed and simulated in Cadence Virtuoso using 180 nm CMOS technology. The network was stimulated by simultaneous trains of inputs $AP_{in,1}$-AP_4 with a period of 30 ns. Other relevant parameters were $r_{RGM} = 0.45$ V, $rg\,dep\,control = 0.4$ V, and $f_{glu} = 1$ V. The output signals during normal operation are shown in figure 11.27(a). $AP_{out,5}$ emits spikes after each input as expected. Figure 11.27(b) shows results when S_8 is disconnected from the circuit to model a synaptic fault and RGM signaling mechanisms are turned off by setting $RGM = 0$ V and $glu_{astro} = 0$ V for all synapses in the network. This effectively removes RGM generation and disconnects the astrocyte circuit. Since S_1–S_4 are not broken, action potentials are still seen in $AP_{out,1}$–$AP_{out,4}$. However, no spikes are seen in $AP_{out,5}$ since N5 does not receive the input $AP_{out,4}$.

Next, RGM signaling mechanisms are turned on and the output signals are plotted in figure 11.27(c). Initially N5 does not fire since the network is damaged. However, it starts to spike at 120 ns when the fourth input spike is given. To explain why this happens, we can look at the neurotransmitter (NT) signals that represent synapse weights, as shown in figure 11.27(d). The green curve plots NT for S_1–S_4. At these synapses, decreases and increases in neurotransmitter concentration due to RG depression and RG potentiation balance each other out, and the NT signal stays relatively constant, representing stable synaptic strengths. Ca^{2+} increases in Microdomain$_1$ and propagates to Microdomain$_2$, inducing glutamate release and potentiation. At synapses connected to N5, the effects of RG potentiation will be greater than those of RG depression, resulting in an increase in synaptic weights. This is shown in the blue curve that plots NT for S_5–S_7. The NT signal slowly increases and after 120 ns it is large enough to allow N5 to fire.

The amount of neural activity required before self-repair occurs can be tuned by varying r_{RGM}, the signal that represents the rate of RGM production. The number

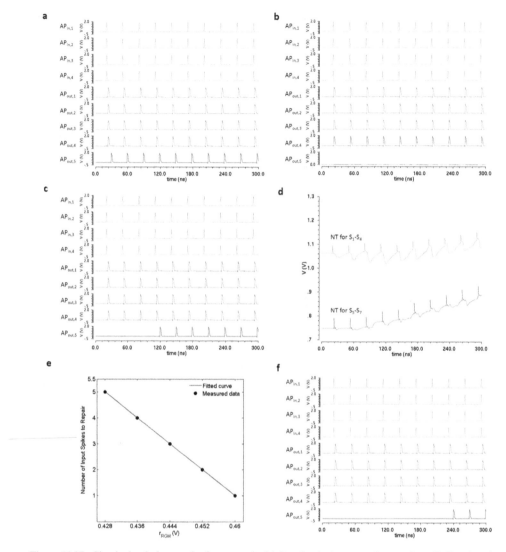

Figure 11.27. Circuit simulation results for network. (a) Results during normal operation. (b) Results when RGM signaling is omitted and one synapse (S_8) is broken. (c) Results when RGM signaling is included and S_8 is broken. (d) Neurotransmitter (NT) signals for the synapses when S_8 is broken. (e) Number of input spikes required before self-repair occurs as a function of r_{RGM} when S_8 is broken. (f) Results when two synapses (S_7 and S_8) are broken [15].

of coincident input spikes before self-repair occurs is plotted as a function of r_{RGM} in figure 11.27(e). It can be seen that higher r_{RGM} values will need less network activity in order to initiate self-repair.

Simulation results for a network with two broken synapses (S_7 and S_8) are shown in figure 11.27(f). Self-repair occurs after seven input spikes have been given, showing that more neural activity is required when more faults are present. This is because more astrocytic Ca^{2+} needs to build up for sufficient amounts of glutamate to be released. The use of this self-repair mechanism is described in [14].

11.7 Chapter summary

This chapter covered circuits implementing the tripartite synapse, neural synchronization, retrograde signaling and self-repair of synapses, all involving astrocytes. The material spanned two dissertations by Irizarry-Valle and Lee.

The next chapter contains circuits for the retina designed by Ko-Chung Tseng.

Certain sections of text in this chapter have been reproduced with permission from [7], [12] and [21]. Copyright IEEE.

References

[1] Allam S L *et al* 2012 A computational model to investigate astrocytic glutamate uptake influence on synaptic transmission and neuronal spiking *Front. Comput. Neurosci.* **6** 70

[2] Carmignoto G and Fellin T 2006 Glutamate release from astrocytes as a non-synaptic mechanism for neuronal synchronization in the hippocampus *J. Physiol. Paris* **99** 98–102

[3] Chaoui H 1995 CMOS analogue adder *Electron. Lett.* **31** 180–1

[4] Hsu C-C 2014 Dendritic computation and plasticity in neuromorphic circuits *PhD Thesis* University of Southern California

[5] Hsu C-C and Parker A C 2014 Dynamic spike threshold and nonlinear dendritic computation for coincidence detection in neuromorphic circuits *2014 36th Annual Int. Conf. of the Engineering in Medicine and Biology Society IEEE* (Piscataway, NJ: IEEE) 461–4

[6] Irizarry-Valle Y 2016 Modeling astrocyte-neural interactions in CMOS neuromorphic circuits *PhD Thesis* University of Southern California

[7] Irizarry-Valle Y and Parker A C 2015 An astrocyte neuromorphic circuit that influences neuronal phase synchrony *IEEE Trans. Biomed. Circuits Syst.* **9** 175–87

[8] Irrizarry-Valle Y, Parker A C and Joshi J 2013 A CMOS neuromorphic approach to emulate neuro-astrocyte interactions *Int. Joint Conf. Neural Networks (IJCNN)*

[9] Joshi J, Parker A C and Hsu C C 2010 A carbon nanotube spiking cortical neuron with tunable refractory period and spiking duration *IEEE 2010 Latin American Symp. on Circuits and Systems (LASCAS 2010)*

[10] Joshi J 2013 Plasticity in CMOS Neuromorphic Circuits *PhD Thesis* University of Southern California

[11] Joshi J, Parker A C and Tseng K-C 2011 An synchronization glial microdomain to invoke excitability in cortical neural networks 2011 *Int. Symp. of Circuits and Systems (ISCAS) IEEE* (Piscataway, NJ: IEEE) 681–4

[12] Joshi J, Parker A C and Tseng K-C 2011 An in-silico glial microdomain to invoke excitability in cortical neural networks *IEEE Int. Symp. Circuits and Systems ISCAS*

[13] Joshi J *et al* 2009 A carbon nanotube cortical neuron with excitatory and inhibitory dendritic computations *2009 IEEE/NIH Life Science Systems and Applications Workshop* (Bethesda, MD: IEEE) 133–6

[14] Lee R K and Parker A C 2019 An electronic neuron with input-specific spiking *2019 Int. Joint Conf. Neural Networks (IJCNN)* (Piscataway, NJ: IEEE) 1–8

[15] Lee R K 2018 Astrocyte-mediated plasticity and repair in CMOS neuromorphic circuits *PhD Thesis* University of Southern California

[16] Lia A *et al* 2021 Calcium signals in astrocyte microdomains, a decade of great advances *Front. Cell. Neurosci.* **15** 177

[17] Parker A C 2013 The biorc biomimetic real-time cortex project University of Southern California URL: http://ceng.usc.eduparker/BioRCresearch.html

[18] Wade J *et al* 2012 Self-repair in a bidirectionally coupled astrocyte-neuron (an) system based on retrograde signaling *Front. Comput. Neurosci.* **6** 76

[19] Wade J J *et al* 2011 Bidirectional coupling between astrocytes and neurons mediates learning and dynamic coordination in the brain: a multiple modeling approach *PLoS One* **6** e29445

[20] Haydon P G and Carmignoto G 2006 Astrocyte control of synaptic transmission and neurovascular coupling *Physiol. Rev.* **86** 1009–1031

[21] Irizarry-Valle Y and Parker A C 2014 Astrocyte on neuronal phase synchrony in CMOS *2014 IEEE International Symposium on Circuits and Systems (ISCAS) (Melbourne)* 261–64

[22] Joshi J, Parker A C and Tseng K-C 2011 An in-silico glial microdomain to invoke excitability in cortical neural networks *Circuits and Systems (ISCAS), 2011 IEEE Int. Symp.* 681–4

[23] Carmignoto G 2000 Reciprocal communication systems between astrocytes and neurones *Neurobiol.* **62** 561–81

Chapter 12

The retina

Ko-Chung Tseng and Alice C Parker

For this chapter, focused on the retina, we implement a portion of the starburst amacrine cell (SAC) and differential motion detection model, drawn from Tseng's thesis [42]. We also investigate the importance of the feedback and lateral connections in implementing these motion sensing functions in a silicon circuit. To validate the importance of the feedback and lateral pathways in the silicon retina, we first build a portion of a retinal network from photoreceptors to ganglion cells that maintains a hierarchical structure similar to that of the biological retina. Lateral connections with horizontal cells and amacrine cells are implemented, along with feedback within the inner and outer plexiform layers of the retina. We then perform demonstrations by comparing the silicon retina tested to one altered by removing these pathways and observing how the behaviors in the silicon retina are changed.

We also compare some of our simulation results with biological data. In this research, we showed that some functions cannot be achieved or performances degrade without feedback and lateral connections. Hence, we concluded that incorporating feedback and lateral connections in the artificial retina helps the performance even though it complicates the retinal network.

This chapter also contains the major results of the dissertation research, directional selectivity, differential motion detection, and the complete retinal pathway from photoreceptor to ganglion cell spiking. These mechanisms are demonstrated with neural compartments that illustrate these particular behaviors, but entire cell designs for the amacrine cells are not included in the research. Since the amacrine cells do not spike, the dendrites designed could be joined easily into complete cells.

12.1 Related retinal neuromorphic research

In an effort to compare our research with other related work, we introduce related work by classifying the related work into three categories: (1) neuromorphic designs of the retina in silicon circuits; (2) neuromorphic models of motion detection in the visual system; and (3) implantable artificial retinas. We describe the related studies and explain the importance of our research by presenting a comparison.

12.1.1 Neuromorphic designs of the retina in silicon circuits

Mead and Mahowald first modeled early visual processing in the retina [33] in analog CMOS using very large-scale integration (VLSI) technology. The computation performed by their silicon retina is based on models of computation in distal layers of the vertebrate retina, which include the cones, the horizontal cells, and the bipolar cells (BCs). Cones have been implemented using parasitic phototransistors and MOS-diode logarithmic current-to-voltage converters. Horizontal cells perform averaging using a hexagonal network of resistors. BCs detect the difference between the average output of the horizontal cells and the output of the cone. The design can perform contrast enhancement and center-surround antagonism. Soon after that, Delbruck and Mead proposed the first adaptive photoreceptor [12] which models light adaptation using feedback in an analog circuit. Mahowald combined these two designs and proposed a more complete artificial outer retina [32] that can also perform contrast enhancement and center-surround antagonism. Delbruck later proposed several improved versions of the adaptive photoreceptor designs [10, 11]. Boahen and Andreou modeled the outer plexiform layer of the vertebrate retina using an analog circuit [6]. They used a current-mode circuit to model the reciprocal synapses between cones and horizontal cells that produce the antagonistic center/ surround receptive field. Delbruck and Liu designed a silicon chip that emulates the neurons in the visual system by using analog very large-scale integration (aVLSI) circuits [13]. Their design aimed at substituting for a live animal in experiment designs and lectures. The model contained photoreceptor cells, horizontal cells, ON–OFF BCs, and ON–OFF ganglion cells. The neurons in Tseng's chip displayed properties that are central to biological vision: receptive fields, spike coding, adaptation, band-pass filtering, and complementary signaling. Due to the lack of feedback from horizontal cells to photoreceptor cells, as well as amacrine cells, their design could only demonstrate limited functions. Hasegawa and Yagi emulated the architecture and functionality of the vertebrate outer retina [21]. Their silicon retina carries out the spatial filtering of input images instantaneously, using embedded resistive networks that emulate the receptive field structure of the outer retinal neurons, and a digital computer carries out temporal filtering of the spatially filtered images to emulate dynamic properties of the outer retinal circuits. The aim of their study was to emulate dynamic neural images produced by BCs in response to natural scenes in real time. Kameda and Yagi modeled the outer retina using an analog neuromorphic multi-chip system to mimic the hierarchical structure of the outer retina [27]. The functional network circuits were divided into two chips: the photoreceptor network chip (P chip) and the horizontal cell network chip (H chip). The output images of the P chip are transferred to the H chip using analog voltages through the bus. An off-chip differential amplifier that models the BC layer takes input from photoreceptors and horizontal cells. Their design realized a receptive field that carries out smoothing and contrast enhancement on input images. Zaghloul and Boahen proposed a silicon retina that reproduces the signals in the optic nerve [50]. Their approach was to design an artificial retina from an information theory point of view. They included both ON and OFF cone pathways in their model. Their model has the corresponding nodes representing the responses of the retinal cells. The retinal cells in their model include photoreceptors, horizontal cells, ON/OFF BCs, wide/narrow field amacrine cells, and 4 types of ganglion cells (namely ON-transient, ON-sustained, OFF-transient, and OFF-sustained ganglion cells). The combination of all these retinal cells in their transistor circuit reproduced the responses of ganglion cells. They tested the silicon retina by applying impulses with different frequencies.

12.1.2 Neuromorphic models of motion detection in the visual system

Andreou and Strohbehn designed an aVLSI processor for computer vision based on the Hassenstein–Reichardt–Poggio model for information processing in the visual system of a fly [2]. In their model, the delayed photoreceptor responses may correlate with the current responses of neighboring receptors and perform directional selectivity. Liu was also inspired by motion computation in the fly's visual system and created a neuromorphic circuit model of global motion processing in the fly [31]. Benson and Delbruck proposed a silicon retinal model for direction selectivity [5]. Their design used inhibitory connections in the null direction to perform the direction selectivity. They included only photoreceptor cells and direction-selective ganglion cells (DSGCs) in their model. Etienne-Cummings assumed primate motion detection is performed in the cortex and analyzed insect and primate visual motion detection in a hardware implementation [15]. However, the comparison does not include motion detection in the retina. Wang and Liu designed an aVLSI network using spiking neurons for motion detection [46] which was based on the model proposed by Rao for explaining the formation of direction- and velocity-selective cells in the visual cortex [41]. Nevertheless, their model was not focusing on the retina.

12.1.3 Implantable artificial retinas

Researchers led by Humayun on the 'Artificial Retina Project' developed an implantable microelectronic retinal prosthesis. Their approach was to develop an implantable microeletronic retinal prosthesis that restores sight to people blinded by retinal diseases. Visually-impaired patients whose conditions are not congenital (namely, the optic nerve and visual cortex remain functional) could undergo a surgical procedure involving surgically implanting a special microchip behind the retina to restore partial sight [25]. Their most recent retinal prosthesis system is Argus II (now bought by Vivant, the status of the produce is unlear). It consisted of five main parts: (1) digital camera built into a pair of glasses which captured images in real time and sent images to a microchip; (2) a video-processing microchip built into a handheld unit that processed images into electrical pulses representing patterns of light and dark and sends the pulses to a radio transmitter in the glasses; (3) a radio transmitter that wirelessly transmitted pulses to a receiver implanted above the ear or under the eye; (4) a radio receiver that sent pulses to the retinal implant by a hair-thin implanted wire; and (5) a retinal implant with an array of 60 electrodes on a chip measuring 1 mm by 1 mm. The camera was implanted in the frame of one's eyeglasses to stimulate an array of electrodes placed on the retinal surface. The moving images are sent along the optic nerve to the brain. The device could provide sight (the detection of light) to people who have become blind from degenerative eye diseases like macular degeneration and *retinitis pigmentosa*. The ultimate goal of the project is to restore reading ability, facial recognition, and unaided mobility for the blind [20]. Due to the vast knowledge required from multiple sources, the 'Artificial Retina Project' requires multidisciplinary collaboration with medical science, material science, neuroscience, biomedical engineering, and electrical engineering. Parker and Azar have proposed a bio-inspired 3D hierarchical pyramidal architecture for a synthetic retina [37]. They proposed that future artificial retinas should maintain a hierarchical structure similar to that of the biological retina. To substitute an artificial retina for a biological retina, an artificial retina should be able to process visual information in a similar way to how a biological retina would. In other words, the future artificial retina should be equipped with the capability of processing visual information including adaptation, dynamic behaviors, and extracting useful and variant information from the scene. Their model aims to mimic the overall structure, connectivity, and functionality of the human retina. They have also raised several challenges for future retinal prostheses which include power consumption, modeling visual information processing, encoding visual information into spikes, and biocompatiblility.

12.2 Comparison of Tseng's research to state of the art

For research described in this chapter, Tseng implemented a portion of the starburst amacrine cell (SAC) and differential motion detection model found in the vertebrate retina. Modeling this aspect of the vision system had not been done by others and may be useful for service robots, autonomous vehicles and other applications that require processing dynamic visual information in real time.

Moreover, Tseng used the circuits to validate the importance of the feedback and lateral pathways in performing motion sensing functions of a silicon retina. In order to achieve this, Tseng implemented many CMOS circuits that model the mechanisms in the biological retinas. The mechanisms that he implemented can be removed by disconnecting feedback or lateral connection among CMOS circuits modeling retinal cells. This allowed him to perform demonstrations by comparing the silicon retina tested to one altered by removing these pathways and observing how the behaviors in the silicon retina are changed. Table 12.1 compares Tseng's research to the related work that we have described.

12.3 The outer retina design

This section presents Tseng's outer retinal circuits as well as their testing results. The outer retina has been modeled by others extensively. In order to be compatible with the inner retinal circuits in the next section, he designed his own outer retinal circuits

Table 12.1. Comparison to state of the art research in neuromorphic designs of the retina. Reproduced from [51].

Name	Target	Approach	Input size	Output	Functionality
BioRC Retina (2012)	Inner and outer retina (the vertebrate retina)	MOS transistors	490 photoreceptors	Spikes	(1) Contrast enhancement (2) Center-surround antagonism (3) Directional selectivity (4) Differential motion detection
Mahowald (1992)	Outer retina	MOS transistors	4096 photoreceptors	Graded potential	(1) Contrast enhancement (2) Center-Surround antagonism
Hasegawa and Yagi (2008)	Outer retina	Digital processing (PC) and FPGA	1840 photoreceptors	Graded potential	Spatiotemporal responses of BCs
Kameda and Yagi (2006)	Outer retina	FPGA	1840 photoreceptors	Graded potential	(1) Contrast enhancement (2) Center-Surround antagonism
Zaghloul and Boahen (2001) Spikes	Inner and outer retina Responses over different frequencies	MOS transistors	5760	Graded potential	phototransistors
Delbruck and Liu (2004)	Inner and outer retina w/o Amacrine cells	MOS transistors	7 photoreceptors	Spikes	(1) Contrast enhancement (2) Center-Surround antagonism
Andreou and Strohbehn (1990)	Fly's visual system	MOS transistors	50 photoreceptors	Graded potential	Directional selectivity
Benson and Delbruck (1997)	Photoreceptors and direction selectivity (DS) cell	MOS transistors	1927 photoreceptors	Graded potential	Directional selectivity
USC Artificial Retina Project (2012)	Implantable artificial retina	Microelectronic prosthesis	60 electrodes	Current	Restore sight to the blind

that performed edge detection, contrast enhancement, and center-surround antagonism. He also created an external control knob (i.e. glutamate reuptake) to control the amount of neurotransmitter from the photoreceptor reaching a postsynaptic site of the horizontal cell. The circuit models include the photoreceptor circuit, the horizontal cell compartment circuits, and the transient on-type BC circuit.

12.3.1 The photoreceptor circuit and testing results

Tseng's photoreceptor design is a modified version of the adaptive photoreceptor design by Delbruck and Mead [10] shown in figure 12.1. With a delayed feedback path, their adaptive photoreceptor provides high gain for transient signals that are centered around the adaptation point. Due to its simple structure and the adaptive property, we used their design and made some changes to meet our requirements, namely modeling the output response of biological photoreceptors. The modifications are as follows: (1) the design was revised to better match the responses of biological photoreceptors; (2) a transistor, whose gate receives feedback from the horizontal cell (i.e. HC_fb) was added; (3) the transistors M1 and M2 were added for adjusting the light sensitivity. Please refer to figure 12.2. When absorbing photons, the photodiode induces a current flow that pulls down the gate voltage of M3. It results in an increase of the gate voltage of M9. And, the output, therefore, drops. After some delay that is produced by M8 and C1, the output response will lower the gate voltage of M6 that pulls down the gate voltage of M9. As a result, the output increases. This adaptive property is due to the negative feedback loop that models the adaptive property of the biological photoreceptor. We can control the sensitivity of the photoreceptor circuit by adjusting the sensitivity control knob. If the voltage level of sensitivity is high, transistor M1 is more resistive and the gate voltage of M3 can be pulled up higher, given the amount of current flowing through the photodiode. If the voltage level of sensitivity is low, transistor M1 is less resistive and requires a stronger light, namely more current flowing

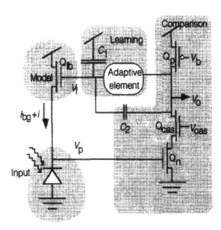

Figure 12.1. The photoreceptor circuit design By Delbruck and Mead. Copyright 1994 IEEE. Reprinted, with permission, from [10].

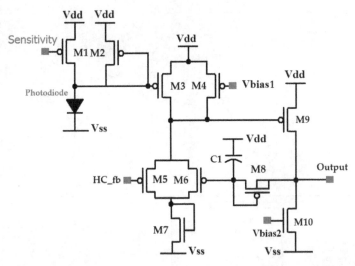

Figure 12.2. The photoreceptor circuit design. Reproduced from [51].

through the photodiode, to pull up the gate voltage of M3 in order to evoke a stronger response at the output.

The simulations of the photoreceptor circuit in figures 12.3 and 12.4 were conducted using TSMC18 CMOS (180 nm) technology in SPECTRE and sensitivity was set to be 0.9 V. (We will explain how changing sensitivity alters the output response later.) We used a current source to model the photocurrent flowing through the photodiode. In figure 12.3, we observed the output response during the time window from 0 to 400 μs. We first applied 200 nA as initial DC input current and changed the current intensity at time 100 μs. We tried different amounts of input changes (200 nA, 220 nA, 240 nA, 260 nA, 280 nA, 300 nA, and 320 nA). As the amount of input change increased, the response of the photoreceptor output increased as well. The overshoots after removal of light were due to the internal feedback of the photoreceptor design. Similar responses are observed in biological photoreceptors as well [8].

Figure 12.4 shows the relationship between the input range and the output range under 13 different amounts of initial photocurrent (including 100 nA, 500 nA, 1000 nA, 1500 nA, 2000 nA, 2500 nA, 3000 nA, 3500 nA, 4000 nA, 6000 nA, 8000 nA, 10 000 nA, and 15 000 nA). The blue trace (labeled by DC) crossing all the other curves represents the output voltage level of the photoreceptor at different amounts of initial photocurrent before changing the photocurrent. Under different amounts of initial photocurrent, we varied the photocurrent intensity, recorded the peak values of the output responses, and formed 13 different curves labeled by their values of initial photocurrent (100 nA, 500 nA, 1000 nA, 1500 nA, 2000 nA, 2500 nA, 3000 nA, 3500 nA, 4000 nA, 6000 nA, 8000 nA, 10 000 nA, and 15 000 nA) shown on the right side of the figure. As the amount of initial photocurrent increases, the input range to cause responses also increased. In other words, the photoreceptor

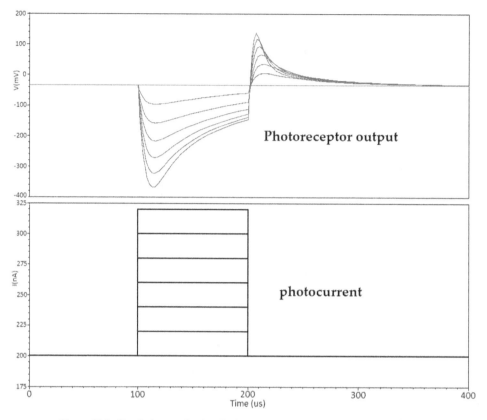

Figure 12.3. Simulation result of an isolated photoreceptor. Reproduced from [51].

was sensitive to a small input change at a relatively dark background while less sensitive to a small input change at a relatively bright background.

We examined the effect of changing the sensitivity of the photoreceptor. We first gave 200 nA of photocurrent as the initial value. Then, we changed the photocurrent and observed the amplitude of the output response under seven different values of the sensitivity input (including 0.6 V, 0.5 V, 0.4 V, 0.36 V, 0.34 V, 0.32 V, and 0.3 V). We used the photocurrent intensity as the x-axis and the response amplitude as the y-axis to plot figure 12.5. In this figure, eight different curves were labeled by their values of the sensitivity input. We observed that the input range (i.e. the range of the photocurrent intensity) is shifting when changing the sensitivity input. Therefore, we concluded that the photoreceptor requires stronger input changes to evoke the output response as the sensitivity input decreases,.

To better analyze the circuit's behavior, we further found the best-fit line (in figure 12.6) illustrating the output response and compared it with the response of the photoreceptor circuit. The equation of the best-fit line is shown in equation (12.1) in which we decomposed the equation into three components, i.e. DC, pull-down, and pull-up.

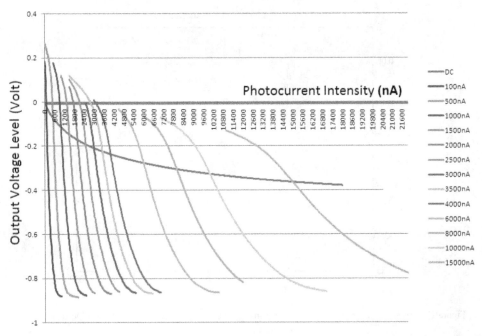

Figure 12.4. Response ranges of the photoreceptor (when sensitivity is 900 mV). Reproduced from [51].

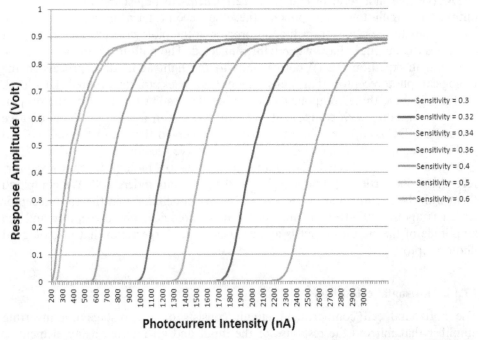

Figure 12.5. The range of the responses of an isolated photoreceptor given different sensitivity values ranging from 0.6 to 0.3 Volt. Reproduced from [51].

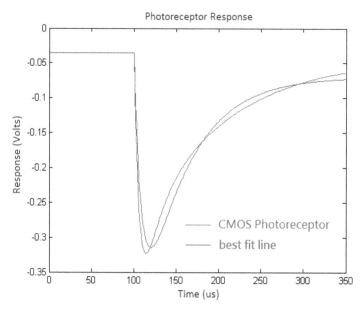

Figure 12.6. Best-fit line representing the response of the photoreceptor circuit. Reproduced from [51].

$$\text{Response}(t) = -0.0689 - (0.4462 \times e^{-0.019\,37 \times t}) + (0.48 \times e^{-0.1062 \times t})(\text{Volts}) \quad (12.1)$$

DC (i.e. the first term in equation (12.1)) helps to adjust the DC level of the output. The pull-down component (i.e. the second term in equation (12.1)) corresponds to the photo-transduction process in the biological photoreceptor that decreases the output voltage when light is injected. The pull-up component (i.e. the last term in equation (12.1)) corresponds to the light adaptation process in the biological photoreceptor that pulls the output back to its original DC level. At time 0, these three components determine the resting potential of the output. To better visualize each component, we plotted them in figure 12.7. Note that we divided the DC component into two parts and merged them into the pull-up and pull-down components, allowing us to easily observe the curves.

Moreover, we collected the output responses of biological photoreceptors recorded from turtles [8], humans [35], and tiger salamanders [18]. We compared them with the circuit's outputs in figure 12.8. We concluded that the photoreceptor circuit is about 4000–10 000 times faster than biological photoreceptors and the amplitude of the circuit output is about 20–50 times larger than that of biological photoreceptors.

12.3.2 Horizontal cell design

The horizontal cell compartment circuit consists of a two-stage non-inverting amplifier that mirrors the response of the input and an internal delay element, a diode-connected PMOS transistor, between two amplifiers, as shown in figure 12.9. To model the horizontal cell layer, the output, horizontal cell (HC) membrane

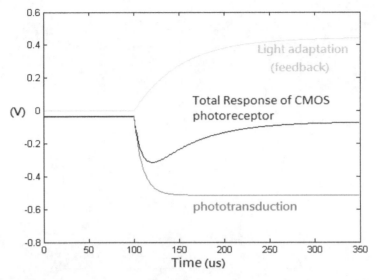

Figure 12.7. Curves representing the decomposed terms of the best-fit line. Reproduced from [51].

potential, is connected to other compartments through pass transistors that are used to model resistors. The pass transistors act like resistors, which has been determined to be a good model for HCs [45, 48].

12.3.3 The outer retina network and testing results

In figure 12.10, we show the circuit implementing the interaction of one photo-receptor and one HC compartment. Between two circuits, we inserted a buffer with a control knob, glutamate reuptake, that models the effect of glutamate reuptake. The input termed 'glutamate reuptake' can be used to demonstrate the impact of glutamate uptake on the HC. The outputs of the photoreceptor and glutamate reuptake control determine the voltage response of glutamate release reaching the postsynaptic site of the HC. The response of the HC compartment mirrors the response of 'glutamate concentration' with the internal delay modeled by transistor M13, and is modulated by the output responses of its neighboring HC compartments. When the voltage of the photoreceptor's output drops, the HC compartment's output drops as well. The response of each HC compartment feeds back to the photoreceptor and helps to perform some functions such as contrast enhancement and center-surround property. As we explained in chapter 1, the feedback from the HC compartment to the photoreceptor is negative. To demonstrate the functions of the feedback, we will compare the outer retina design tested to one altered by removing the HC layer in this section.

To explain the connections of the outer retina, a one-dimensional outer-retinal network structure is shown in figure 12.11. One photoreceptor connects to one HC compartment. A complete HC is formed by connecting a few compartments with pass transistors. Each photoreceptor influences others through the HC compartments and the resistor network. To demonstrate the properties of the outer retina

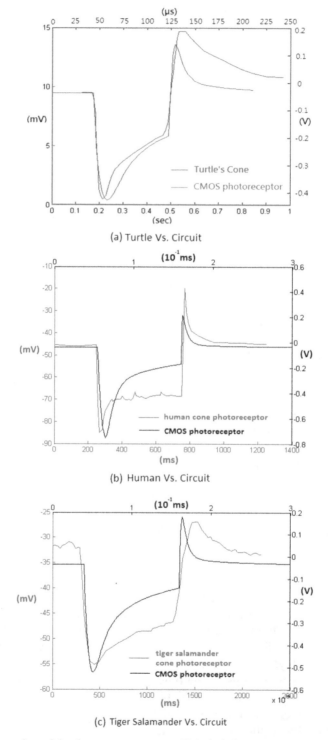

Figure 12.8. Comparison of the photoreceptor output to biological photoreceptors. Reproduced from [51].

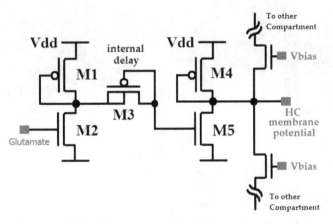

Figure 12.9. The HC compartment design. Reproduced from [51].

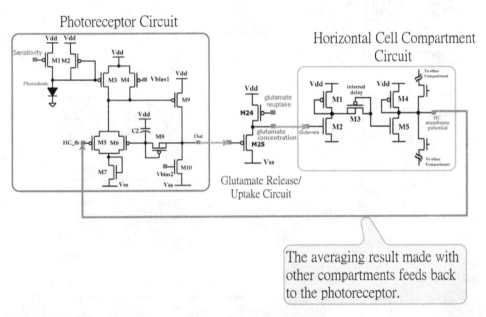

Figure 12.10. The interaction between a photoreceptor design and an HC compartment design. Reproduced from [51].

network, we constructed a two-dimensional network structure and did some experiments which will be shown in the following section.

12.3.4 Glutamate reuptake

As we described in the previous section, we inserted a buffer with a control knob, glutamate reuptake, that models the effect of glutamate reuptake. The rate of glutamate reuptake is represented by the voltage level of the input, glutamate reuptake. To examine changing the input of glutamate reuptake, we used the circuit

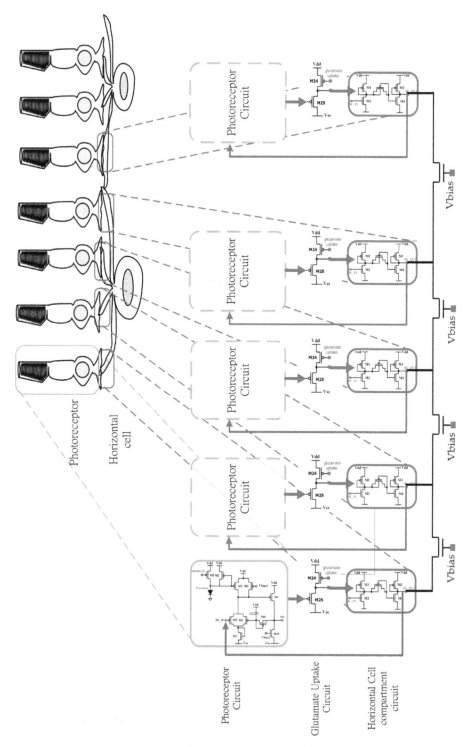

Figure 12.11. A one-dimensional photoreceptor-HC network. Reproduced from [51].

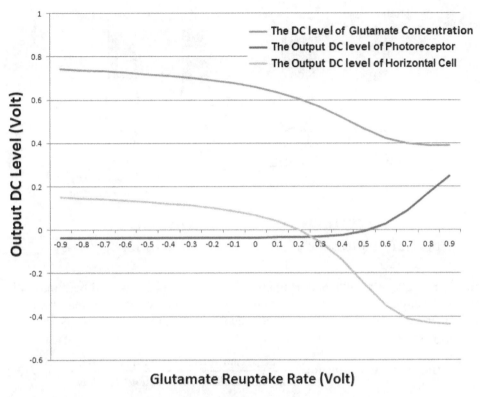

Figure 12.12. Simulation result for changing glutamate reuptake from −0.9 to 0.9 V. Reproduced from [51].

shown in figure 12.10 that contains a photoreceptor circuit and an HC compartment circuit. We gave 200 nA of photocurrent and varied the glutamate reuptake rate from low to high by sweeping glutamate reuptake from −0.9 to 0.9 Volt in the circuit. We observed the change of glutamate concentration, along with the output DC levels of the photoreceptor and HC. Note that the voltage level of glutamate concentration corresponds to the glutamate concentration in the synaptic cleft. The higher the voltage level is, the higher the glutamate concentration is. And, we used the glutamate reuptake rate as the *x*-axis and the output DC level as the *y*-axis to plot the results shown in figure 12.12. As the glutamate reuptake rate increased, the DC level of glutamate concentration was reduced. The DC level of the HC output will decrease due to less excitation provided by glutamate. The DC level of the photoreceptor will increase due to less inhibition from the HC.

12.3.5 Contrast enhancement

To demonstrate that the interaction of photoreceptors and HCs can enhance the contrast of two inputs, we used two configurations to perform the experiments as shown in figure 12.13: one has two photoreceptors; the other has two photo-receptors interacting with an HC. We used eight different amounts of photocurrents

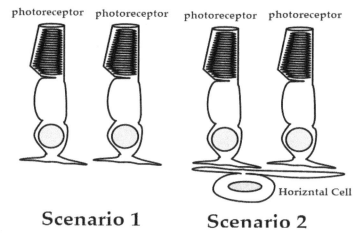

Figure 12.13. Two configurations for testing contrast enhancement. Reproduced from [51].

(i.e. 0, 100, 200, 300, 400, 500, 600, and 700 nA) as the background light intensities to test the circuits. In each case, we increased the amount of photocurrent, measured the difference of the two outputs, and calculated the amount of contrast enhancement by using the following equation.

$$\text{Contrast enhancement} = \frac{\textbf{The output difference with feedback}}{\textbf{The output difference without feedback}} \quad (12.2)$$

Note that the output differences in both cases are measured from resting level to peak. The simulation results of the eight cases are plotted in figure 12.14, where eight different amounts of photocurrents (i.e. 0, 100, 200, 300, 400, 500, 600, and 700 nA) as the background light intensities are used, respectively. In each plot, x- and y-axis represent the two inputs and z-axis represents the amount of contrast enhancement. For all the cases shown in the figure, the amount of contrast enhancement increased as the amount of the two inputs are getting closer (namely along the diagonal line). However, when the difference of the two inputs is really small, the amount of contrast enhancement will quickly drop to one. Therefore, we can infer that the difference of the two inputs must pass a certain amount of threshold to exhibit contrast enhancement. Based on the simulation results in figure 12.14, the threshold increased as the background light intensity increased.

To explain the contrast enhancement in the circuit, please refer to figure 12.10. When the light shines on the photodiode, the gate voltage of transistor M3 increases and then the output of the photoreceptor decreases. The output of the HC also decreases and averages with the responses of its neighboring HC compartments. The averaging output response from the HC compartment then feeds back to the gate of transistor M5 which pulls down the source voltage of transistor M3. As you notice, transistor M3 whose conductivity is proportional to the light intensity is competing against transistor M5 which receives the feedback from the HC compartment. If the light intensity is weak, the feedback can easily increase the output response of the

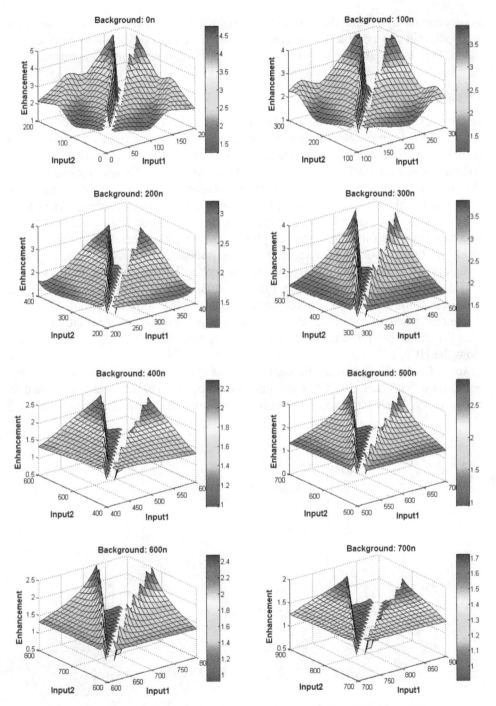

Figure 12.14. Simulation results of contrast enhancement. Reproduced from [51].

photoreceptor and make the output more positive. If the light intensity is strong, the feedback will not be able to increase the output voltage of the photoreceptor too much. Due to this property, the circuit can exhibit contrast enhancement.

12.3.6 Center-surround property

In the previous section, we demonstrated that the neuromophic design can exhibit contrast enhancement. In this section, we constructed a larger network to further demonstrate the center-surround property. As we explained in chapter 1, HC-to-cone feedback helps establish the center-surround arrangement of visual receptive fields. We will demonstrate the complete retinal pathway performing center-surround property. In this section, we observed the response of center photoreceptors instead. In the case of dark center bright surround, the center photoreceptors receive a strong feedback from the surround photoreceptor due to the HCs. Therefore, when the light shines on the surrounding photoreceptors, one should expect that the center photo-receptors will be depolarized due to the strong feedback from the HC. In the case of a bright center and dark surrounding, the surrounding photoreceptors receive a strong feedback from the center photoreceptors due to the feedback from the HCs. Therefore, when the light shines on the center photoreceptors, one should expect that the center photoreceptors would be hyperpolarized due to the weak feedback from the HCs.

In order to demonstrate the center-surrounding property in the outer retinal circuit, we constructed a 14-by-14 photoreceptor-HC (PHC) array as shown in figure 12.15. Each photoreceptor receives feedback from the HC compartment it

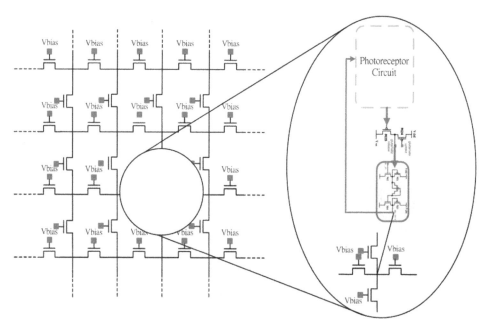

Figure 12.15. The configuration of the 14-by-14 PHC array. Reproduced from [51].

connects to. The output of each HC compartment is connected with its neighboring compartments using pass transistors. To test the 14-by-14 PHC array, we used two different input patterns, dark-center-bright-surround and bright-center-dark-surround. The simulation results are shown in figure 12.16. The left column and right column show the case of dark-center-bright-surround and bright-center-dark-surround, respectively. We also measured the difference of the response across the edge. In each plot, x- and y-axis indicate the index along the x and y direction, respectively. The location of each photoreceptor can be decided by these two indexes. The z-axis represents the voltage level of the corresponding photoreceptor. The six plots in figure 12.16 are recorded at the moment when the responses of the

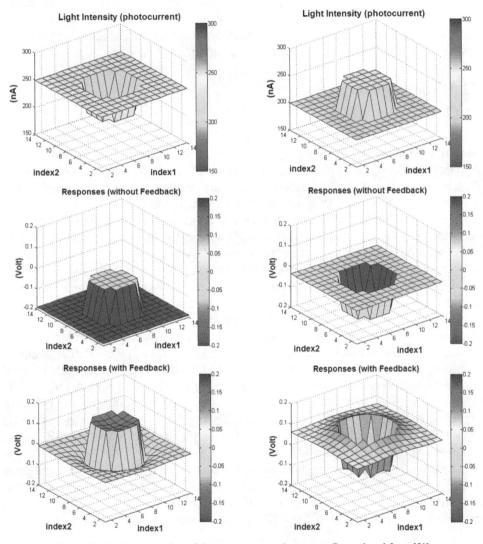

Figure 12.16. Demonstration of the center surround property. Reproduced from [51].

photoreceptors reach their maximum/minimum value. In both cases (left column and right column), the differences in the case of having the HC are 0.191 Volt and 0.192 Volt, respectively while the difference in the case of having no HC is only 0.15 Volt.

12.3.7 Edge detection

We tested the 14-by-14 PHC array. Initially, the input photocurrents are all 200 nA. At time 150 ns, we injected an input stimulus which formed an edge, as shown in figure 12.17(a), and we observed the responses of the photoreceptors over time, which are plotted in figure 12.17(b). The photoreceptors along the bright edge are strongly hyperpolarized because they receive less feedback from the photoreceptors along the dark edge. On the other hand, the photoreceptors along the dark edge receive strong feedback from the photoreceptors along the bright edge. It results in a strong depolarization of the photoreceptors along the dark side.

12.4 The inner retina design

12.4.1 On-type BC design

BCs relay the signals from the outer retina to the inner retina; they are considered an important stage from which segregation of visual signal occurs and initiate a chain of parallel processing for higher visual areas in the brain [47] [1]. BCs have two types: ON BC and OFF BC. Both receive glutamate released from photoreceptors but respond differently. ON BCs are mediated by metabotropic glutamate receptors (mGluR6) on the dendrite while OFF BCs are mediated by ionotropic glutamtate receptors (iGluRs). When light hits a photoreceptor, the photoreceptor hyperpolarizes and causes less glutamate release. ON BCs react to this change by depolarizing while OFF BCs react by hyperpolarizing. ON type BCs have two sub-types: transient and sustained. Different types of BCs connect to specific types of ganglion cells to carry out various retinal computations [3].

Transient-ON BCs are involved in the computation of differential motion detection [4]. ON BCs receive glutamate released from the photoreceptors. Recent studies have revealed that a transient receptor potential-like (TRP/TRPL) channel is necessary for the depolarizing light response of ON-BCs, and further that the TRP channel is a component of the channel that generates this light response [34, 39, 40]. The identification of TRPM1 in particular as the channel gated by the mGluR6 signaling cascade in ON BCs reveals a major role for TRP channels in vertebrate vision [39]. Despite intensive research, the molecular nature of the mGluR6-gated channel has remained elusive [39].

The mGluR6 cascade starts with the opening of the mGluR6 receptor through an indirect metabotropic process and ends up with the closure of mGluR6-gated channel (i.e. TRP channel) as shown in the left drawing of figure 12.18. (The left part of figure 12.18 is taken from [29].) This process enables the conversion of a

---

[1] The majority of figures in this section on the inner retina are from [42] unless otherwise specified.

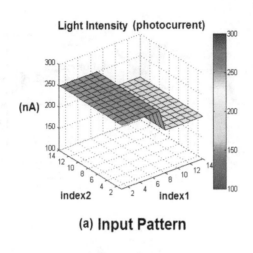

(a) Input Pattern

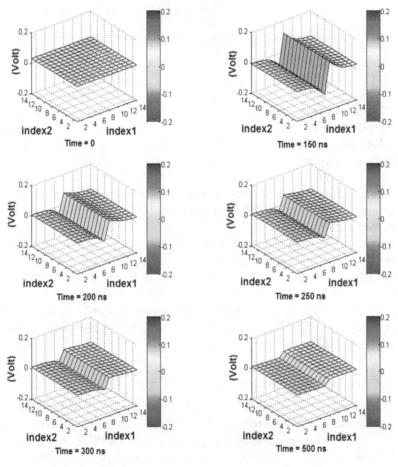

(b) The Responses over Time

Figure 12.17. The responses of photoreceptors to an edge over time. Reproduced from [51].

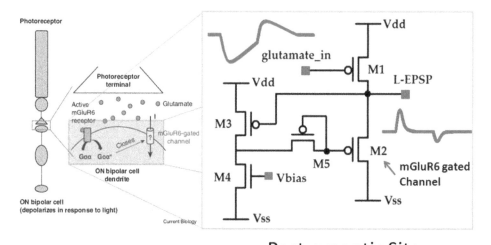

Post-synaptic Site

Figure 12.18. The postsynaptic circuit of the transient-ON BC. Reproduced from [51].

sustained input from photoreceptors into a more transient output. The response at the postsynaptic site is called light-evoked excitatory postsynaptic potential (L-EPSP). Like other neurons, the L-EPSPs on the dendrite sum nonlinearly and produce a potential output at its axon terminal. Moreover, the voltage-gated ion channels located on either their dendrites or somas can enhance the BC L-EPSPs by amplifying the transient component of the response [24]. At the axon terminal, one observes the output is rectified [14]. Each BC's rectified response ensures that its vote will be counted, because it cannot be vetoed by signals of equal magnitude but opposite sign in other parts of the receptive field [14]. A simplified transient-ON BC model is shown in figure 12.20.

The circuit on the right shown in figure 12.18, namely the postsynaptic circuit of transient-ON BC, has negative feedback that controls the gate voltage of M2. As a result, the L-EPSP output will be quickly pulled down as shown in the simulation result in figure 12.19. The ON BC synapse circuit models the mGluR6 cascade process that converts a sustained input from photoreceptors into a more transient output, namely L-EPSP. The output will be further processed to achieve various retinal computations in the inner retina.

12.4.2 A directionally-selective neuromorphic circuit

The starburst amacrine cell (SAC), found in the mammalian retina and with a characteristic radially symmetric morphology, is thought to provide directional inhibitory input to direction-selective ganglion cells (DSGCs) [1, 17, 49]. It is generally believed that SACs first perform the neural computations that induce directional selectivity in the ganglion cell. The computation of direction selectivity (DS) occurs at individual dendritic branches of each SAC and each dendritic branch acts as an independent computation module [16]. Both the dendritic

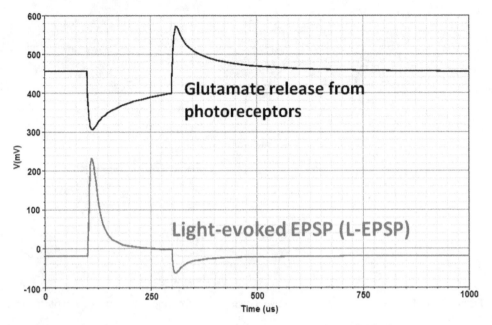

Figure 12.19. Simulation result of the postsynaptic circuit of the transient-ON BC. Copyright 2012 IEEE. Reprinted, with permission, from [42].

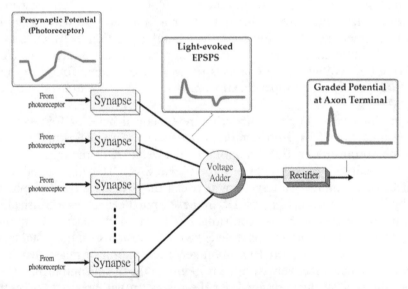

Figure 12.20. Simplified transient-ON BC model with dendritic computation. Reproduced from [51].

calcium signal and membrane voltage in the dendritic tip generate a stronger response by the stimuli moving from the soma towards the dendritic tip (namely centrifugal motion) than moving the opposite direction (namely centripetal motion) [16]. To explain the DS observed in the SACs, neuroscientists have

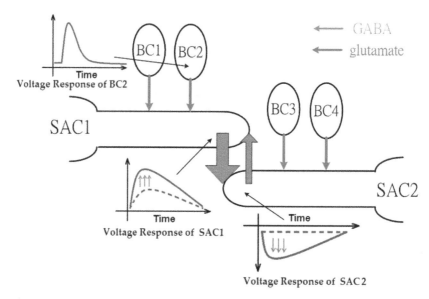

Figure 12.21. The inhibitory interaction between two SACs. Copyright 2011 IEEE. Reprinted, with permission, from [43].

proposed at least two fundamentally different mechanisms [22]: dendrite-intrinsic electrotonics [38, 44] and lateral inhibition [7, 30]. Hausselt *et al* demonstrated that the intrinsic electrical mechanisms of SACs may produce DS without inhibitory network interactions [22]. However, the lateral inhibition between two SACs enhances the difference in response and generates a robust directional selectivity [30]. Moreover, voltage-gated channels (possibly Ca^{2+}) being found in the distal dendrite [22] imply that a super-linear summation may occur in the distal dendrite of the SAC.

The mechanisms thought to underlie are explained here. SACs receive glutamate released from BCs. Furthermore, the dendritic tip releases and receives the GABA neurotransmitter. Euler *et al* observed a weak DS at the soma but a strong DS in the dendritic tips [16]. They also found that SACs have directional responses even if GABA inhibitory interactions between the SACs are blocked pharmacologically [16]. Their results suggest DS in the starburst cell arises intrinsically from its distinctive morphology. A centrifugal (CF) motion generates an in-phase response which can be summed effectively with the response in the distal compartment. However, centripetal (CP) motion generates an out-of-phase response that cannot be summed effectively with the response in the distal compartment. Hence, SAC produces a stronger response in the distal tip with respect to centrifugal motion.

The lateral inhibition between two overlapping SACs makes the DS response more robust [30]. The distal dendrite of SACs releases GABA neurotransmitters and GABA receptors are also found in the SAC dendrites. Therefore, as long as the processes of two neighboring starburst cells overlap, they are likely to form

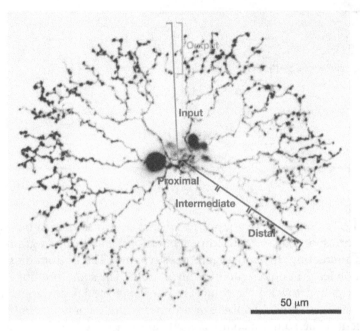

Figure 12.22. Starburst amacrine cell. Reproduced from [16], copyright (2002), with permission from Springer Nature.

reciprocal connections. The reciprocal synapse, which is a positive feedback loop, can enhance the difference in responses between the two SACs. The interactions between SACs are illustrated in figure 12.21. When the light moves to BC2, the distal dendrite of SAC1 produces a voltage response and releases more GABA which inhibits the response of distal dendrite in SAC2. SAC2 in turn produces less GABA release which enhances the response of the distal dendrite in SAC1.

Figure 12.22 illustrates the morphology of the amacrine cell, taken from [16]. The authors compartmentalize an SAC into three compartments in a branch: distal, intermediate, and proximal compartments. Therefore, we modeled these three compartments in the same fashion. The distal compartments receive glutamate release from BCs as well as GABA release from other SACs. To model the distal compartment, we need to have two inputs: one for glutamate; the other for GABA. The basic distal compartment design is presented in figure 12.23. The gate of the lower NMOS, M2, connects to GABA input from other SAC while the gate of the upper NMOS connects to glutamate input from BC. The output represents the membrane potential of the distal compartment of SAC The circuit can model the responses caused by the changes of glutamate and GABA. (Glutamate, an excitatory neurotransmitter, depolarizes the output while GABA, an inhibitory neurotransmitter, hyperpolarizes the output.) From transistor M1's perspective, the basic distal compartment is a source follower. From transistor M2's perspective, the basic distal compartment is a common source amplifier.

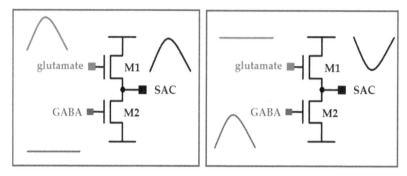

Figure 12.23. Basic distal compartment of the SAC. Reproduced from [51].

Figure 12.24 shows two overlapped branches of two simplified biological SACs and the corresponding circuit implementation. The top diagram represents two SACs interacting through a reciprocal synapse. The bottom diagram depicts the correspondence in our circuit implementation. The somatic compartments and signal propagation toward the soma are not being modeled in our circuit. Each branch of the SAC model consists of an intermediate compartment and a distal compartment. (The somatic compartments are not included in our model.) Both compartments receive glutamate inputs from the BCs. The signals will first go through the wave-shaping circuits that convert the glutamate input into cation concentration inside the cell. The cation concentration at the intermediate compartment will propagate to the distal compartment through a delay circuit and be summed with the cation concentration at the distal compartment. A fully-functional SAC would have a feedback path. We only consider propagation towards the dendritic tip for this simplified SAC.

The summation is implemented by using a voltage adder. In figure 12.24, the subscript of the parameters for the left SAC is 1 and the subscript of the parameters for the right SAC is 2. Here, we only use the name of the parameters without the subscripts to explain these parameters. The output of the voltage adder labeled [*Cation*] represents intra-cellular cation concentration at the distal compartment. The membrane potential of the distal compartment labeled V_d is influenced by [*Cation*] and *GABA IN*. *GABA IN* represents GABA from another SAC. *GABA release* is the voltage output modulated by V_d and *GABA reuptake*. The voltage adder circuit is a modified version of Chaoui's Circuit [9] and is capable of performing nonlinear summations of intra-cellular [*Cation*]. In the wave-shaping circuit, the rise of glutamate induces more current to charge the output capacitor C quickly to $V_{glutamate} - V_{th}$, where V_{th} is the threshold voltage of the pull-up transistor in the wave-shaping circuit. The pull-down transistor provides a resistive path for discharging the output capacitor C when glutamate input decreases. Therefore, the wave-shaping circuit can produce an output with smaller response than the input and longer duration. The delay circuit uses a current-mirror structure to model the propagation delay along the branch of the SAC.

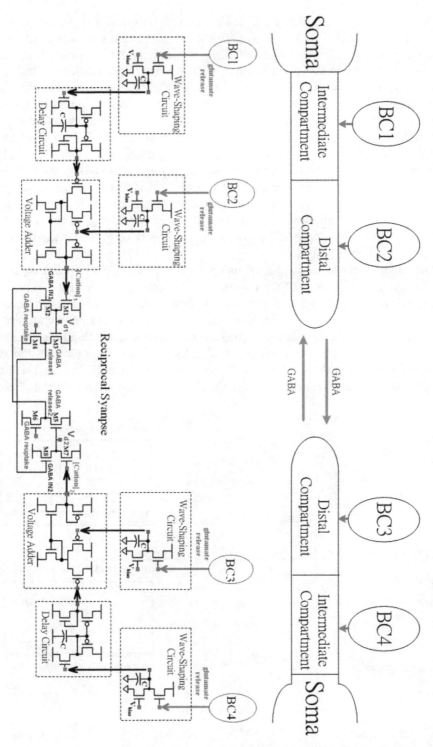

Figure 12.24. Overlapped branches of two simplified biological SACs. Reproduced from [51].

Next, we demonstrated an SAC model with a reciprocal synapse. Figure 12.24 illustrates the scenario we set up to perform the experiments. Consider the case in which $[Cation]_2$ remains the same and $[Cation]_1$ increases. At the outset, both V_{d1} and *GABA release1* increase. The increase of *GABA release1* pulls down V_{d2} and *GABA release2*. The decrease of *GABA release2* pulls up V_{d1}. As a result, V_{d1} is increased due to the positive feedback loop. During this operation, transistor M8 enters the linear region as *GABA IN2* increases. Therefore, the gain of the common source amplifier consisting of M8 and M7 decreases. Meanwhile, transistor M2 soon enters the subthreshold region that allows V_{d1} to increase more quickly than transistor M1 is in the saturation region. However, the amount of increase is limited by the decrease in gain of the common source amplifier consisting of M8 and M7. Eventually, the whole loop reaches a stable state without divergences or oscillations. V_{d1} is still proportional to the amplitude of $[Cation]_1$. We may conclude that the SAC design with the reciprocal synapse still possesses the property of graded potential output and the operation is stable.

The experiments were conducted using TSMC 18 CMOS (180 nm) technology using Cadence SPECTRE software simulating the configuration with two branches, as shown in figure 12.24, and also the configuration with only one branch. To demonstrate the dendrite-intrinsic electrotonics of the SAC design, we applied two kinds of moving stimuli, namely centripetal motion and centrifugal motion, to the configuration with only one branch and measured the responses of the distal compartment for both cases. The results are plotted in figure 12.25. The black trace and purple trace represent the inputs to the simulation that are the outputs from the

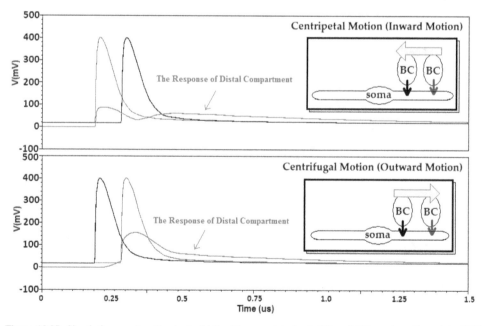

Figure 12.25. Simulation results of a single SAC with respect to both CP and CF motion. Copyright 2011 IEEE. Reprinted, with permission, from [43].

BCs connecting to the intermediate compartment and distal compartment, respectively. The red trace is the response of the distal compartment. The glutamate inputs are generated by the outer retina circuit that we made. The moving stimulus from the intermediate compartment to the distal compartment will first evoke a response at the intermediate compartment. After some delay, the signal reaches the distal compartment. Meanwhile, the moving stimulus has reached the distal compartment and the evoked response can therefore be summed with the response from the intermediate compartment. This results in a larger voltage response at the distal compartment than at the intermediate compartment. For the opposite moving stimulus, the response cannot be optimally summed because the signal from the intermediate compartment cannot reach the distal compartment on time. The simulation results demonstrate that the stimulus moving centrifugally evokes a stronger response than moving centripetally.

To demonstrate the lateral inhibition between the SACs, which enhances the difference in response of the distal dendrite, we tested the two configurations described before and compared their responses. We applied a stimulus moving centrifugally to both configurations. We measured the responses of the distal compartments for both configurations that are plotted in figure 12.26. The black trace and purple trace in the upper figure represent the inputs to the simulation that are the outputs from the BCs connecting to the intermediate compartment and distal compartment, respectively. The blue trace and red trace represent the responses of the distal compartment with a reciprocal synapse and having no reciprocal synapse,

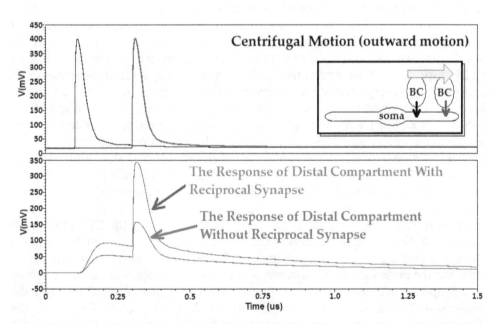

Figure 12.26. Comparison of the simulation results both with and without reciprocal synapse to CF motion. Copyright 2011 IEEE. Reprinted, with permission, from [43].

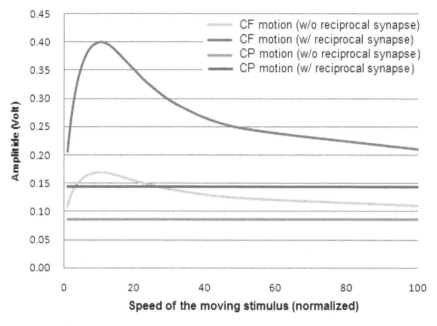

Figure 12.27. Amplitude of the SAC distal compartment versus speed of the stimulus. Copyright 2011 IEEE. Reprinted, with permission, from [43].

respectively. The results indicate that the positive feedback of the reciprocal synapse effectively enhances the response of the distal compartment.

To characterize the circuit's behaviors, we applied a moving stimulus at different speeds and different input intensities. We observed the responses of the distal compartment and the simulation results are plotted in figures 12.27 and 12.28, respectively. Both figures record the maximum amplitude of the response. In figure 12.27, the responses are measured by using a stimulus with photocurrent of 250 nA and the speed (as shown in the x-axis) has been normalized on a scale from 1 through 100. For CP motion, the evoked responses are not sensitive to the speed in either case of having a reciprocal synapse or having no reciprocal synapse. For CF motion, the evoked response is small when the speed is slow and fast. The results imply that CF motion evokes a larger response than CP motion within a range of speed and the amplitude is enhanced by the presence of the reciprocal synapse.

In figure 12.28, the simulations are conducted by sweeping the CF motion with different amounts of photocurrents as the input along the CF direction. We used the moving stimulus at two speeds, 1 and 10. In each case, we plotted two curves reflecting the presence and no presence of a reciprocal synapse. Given the presence of a reciprocal synapse and the moving stimulus at a proper speed (i.e. 10), the response of the distal compartment is stronger than other cases. Moreover, the response is enhanced by the presence of the reciprocal synapse across the entire input range that we swept.

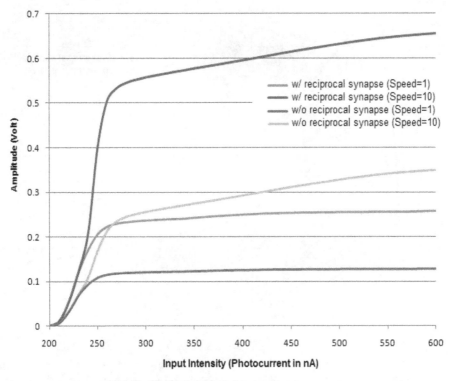

Figure 12.28. Amplitude of the SAC distal compartment versus input intensity. Copyright 2011 IEEE. Reprinted, with permission, from [43].

Next, we further quantified starburst DS by calculating a DS index (DSI) used in a SAC model [44].

$$\text{DSI} = \frac{V_{cf} - V_{cp}}{V_{cf} + V_{cp}} \tag{12.3}$$

where V_{cf} and V_{cp} are the peak responses measured at the distal compartment in the CF and CP directions, respectively. A DSI of 0 indicates no DS, 1 indicates maximal DS with the preferred direction being CF, and −1 indicates maximal DS with a CP preference [44]. We plotted the results in figure 12.29 in which DSI is measured and calculated with respect to the moving stimulus at different speeds (given a photocurrent of 250 nA as the input). The maximum DSIs occur for both curves when the peak DSI speed is equal to the propagation speed of the moving stimulus (the speed is about 10) and the presence of the reciprocal synapse leads to a higher DSI.

12.4.3 A neuromorphic circuit that computes differential motion

Detecting moving objects in a moving background or a dynamic scene is essential to the survival of some animals. Circuitry computing differential motion is found in the biological retina. An object-motion-sensitivity (OMS) ganglion cell remains silent

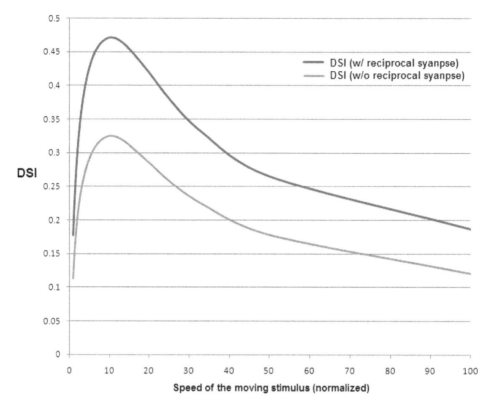

Figure 12.29. DSI. Reproduced from [51].

under global motion of the entire image but fires when the image patch in its receptive field moves differently from the background. The differential motion neuromorphic circuit that we built compares the motion speeds of the central receptive field and peripheral receptive field. In this section, we demonstrate that there is a response if motion speeds of the central and peripheral receptive fields are different. However, the response is suppressed if motion speeds of the central and peripheral receptive fields are the same.

The OMS neurons are highly tuned to detect differential motion between the receptive field center and the periphery. The polyaxonal amacrine cell appears to be a plausible candidate to transmit inhibition from the background region [4]. The inhibition signal may be derived from polyaxonal amacrine cells that inhibit the BC synaptic terminal, close to the site of transmission but at some electrotonic distance from the soma. In the salamander, the BCs involved in the computation of differential motion detection are mainly transient OFF-type BCs [4]. Transient ON-type BCs are believed to be involved in this computation as well [4, 19]. The transient ON-type BC produces a positive response lasting a short duration of time when increasing the light intensity. The transient OFF-type BC produces a positive response lasting a short duration of time when decreasing the light intensity. Compared to the sustained BCs, the transient BCs

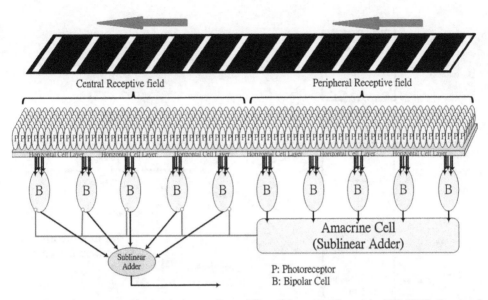

Figure 12.30. A neuromorphic circuit that performs differential motion. Copyright 2011 IEEE. Reprinted, with permission, from [43].

have a shorter duration of the response. The BCs not only relay the visual information from photoreceptors but also shape visual response before transmitting to the inner retina. The details of the signaling cascade in the BCs are given by several researchers [34, 39, 40]. The signaling cascade can be considered a feedback effect that enables the conversion of a sustained input from photoreceptors into a more transient output [28].

We constructed a neuromorphic circuit that computes retinal differential motion (figure 12.30). The network consists of a 7-by-70 photoreceptor array, a layer of HCs, 10 BCs, and one sublinear voltage adder that models an amacrine cell. The photoreceptors and the HC layer that perform contrast enhancement have been presented in the previous chapter. In our circuit, each receptive field is covered by five BCs. One BC connects postsynaptically with five photoreceptors and the amacrine cell connects postsynaptically with five BCs and presynaptically to axonal terminals in five other BCs belong to a different receptive field. The amacrine cell is modeled by using a voltage adder circuit [9] that performs nonlinear summations as before. Modeling the ganglion cells is presented in the next section. In this section, we used a sublinear voltage adder to sum up the BCs' responses from the central receptive field and measured the output response of the summation of the BCs. Therefore, we may easily observe the effect of inhibition from the peripheral receptive field under different cases. The BCs that we modeled in the network are transient ON-type BCs in which the mGluR6 (glutamate receptor) cascade causes conversion of a sustained input from photoreceptors into a more transient output [28]. The postsynaptic circuit of the transient-ON BC has been presented in the previous section and shown in figure 12.31. The L-EPSPs are

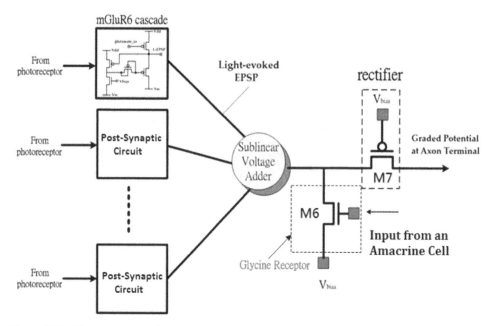

Figure 12.31. The postsynaptic circuit of the transient-ON BC. Copyright 2012 IEEE. Reprinted, with permission, from [42].

summed and rectified at the output. Transistor M6 pulls down the output voltage if the input from an amacrine cell is asserted. Transistor M6 models the glycine receptor that receives the inhibition from the amacrine cell. Transistor M7, rectifying the negative response, ensures that each BC's vote will be counted and cannot be vetoed by signals of equal magnitude but opposite sign in other parts of the receptive field.

The simulations were conducted with TSMC18 CMOS (180 nm) technology using the SPECTRE simulator. We used the circuit configuration shown in figure 1.36 and applied grating stimuli moving from the right to the left of the receptive field. Grating stimuli consist of black and white bars that are represented by the photocurrent of 200 nA and 250 nA, respectively. The black bars span four photoreceptors while the white bars span only one photoreceptor. We tried two different cases of moving grating stimuli (i.e. the same speed and different speeds). The results are shown in figure 12.32. The responses shown in figure 12.32 record the summation of the BCs' responses in the central receptive field during the first 8 ms. When the moving grating stimuli are moving at the same frequency, the responses are much smaller than those moving at different frequencies. The smaller response in the upper waveforms of figure 12.32 is due to the timely inhibition from the peripheral receptive field. The responses of both cases are small at the beginning of the simulation (before 1 ms) because the moving bars have not spanned the entire receptive field.

We simulated the circuit using different speed combinations of the central and peripheral receptive field (both from 50 kHz to 5 kHz) and measured the maximum

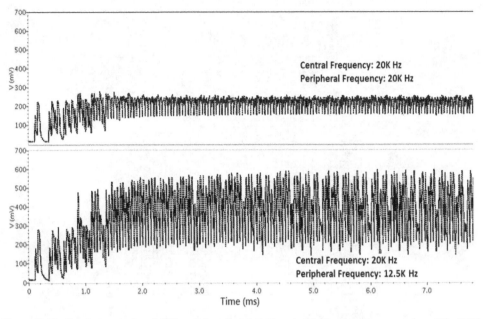

Figure 12.32. Simulation results of differential motion detection circuit, showing the summation of the BCs' responses over time as a grating is shifted. Copyright 2012 IEEE. Reprinted, with permission, from [42].

output response during the first 10 ms. The black and white bars are represented by the photocurrents of 200 nA and 250 nA, respectively. The results are shown in figure 12.33. The *x*-axis and *y*-axis represent the speeds of moving bars in the peripheral and central receptive fields. The cells falling on the diagonal line are the cases having the same speed of moving bars in the peripheral and central receptive fields. The responses recorded from those cells are smaller due to the timely inhibition from the peripheral receptive field that suppresses the responses of the BCs in the central receptive field. We also observed that the different speeds of moving bars may still produce small responses in certain cases, i.e. the highlighted cells not falling on the diagonal line. Those cases occur when the speed of the moving bars in the peripheral receptive field is a multiple of that in the central receptive field or when the bars in the peripheral receptive field are moving much faster than the bars in the central receptive field. In the latter case, the cells close to the lower left corner of figure 12.33, the inhibition from the peripheral receptive field is too strong to generate the response at the output. The highlighted cells in figure 12.33 indicate the responses less than 0.35 V. Hence, we concluded that an output response above a certain value (i.e. 0.35 V in the case we presented in figure 12.33) indicates that the motions from the central receptive field and peripheral receptive field are at different speeds. However, an output response below that certain value does not necessarily imply the motions from the central receptive field and the peripheral receptive field are at the same speed due to a few failing cases that we found. Moreover, the amplitude of the output response does not indicate the magnitude of the speed difference according to the results we observed.

Speed of the Moving Bars
in Central Receptive Field (Hz)

Speed of the Moving Bars in Peripheral Receptive Field (Hz)

	50k	33.33k	25k	20k	16.66k	14.28k	12.5k	11.11k	10k	9.09k	8.33k	7.69k	7.14k	6.66k	6.25k	5.88k	5.55k	5.26k	5k
50k	0.2963	0.4911	0.3876	0.5169	0.4840	0.5323	0.5230	0.5456	0.5393	0.5546	0.5552	0.5573	0.5589	0.5573	0.5618	0.5623	0.5623	0.5632	0.5588
33.33k	0.4729	0.2686	0.4963	0.5157	0.4457	0.5393	0.5475	0.5367	0.5533	0.5603	0.5581	0.5645	0.5649	0.5629	0.5682	0.5684	0.5683	0.5699	0.5686
25k	0.4265	0.5012	0.2615	0.5216	0.5131	0.5493	0.5055	0.5700	0.5772	0.5797	0.5799	0.5857	0.5885	0.5919	0.5906	0.5923	0.5934	0.5938	0.5830
20k	0.4705	0.5239	0.5239	0.2569	0.5524	0.5571	0.5721	0.5774	0.5457	0.5832	0.5913	0.5919	0.5921	0.5934	0.5956	0.5923	0.5954	0.5981	0.5975
16.66k	0.4098	0.3349	0.4638	0.5512	0.2541	0.5619	0.5577	0.5621	0.5718	0.5849	0.5623	0.5875	0.5858	0.5928	0.5937	0.5895	0.5939	0.5908	0.5934
14.28k	0.4564	0.4860	0.5082	0.5300	0.5500	0.2514	0.5652	0.5663	0.5768	0.5801	0.5838	0.5826	0.5692	0.5853	0.5888	0.5858	0.5855	0.5908	0.5876
12.5k	0.3882	0.4747	0.2555	0.5062	0.4941	0.5419	0.2488	0.5631	0.5613	0.5752	0.5728	0.5800	0.5824	0.5821	0.5719	0.5827	0.5824	0.5830	0.5862
11.11k	0.4352	0.2983	0.4964	0.4971	0.4332	0.5338	0.5444	0.2465	0.5608	0.5705	0.5703	0.5692	0.5767	0.5740	0.5749	0.5765	0.5725	0.5806	0.5816
10k	0.3654	0.4634	0.4217	0.2078	0.4769	0.5210	0.5279	0.5603	0.2446	0.5677	0.5645	0.5647	0.5727	0.5688	0.5729	0.5771	0.5768	0.5738	0.5709
9.09k	0.4217	0.4497	0.4888	0.5155	0.5081	0.5451	0.5370	0.5495	0.5633	0.2422	0.5561	0.5598	0.5706	0.5642	0.5690	0.5656	0.5665	0.5677	0.5740
8.33k	0.3467	0.2750	0.2290	0.4811	0.2026	0.5068	0.4700	0.5306	0.5523	0.5552	0.2414	0.5596	0.5606	0.5566	0.5585	0.5648	0.5643	0.5674	0.5626
7.69k	0.4099	0.4400	0.4577	0.4685	0.4895	0.5019	0.5246	0.5448	0.5415	0.5416	0.5523	0.2408	0.5606	0.5566	0.5585	0.5596	0.5644	0.5654	0.5630
7.14k	0.3313	0.4387	0.3943	0.4651	0.4527	0.2005	0.5187	0.5225	0.5255	0.5516	0.5523	0.5500	0.2399	0.5606	0.5563	0.5584	0.5596	0.5589	0.5607
6.66k	0.4022	0.2617	0.4474	0.1854	0.3837	0.4921	0.5155	0.5172	0.4846	0.5421	0.5316	0.5468	0.5541	0.5417	0.2392	0.5563	0.5629	0.5566	0.5622
6.25k	0.3183	0.4373	0.2123	0.4801	0.4256	0.5195	0.2005	0.5388	0.5185	0.5461	0.5403	0.5424	0.5335	0.5497	0.5455	0.2374	0.5585	0.5690	0.5626
5.88k	0.3955	0.4240	0.4415	0.4545	0.4800	0.4827	0.5091	0.5100	0.5356	0.5169	0.5281	0.5367	0.5434	0.5347	0.5313	0.5476	0.2375	0.5738	0.5677
5.55k	0.3064	0.2509	0.3586	0.4488	0.1811	0.5061	0.4807	0.2007	0.5139	0.5310	0.4948	0.5438	0.5307	0.5475	0.5486	0.5335	0.5433	0.2364	0.5740
5.26k	0.3820	0.4190	0.4446	0.4466	0.1620	0.4575	0.4824	0.4906	0.5079	0.5247	0.5246	0.5325	0.5381	0.5319	0.5295	0.5468	0.5493	0.5218	0.2359
5k	0.2970	0.4177	0.2012	0.1711	0.4204	0.4135	0.4347	0.5226	0.2009	0.5258	0.5318	0.5232	0.5223	0.5166	0.5188	0.5451	0.5317	0.5447	0.2354

Figure 12.33. Maximum BC responses under different speed combinations. Copyright 2012 IEEE. Reprinted, with permission, from [42].

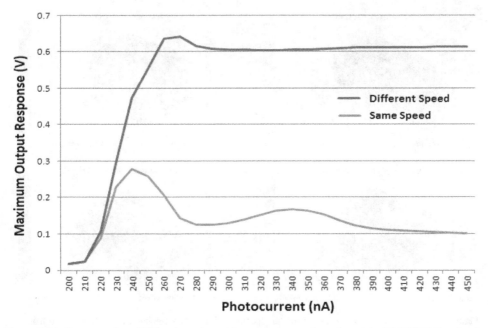

Figure 12.34. Responses over different input intensities to moving gratings. Copyright 2012 IEEE. Reprinted, with permission, from [42].

We then fixed the input intensity of black bars and swept different input intensities of white bars. We have tried two different combinations of the speeds, i.e. at the same speed and at different speeds. For the case having the same speed, we used 20 kHz for both the central and peripheral receptive fields. For the case having different speeds, we used 20 kHz and 12.5 kHz for the central and peripheral receptive field, respectively. The maximum output responses by the sweeping input photocurrent of the white bars from 200 nA to 450 nA are shown in figure 12.34. The black bars are represented by injecting a fixed photocurrent of 200 nA. For the case having the same speed, we used 20 kHz for both the central and peripheral receptive fields. For the case having different speeds, we used 20 kHz and 12.5 kHz for the central and peripheral receptive field, respectively. Among the range we swept, the output responses are suppressed if the speeds are the same.

We repeated the simulations that we used for constructing figure 12.33 by applying different bar spacings and bar widths as inputs. To better visualize the output response under different speed combinations, we plotted bar charts that record the responses of each case shown in figure 12.35, figure 12.36, figure 12.37, and figure 12.38. In figure 12.35, we varied the bar width from 1 to 4 given bar spacing of 5. In figure 12.36, we varied the bar spacing from 6 to 12 given bar width of 1. In figure 12.37, we varied the bar spacing from 6 to 12 given bar width of 2. In figure 12.38, we varied the bar spacing from 6 to 12 given bar width of 3. In these figures, we observed that: (1) the diagonal lines where the speeds are the

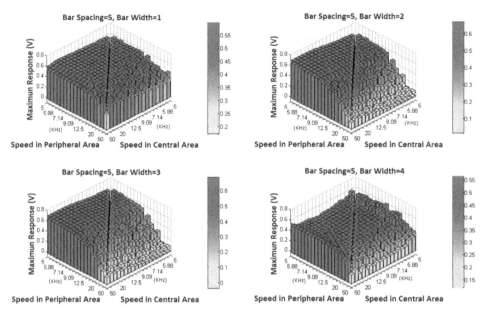

Figure 12.35. Responses in bar Chart I: the bar spacing is 5 and vary the bar width. Reproduced from [51].

same have lower response; (2) the average responses are maximum when the bar spacing is 7 which is also the spacing of the BCs; and (3) the average response decreases when the bar spacing increases due to less input stimuli across the receptive fields.

Since we are interested in knowing how the outer retina circuits impact the computation, we removed the feedback from the HC layer to photoreceptors and observed how the responses are altered. After disconnecting the feedback pathways by removing the HC layer, we repeated the simulations that we used for constructing figures 12.35, 12.36, 12.37, and 12.38 and compared the simulation results. To more easily compare two sets of results, we converted these bar charts into two-dimensional plots and took the speed difference of each speed combination as the x-axis and response as the y-axis. The results are shown in figures 12.39, 12.40, 12.41, and 12.42, respectively. Note that HC denotes horizontal cell layer. In figure 12.39, we varied the bar width from 1 to 5 given the bar spacing of 5. In figure 12.40, we varied the bar spacing from 6 to 12 given the bar width of 1. In figure 12.41, we varied the bar spacing from 6 to 12 given the bar width of 2. In figure 12.42, we varied the bar spacing from 6 to 12 given the bar width of 3. The blue traces indicate the results with the presence of the feedback in the outer retina while the red traces indicate the results without the presence of the feedback in the outer retina. From these figures, we observed that the amplitude of the response does not vary dorectly with the different speeds of two receptive fields. Also, we observed that the response with the HC layer is higher than the responses without the HC layer in most cases.

Next, we need to quantify the amount of performance enhancement. We made equation (12.4) to quantify the performance enhancement.

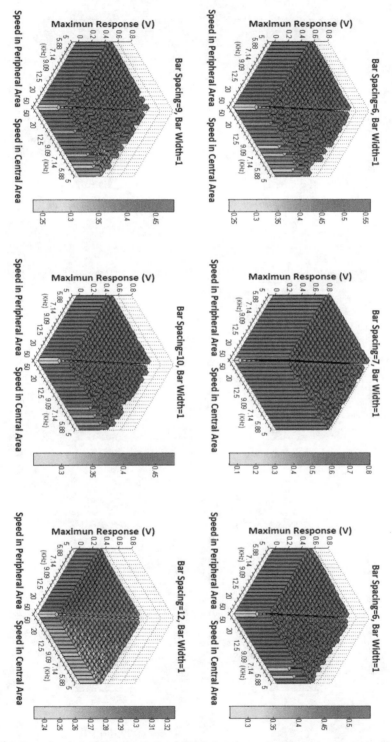

Figure 12.36. Responses in bar Chart II: the bar width is 1 and vary the bar spacing. Reproduced from [51].

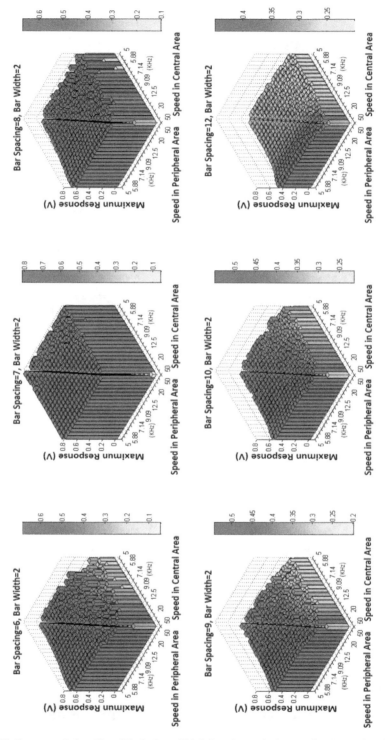

Figure 12.37. Responses in bar Chart III: the bar width is 2 and vary the bar spacing. Reproduced from [51].

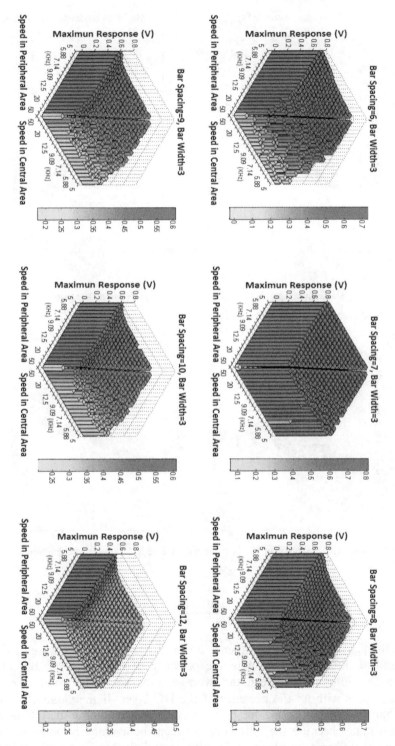

Figure 12.38. Responses in bar Chart IV: the bar width is 3 and vary the bar spacing. Reproduced from [51].

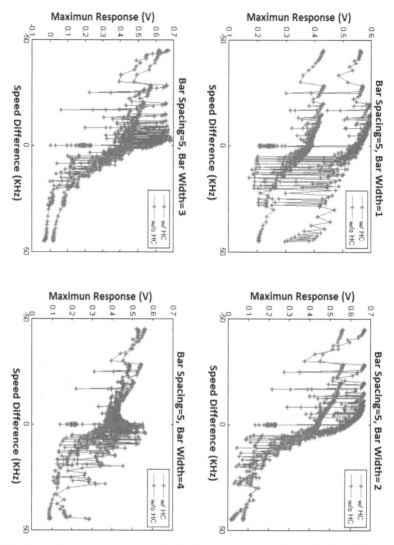

Figure 12.39. Comparing responses in curves I: the bar spacing is 5 and vary the bar width. Reproduced from [51].

$$\text{Enhancement} = \frac{\text{Diff}_{w/\ HC} - \text{Diff}_{w/o\ HC}}{\text{Diff}_{w/o\ HC}}, \qquad (12.4)$$

where $\text{Diff}_{w/\ HC}$ indicates the difference between the average response at the same speed and at different speeds with the presence of the HC layer and $\text{Diff}_{w/o\ HC}$ indicates the difference between the average response at the same speed and at different speeds without the presence of the HC layer. If the value of $\text{Diff}_{w/\ HC}$ is larger than that of $\text{Diff}_{w/o\ HC}$, one may conclude that including the HC layer helps the performance because the difference between the average response at the same speed and at different speeds increases after including the HC layer.

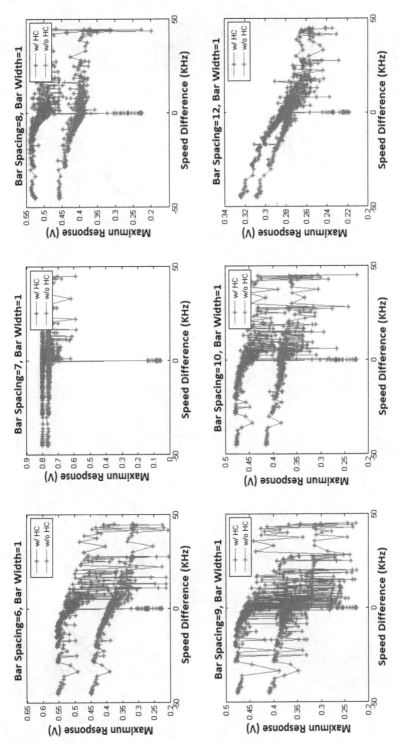

Figure 12.40. Comparing responses in curves II: the bar width is 1 and vary the bar spacing. Reproduced from [51].

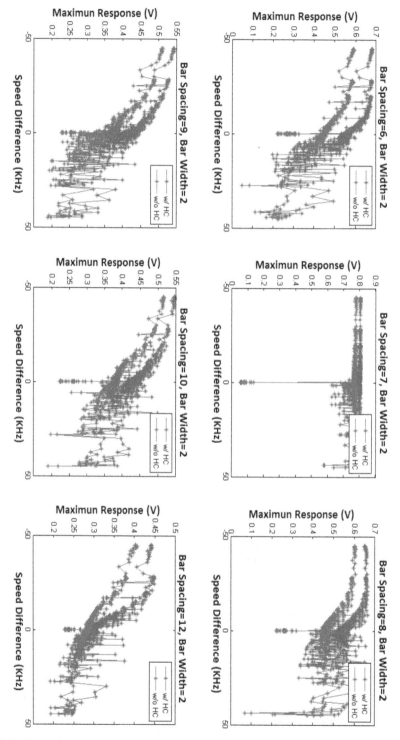

Figure 12.41. Comparing responses in curves III: the bar width is 2 and vary the bar spacing. Reproduced from [51].

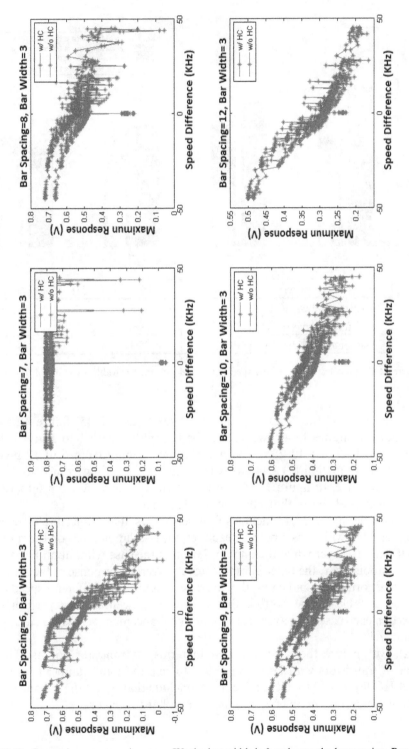

Figure 12.42. Comparing responses in curves IV: the bar width is 3 and vary the bar spacing. Reproduced from [51].

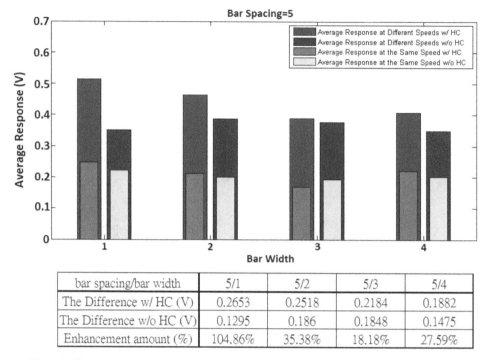

bar spacing/bar width	5/1	5/2	5/3	5/4
The Difference w/ HC (V)	0.2653	0.2518	0.2184	0.1882
The Difference w/o HC (V)	0.1295	0.186	0.1848	0.1475
Enhancement amount (%)	104.86%	35.38%	18.18%	27.59%

Figure 12.43. Enhancement I: the bar spacing is 1 and vary the bar width. Reproduced from [51].

We then plotted the results in figure 12.43, figure 12.45, figure 12.44, and figure 12.46. In figure 12.43, we varied the bar width from 1 to 5 given the bar spacing of 5. In figure 12.45, we varied the bar spacing from 6 to 12 given the bar width of 1. In figure 12.44, we varied the bar spacing from 6 to 12 given the bar width of 2. In figure 12.46, we varied the bar spacing from 6 to 12 given the bar width of 3. Note that HC denotes HC layer.

For example, figure 12.43 includes four sets of results by injecting different bar spacings and bar widths as inputs. In each set, the overlapping bar on the right is the case with an HC layer while the one on the left is the case without an HC layer. In each overlapping bar, the taller bar indicates the average response at the same speed while the shorter bar indicates the average response at different speeds. Each figure has a table in the bottom that calculates how much the performance is enhanced in each case. The average amount of enhancement across the cases studied is about 27.1%.

Next, we analyze the hardware cost in terms of transistor counts. The total number of transistors with HC layer is 9599 while the total number of transistors without HC layer is 6246. Hence, we may conclude that to get the enhancement we need to invest approximately a 33% increase in hardware cost.

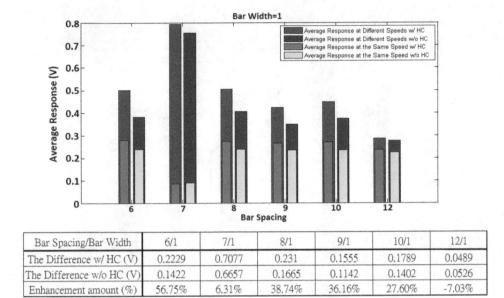

Bar Spacing/Bar Width	6/1	7/1	8/1	9/1	10/1	12/1
The Difference w/ HC (V)	0.2229	0.7077	0.231	0.1555	0.1789	0.0489
The Difference w/o HC (V)	0.1422	0.6657	0.1665	0.1142	0.1402	0.0526
Enhancement amount (%)	56.75%	6.31%	38.74%	36.16%	27.60%	-7.03%

Figure 12.44. Enhancement II: the bar width is 1 and vary the bar spacing. Reproduced from [51].

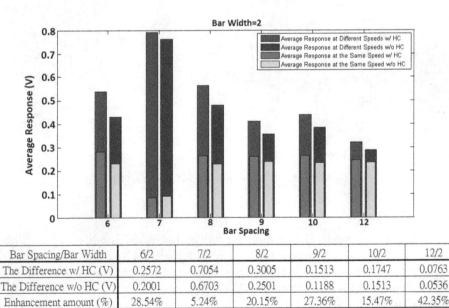

Bar Spacing/Bar Width	6/2	7/2	8/2	9/2	10/2	12/2
The Difference w/ HC (V)	0.2572	0.7054	0.3005	0.1513	0.1747	0.0763
The Difference w/o HC (V)	0.2001	0.6703	0.2501	0.1188	0.1513	0.0536
Enhancement amount (%)	28.54%	5.24%	20.15%	27.36%	15.47%	42.35%

Figure 12.45. Enhancement III: the bar width is 2 and vary the bar spacing. Reproduced from [51].

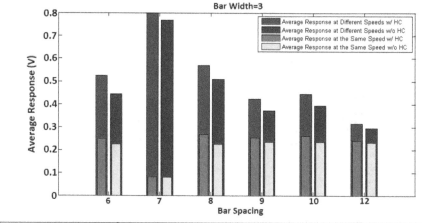

bar spacing/bar width	6/3	7/3	8/3	9/3	10/3	12/3
The Difference w/ HC (V)	0.2731	0.7163	0.3034	0.1681	0.1822	0.0732
The Difference w/o HC (V)	0.22	0.6886	0.2843	0.1369	0.1596	0.0623
Enhancement amount (%)	24.14%	4.02%	6.72%	22.79%	14.16%	17.50%

Figure 12.46. Enhancement IV: the bar width is 3 and vary the bar spacing. Reproduced from [51].

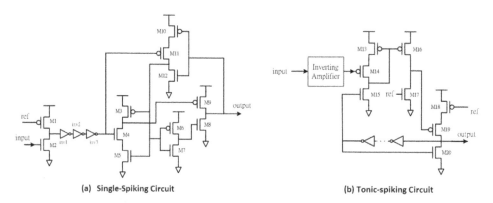

(a) Single-Spiking Circuit   (b) Tonic-spiking Circuit

Figure 12.47. Spiking circuits. Reproduced from [51].

12.4.4 Retinal pathways

In this section, we modeled complete retinal pathways by modifying the BioRC spiking circuits previously published [23, 26]. In figure 12.47(a), the circuit produces one single spike if the input voltage passes the threshold voltage of transistor M2. The circuit formed by transistors M5–M12 produces a single spike at the positive edge of the input. Transistor M1 and M2 are used to detect the input voltage. When the input passes the threshold voltage of transistor M2, the drain voltage of M2 is pulled down to about 0 V. The inverters, inv1, inv2, and inv3, are used to stabilize the input and form a stable pulse for the rest of the circuit formed by transistors M5–M12. In figure 12.47(b), the circuit produces tonic spikes if the input is 0 V. If the input increases, the output generates spikes at a faster rate. The circuit formed by transistors M13–M20 produces tonic spikes, i.e. a oscillator. The original tonic spiking circuit [26] is able to change spiking frequency by adjusting the gate voltage of transistor M14. The spiking frequency is inversely proportional to the gate voltage of transistor M14. Hence, we added an inverting amplifier to make the spiking frequency proportional to the input level. If the input increases, the spiking rate of the circuit increases, as compared to the spontaneous spiking rate. Meanwhile, the output produces tonic spikes whose frequency is about 3.3 kHz when there is no input, i.e. 0 V.

12.4.4.1 Object-motion-sensitivity (OMS) ganglion cell pathway

An object-motion-sensitivity (OMS) ganglion cell remains silent under global motion of the entire image but fires when the image patch in its receptive field moves differently from the background [4, 36]. The OSM ganglion cell pathway performs differential motion detection, which has been presented in the previous section. In this section, we demonstrate the complete OSM ganglion cell pathway by adding the single-spiking circuit (figure 12.47(a)) to the output of the differential motion detection model. The complete OSM ganglion cell circuit model consists of a voltage adder and a single-spiking circuit. The voltage adder sums BC inputs. The single-spiking circuit produces one single spike at a time if the input from the voltage adder passes the threshold voltage of transistor M2.

The simulations were conducted with TSMC18 CMOS (180 nm) technology using Cadence SPECTRE simulator. We used the circuit configuration shown in figure 12.30 plus the OSM ganglion cell circuit model and applied grating stimuli moving from the right to the left to the receptive field. The grating stimuli consists of black and white bars that are represented by a photocurrent of 200 nA and 250 nA, respectively. The black bars span four photoreceptors while the white bars span only one photoreceptor. We recorded the responses from the voltage adder's output labeled by 1 and the OMS ganglion cell's output labeled by 2 shown in figure 12.48. The simulation results are presented in figure 12.49 and figure 12.50. In figure 12.49, we observed that the output remains silent when both speeds are the same. In figure 12.50, the output produces spikes when the speeds are different. The circuit without the OMS ganglion cell circuit testing has been fully described in the previous section. Hence, we only presented two speed combinations that demonstrate the OMS ganglion cell pathway in this section.

Comparing the behaviors of the biological OMS ganglion cell pathway, we applied five periodic jittering bars to each receptive field in the circuit model. The results are shown in figure 12.51. Note that the neuronal recordings of the biological OSM ganglion cell are taken from the paper [4].

12.4.4.2 On-center ganglion cell pathway

In the retina, BCs and ganglion cells are organized in such a way that each cell responses to a small circular patch of the retina that defines the receptive field. The receptive field of the retinal ganglion cell consists of a roughly circular central area and a surrounding ring. Retinal ganglion cells have two basic types of receptive

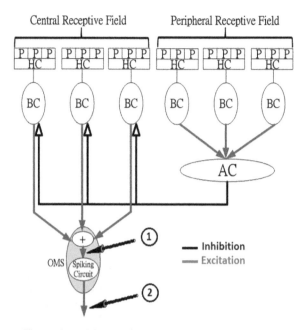

Figure 12.48. Measure the outputs. Reproduced from [51].

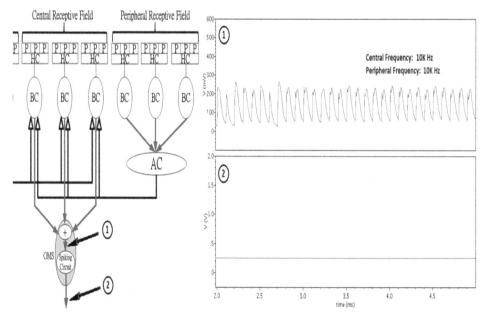

Figure 12.49. Responses at the same speed. Reproduced from [51].

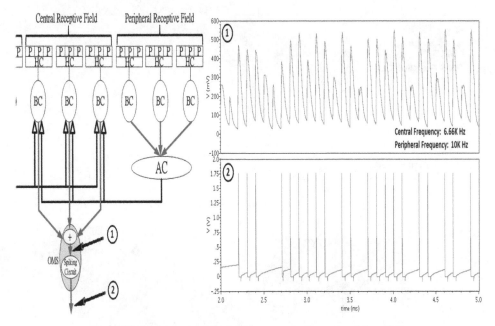

Figure 12.50. Responses at the different speeds. Reproduced from [51].

fields, on-center/off-surround and off-center/on-surround. The center and its surround are always antagonistic and tend to cancel each other's activity. When no light spikes on the receptive field, a spontaneous (tonic) level of spiking activity is recorded from the ganglion cell. Figure 12.52 explains the operation of an on-center ganglion cell pathway. Note that we only show three photoreceptors in the figure for simplicity. The actual number of photoreceptors appearing in the receptive field of a biological retina may be much more than what we show in the figure. In figure 12.52(a), the light shines on the center photoreceptor. The center photoreceptor hyperpolarizes due to the light during t1–t2. The on BC also hyperpolarizes in response to the center photoreceptor. The on ganglion cell generates spikes during t1–t2 due to the hyperpolarization of the on BC. In figure 12.52(b), the light shines on the surround photoreceptors. The center photoreceptor depolarizes due to the inhibition from the surround photoreceptors through the HC during t1–t2. The on BC also depolarizes in response to the center photoreceptor. The on ganglion cell is inhibited from firing during t1–t2 due to the depolarization of the on BC.

In this section, we constructed a on-center ganglion cell pathway from photoreceptors to the ganglion cell and demonstrate the responses in figure 12.53 and figure 12.54. The photoreceptor array consists of 7-by-7 photoreceptors. The central 3-by-3 photoreceptors is the center receptive field and the rest of the photoreceptors are the surround receptive field. The BC circuit model consists of a voltage adder and an inverting amplifier shown in figure 12.55 and connects with the central 3-by-3 photoreceptors. The ganglion cell circuit is shown in figure 12.47(b). The simulations were conducted with TSMC18 CMOS (180 nm) technology using the SPECTRE simulator. In figure 12.53, both receptive fields are dark before 0.1 ms. At time 0.1 ms,

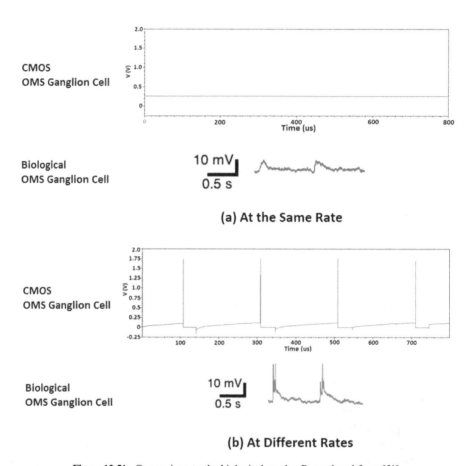

Figure 12.51. Comparison to the biological results. Reproduced from [51].

we shine a light on the center receptive field till 0.5 ms. After 0.5 ms, both receptive fields remain dark till the end of the simulation. We observed the response of the BC and ganglion cell over the time. The ganglion cell generates more spikes when the light strikes the center receptive field. In figure 12.54, both receptive fields are dark before 0.1 ms. At time 0.1 ms, we shine a light on the surround receptive field till 0.5 ms. After 0.5 ms, both receptive fields remain dark till the end of the simulation. We again observed the response of the BC and ganglion cell over the time. The ganglion cell is prevented from spiking during 0.1 m–0.5 ms due to the inhibition from the surround receptive field and produces spikes vigorously due to less inhibition (i.e. more excitation to the center receptive field) from surround receptive field after 0.5 ms.

Note that the HC plays an important role in the on-center ganglion cell pathway. Without the HC, the communication among photoreceptors cannot happen. Hence, we cannot demonstrate the spiking behaviors without the HC.

12.4.4.3 Directionally-selective ganglion cell pathway

The DSGC is the output neuron that computes motion direction in the retina. It codes motion direction by generating more spikes when there is motion in a

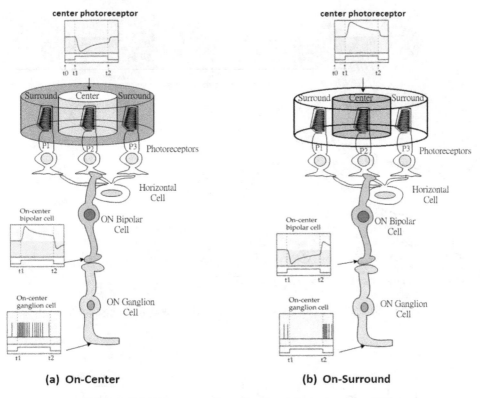

Figure 12.52. On-center ganglion cell pathway. Reproduced from [51].

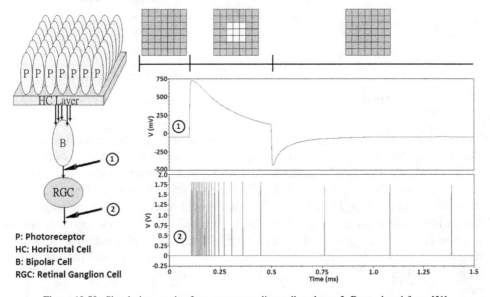

Figure 12.53. Simulation result of on-center ganglion cell pathway I. Reproduced from [51].

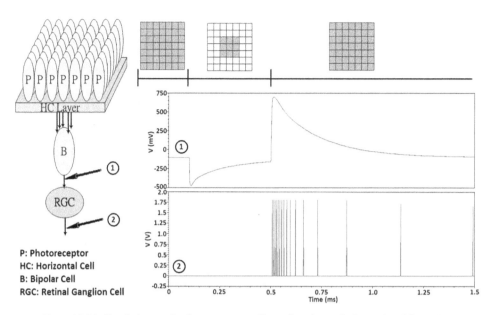

Figure 12.54. Simulation result of on-center ganglion cell pathway II. Reproduced from [51].

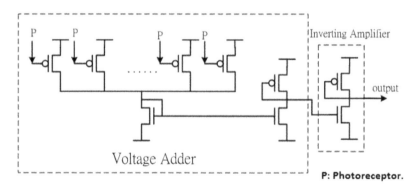

Figure 12.55. On center BC circuit model. Reproduced from [51].

particular direction and generating less spikes (or no spikes) when there is motion in the opposite direction. The underlying neural circuit and its operations is presented in figure 12.56. The SAC responds differently with respect to different moving stimuli and provides inhibition to DSGC while BC excites DSGC. In figure 12.56(a), A moving light from BC1 to BC2 produces a stronger response in the dendritic tip of SAC which cancels the excitation from BC1. Hence, DSGC does not produce spikes vigorously. In figure 12.56(b), the moving light from BC2 to BC1 produces a weaker response in the dendritic tip of SAC which is not enough to cancel the excitation from BC1. Hence, DSGC generates more spikes, as compared to the tonic spiking rate.

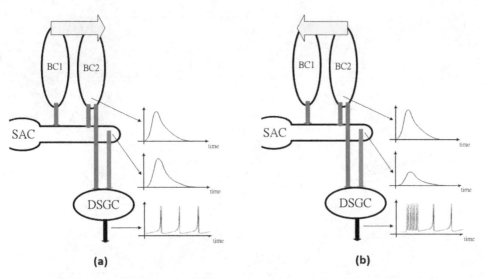

Figure 12.56. DSGC pathway. Reproduced from [51].

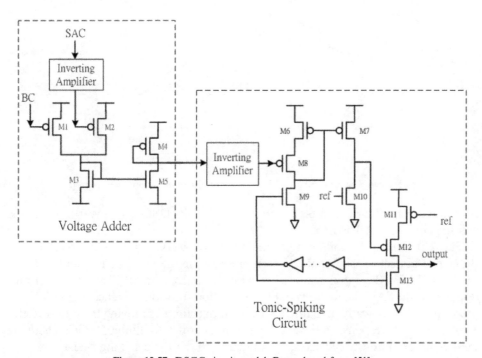

Figure 12.57. DSGC circuit model. Reproduced from [51].

The simulations were conducted with TSMC18 CMOS (180 nm) technology using the SPECTRE simulator. The SAC circuit model has been explained in the previous section. The DSGC circuit model is presented in figure 12.57. DSGC circuit model consists of a voltage adder and the tonic-spiking circuit. The voltage adder

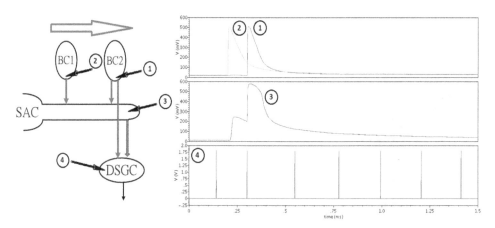

Figure 12.58. The response of DSGC to centrifugal motion. Reproduced from [51].

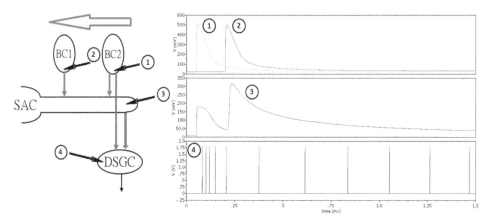

Figure 12.59. The response of DSGC to centripetal motion. Reproduced from [51].

takes input from the BC and SAC. Since SAC inhibits DSGC, an inverting amplifier whose gain is about 1 is necessary.

The retinal network in figure 12.58 and figure 12.59 contains two BCs (i.e. BC1 and BC2), one branch of SAC that has been presented in previous section, and a DSGC. In figure 12.58, the input stimulus moving from BC1 to BC2 evokes a stronger response in the SAC that cancels out the excitation from BC1. Hence, the DSGC still produces spikes tonically. In figure 12.59, the input stimulus moving from BC1 to BC2 evokes a weaker response in the SAC that is not enough to inhibit DSGC. Therefore, the DSGC produces more spikes, as compared to the tonic spiking rate.

12.5 Chapter summary

This chapter covered circuits involving the human retina, found in the dissertation by Tseng. The next chapter covers neurons spiking in a variety of manners, implementing a neural code, as designed by Alzahrani.

Certain sections of text in this chapter have been reproduced with permission from [42] and [43]. Copyright IEEE.

References

[1] Amthor F R, Keyser K T and Dmitrieva N A 2002 Effects of the destruction of starburst-cholinergic amacrine cells by the toxin AF64A on rabbit retinal directional selectivity *Vis. Neurosci.* **19** 495–509

[2] Andreou A G and Strohbehn K 1990 Analog VLSI implementation of the Hassenstein-Reichardt-Poggio models for vision computation *Systems, Man and Cybernetics, 1990. Conf. Proc., IEEE Int. Conf. (Los Angeles, CA)* 707–10

[3] Awatramani G B and Slaughter M M 2000 Origin of transient and sustained responses in ganglion cells of the retina *J. Neurosci.* **20** 7087–95

[4] Baccus S A *et al* 2008 A retinal circuit that computes object motion *J. Neurosci.* **28** 6807–17

[5] Benson R G and Delbrück T 1991 Direction selective silicon retina that uses null inhibition *Advances in Neural Information Processing Systems 4* 756–63 http://citeseerx.ist.psu.edu/viewdoc/summary?doi=10.1.1.86.9407

[6] Boahen K A and Andreou A G 1991 A contrast sensitive silicon retina with reciprocal synapses *Advances in Neural Information Processing Systems 4* 764–72 http://citeseerx.ist.psu.edu/viewdoc/summary?doi=10.1.1.43.8246

[7] Borg Graham L J and Grzywacz N M 1992 *A Model of the Directional Selectivity Circuit in Retina: Transformations by Neurons Singly and in Concert* (San Diego, CA: Academic) pp 347–75

[8] Burkhardt D A 1994 Light adaptation and photopigment bleaching in cone photoreceptors *in situ* in the retina of the turtle *J. Neurosci.* **14** 1091–105

[9] Chaoui H 1995 CMOS analogue adder *Electron. Lett.* **31** 180–1

[10] Delbruck T and Mead C A 1994 Adaptive photoreceptor with wide dynamic range *Circuits and Systems IEEE Int. Symp. (London)* 339–42

[11] Delbruck T and Oberhoff D 2004 Self-biasing low power adaptive photoreceptor *Circuits and Systems IEEE Int. Symp. (Vancouver, BC)* 844–7

[12] Delbrück T and Mead C A 1989 An electronic photoreceptor sensitive to small changes in intensity *Neural Information Processing Systems* 720–7 http://portal.acm.org/citation.cfm?id=89946

[13] Delbrück T and Liu S-C 2004 A silicon early visual system as a model animal *Vis. Res.* **44** 2083–9

[14] Demb J B *et al* 2001 Bipolar cells contribute to nonlinear spatial summation in the brisk-transient (Y) ganglion cell in mammalian retina *J. Neurosci.* **21** 7447–54

[15] Etienne-Cummings R 2001 Biologically inspired visual motion detection in VLSI *Int. J. Comput. Vis.* **44** 175–98

[16] Euler T, Detwiler P B and Denk W 2002 Directionally selective calcium signals in dendrites of starburst amacrine cells *Nature* **418** 845–52

[17] Fried S I, Münch T A and Werblin F S 2002 Mechanisms and circuitry underlying directional selectivity in the retina *Nature* **420** 411–4

[18] Gaal L *et al* 1998 Postsynaptic response kinetics are controlled by a glutamate transporter at cone photoreceptors *J. Neurophysiol.* **79** 190–6

[19] Geffen M N, de Vries S E J and Meister M 2007 Retinal ganglion cells Can rapidly change polarity from off to on *PLoS Biol.* **5** e65

[20] Greenwald S H *et al* 2009 Brightness as a function of current amplitude in human retinal electrical stimulation *Invest. Ophthalmol. Vis. Sci.* **50** 5017–25

[21] Hasegawa J and Yagi T 2008 Real-time emulation of neural images in the outer retinal circuit *J. Physiol. Sci.* **58** 507–14

[22] Hausselt S E *et al* 2007 A dendrite-autonomous mechanism for direction selectivity in retinal starburst amacrine cells *PLoS Biol.* **5** e185

[23] Hsu C-C, Parker A C and Joshi J 2010 Dendritic computations, dendritic spiking and dendritic plasticity in nanoelectronic neurons *2010 53rd IEEE Int. Midwest Sympos. on Circuits and Systems* (Seattle, WA: IEEE) pp 89–92

[24] Ichinose T, Shields C R and Lukasiewicz P D 2005 Sodium channels in transient retinal bipolar cells enhance visual responses in ganglion cells *J. Neurosci.* **25** 1856–65

[25] Javaheri M *et al* 2006 Retinal prostheses for the blind *Ann. Acad. Med. Singap.* **35** 137–44

[26] Joshi J, Parker A C and Hsu C-C 2010 A carbon nanotube spiking cortical neuron with tunable refractory period and spiking duration *IEEE Latin American Sympos. on Circuits and Systems (LASCAS)*

[27] Kameda S and Yagi T 2006 An analog silicon retina with multichip configuration *IEEE Trans. Neural Netw.* **17** 197–210

[28] Kaur T and Nawy S 2012 Characterization of Trpm1 desensitization in ON bipolar cells and its role in downstream signalling *Physiol. J.* **590** 179–92

[29] Koike C *et al* 2010 TRPM1 is a component of the retinal ON bipolar cell transduction channel in the mGluR6 cascade *Proc. Natl. Acad. Sci.* **107** 332–7

[30] Lee S and Jimmy Zhou Z 2006 The synaptic mechanism of direction selectivity in distal processes of starburst amacrine cells *Neuron* **51** 787–99

[31] Liu S-C 2000 A neuromorphic aVLSI model of global motion processing in the fly *IEEE Trans. Circuits Syst.* II **47** 1458–67

[32] Mahowald M A 1992 VLSI analogs of neuronal visual processing: a synthesis of form and function *PhD Thesis* California Institute of Technology http://portal.acm.org/citation.cfm?id=168951

[33] Mead C and Mahowald M 1988 A silicon model of early visual processing *Neural Netw.* **1** 91–7

[34] Morgans C W 2009 TRPM1 is required for the depolarizing light response in retinal ON-bipolar cells *Proc. Natl Acad. Sci.* **106** 19174–8

[35] Ohkuma M *et al* 2007 Patch-clamp recording of human retinal photoreceptors and bipolar cells *J. Photochem. Photobiol.* **83** 317–22

[36] Olveczky B P, Baccus S A and Meister M 2003 Segregation of object and background motion in the retina *Nature* **423** 401–8

[37] Parker A C and Azar A N 2009 A hierarchical artificial retina architecture *Proc. Bioengineered and Bioinspired Systems IV SPIE Europe Microtechnologies for the New Millennium* **7365** 736503

[38] Poznanski R R 1992 Modelling the electrotonic structure of starburst amacrine cells in the rabbit retina: a functional interpretation of dendritic morphology *Bull. Math. Biol.* **54** 905–28

[39] Ribelayga C 2010 Vertebrate vision: TRP channels in the spotlight *Curr. Biol.* **2010** R278–80

[40] Shen Y *et al* 2009 A transient receptor potential-like channel mediates synaptic transmission in rod bipolar cells *J. Neurosci.* **29** 6088–93

[41] Shon A P, Rao R P and Sejnowski T J 2004 Motion detection and prediction through spike-timing dependent plasticity *Network* **15** 179–98

[42] Tseng K-C and Parker A C 2012 A neuromorphic circuit that computes differential motion *2012 55th Int. Midwest Symp. Circuits and Systems (MWSCAS) IEEE* (Piscataway, NJ: IEEE) 89–92

[43] Tseng K-C, Parker A C and Joshi J 2011 A directionally-selective neuromorphic circuit based on reciprocal synapses in Starburst Amacrine Cells *2011 Annual Int. Conf. of the IEEE Engineering in Medicine and Biology Society* (Piscataway, NJ: IEEE) 5674–7

[44] Tukker J J, Rowland Taylor W and Smith R G 2004 Direction selectivity in a model of the starburst amacrine cell *Vis. Neurosci.* **21** 611–25

[45] Usui S *et al* 1996 Reconstruction of retinal horizontal cell responses by the ionic current model *Vis. Res.* **36** 1711–9

[46] Wang Y and Liu S-C 2010 Motion detection using an a VLSI network of spiking neurons *Circuits and Systems (ISCAS), Proc. 2010 IEEE Int. Symp. (Paris)* 93–6

[47] Wu S M, Gao F and Maple B R 2000 Functional architecture of synapses in the inner retina: segregation of visual signals by stratification of bipolar cell axon terminals *J. Neurosci.* **20** 4462–70

[48] Yagi T 1986 Interaction between the soma and the axon terminal of retinal horizontal cells in Cyprinus carpio *J. Physiol.* **375** 121–35

[49] Yoshida K *et al* 2001 A key role of starburst amacrine cells in originating retinal directional selectivity and optokinetic eye movement *Neuron* **30** 771–80

[50] Zaghloul K A and Boahen K 2006 A silicon retina that reproduces signals in the optic nerve *J. Neural Eng.* **3** 257

[51] Tseng K-C 2012 Neuromorphic motion sensing circuits in a silicon retina *PhD Thesis* University of Southern California

IOP Publishing

Neuromorphic Circuits
A constructive approach
Alice C Parker and Rick Cattell

Chapter 13

The neural code

Rami Alzahrani and Alice C Parker

Temporal coding is one of the two major theories about how neural information is encoded in neural signals, proposing that the temporal structure of the spike train carries additional information beyond the mean firing rate in cortical neurons. For example, recent studies have suggested that in the neocortex and hippocampus, the neural information is reliably conveyed by the precisely-timed action potentials (APs) at the neuron's output [5]. This example and many other pieces of evidence suggest that biological neurons signal each other in a rich and complex manner to perform complex cognitive computing tasks in real time. The implementation of such capabilities using electronic circuits is a difficult task. Many neuromorphic circuits mimic different aspects of a biological neuron, yet neuronal modulation has received little focus. You may ask, *what is neuronal modulation?* Neuronal modulation describes the physiological process by which a neuron encodes various input properties into various output properties in the form of different AP patterns and shapes. In other words, neuronal modulation is a determining factor in understanding what neuronal code to use when modeling biological neurons and comprehending how neurons process and interpret information.

We posit throughout this chapter that each neuron may have a unique built-in modulation function depending on its role. Therefore, this chapter introduces a new technique to convert continuous stimulus shapes into modulated AP spiking/ bursting patterns to build rich behavioral electronic neurons. We test the hypothesis using the most straightforward modulation function (direct correlation). The results show plausible excitatory spiking patterns consistent with spiking patterns produced by the Izhikevich mathematical model reflecting various biological neuronal behaviors [12]. The difference between our circuit model approach and Izhikevich's mathematical model is that our model uses various biological voltage-gated ion channel properties to describe different AP patterns. Thus, a good grasp of how various biological voltage-gated ion channels at the axon initial segment (AIS) region work is essential in understanding the working principle of our neuromorphic work.

13.1 Introduction to dynamic neuronal coding circuits

In general, neuromorphic systems rely on very large-scale integration (VLSI) of interconnected electronic devices, which allows these systems to resemble various biological neuronal mechanisms [10]. Such systems are considered to be fault-tolerant and usually follow a distributed memory-computational architecture using different synaptic weights as memory [8]. The BioRC group and many others have shown various electronic implementations of neurons, synapses, and other related mechanisms [6, 9, 11, 16, 20]. Our previous neuromorphic Biomimetic Real-time Cortex (BioRC) group work has demonstrated capabilities such as the implementation of spike/timing/dependent plasticity to mimic learning mechanisms in biological neurons [13, 14, 21], learning without forgetting [22], using dopamine signaling as a reward in learning [3], spiking with a particular set of inputs [15], and recently, spiking in response to specific frequencies [23]. With the library of neuromorphic circuits that we have implemented and as part of our investigation of how the human brain might learn new tasks without forgetting old ones, we have begun to examine neuronal signaling and how different patterns may convey different information. The most widely accepted neuronal computation scheme views neurons as a centralized unit at which an AP takes place if the summation of the synaptic inputs at the soma exceeds a certain threshold, whether the summation is performed linearly or non-linearly (current or conductance-based, respectively) [4]. Dendritic computation has shown to play a significant role in neuronal signaling. In 2004, Polsky *et al* discussed how the locations of the synapses in pyramidal neurons play a significant role in the summation of the received presynaptic inputs [18]. The BioRC group has demonstrated various neuromorphic dendritic computations [6]. In 2017, Sardi *et al* conducted an experiment concluding that a biological neuron consists of multiple independent threshold units [19]. Motivated by the realizations described in [19], we built an electronic neuron consisting of two dendritic branches to encode information about the origin of the stimulus by observing the variability of the repolarization time of a single spike [15].

Our modeling hypothesis suggests that the influence of stimulus dynamics on the induced APs may follow an unknown type of neuronal modulation. Here, the term *neuronal modulation* refers to the process by which a neuron translates its synaptic inputs to a distinct AP pattern. Although such modulation has not been well discussed in the literature, a biological basis is proposed [17]. The proposed model can be used in building a rich behavioral neuromorphic neuron to perform complex tasks. Figure 13.1 shows the general block diagram of the proposed model. To investigate the behavioral capabilities, (1) we modeled the output of various dendritic computations using the parameter *Vsoma*, in which *Vsoma* can be any analog or digital signal, and (2) a direct correlation is used between *Vsoma* and the AIS modulation block. A direct correlation means there is no modulation function; hence the modulation function is shown as a dashed box (figure 13.1), to show that even with the simplest type of modulation, the neuronal computation can be

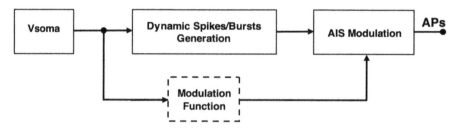

Figure 13.1. The general block diagram of the BioRC dynamic encoding neuronal model. To test the model hypothesis, a simple modulation function is used where the modulation function block is a simple direct path from the *Vsoma* block to the AIS modulation block, hence the dotted border line is used for the modulation function block. Reproduced from [2]. Published by Association for Computing Machinery. Copyright 2020 Owner/Author.

increased, although other types of modulation function can be used to perform neuronal arithmetic operations (e.g. differentiation or integration). We demonstrate the circuit using Cadence Virtuoso simulator tools.

13.2 Dynamic neuronal coding circuit implementations

The BioRC dynamic encoding neuronal model given here is a modified version of the previous BioRC voltage-based axon hillock design [6], to support dynamic activation–deactivation of C_{av} channels and provide a direct stimulus to AP modulation using a direct path from Vsoma to AIS block. The model's schematic diagram consists of *Somatodendtritic*, *Amp*, *Cav*, *Nav*, *Kv*, *Spiking Generator*, and *AIS Modulation* sub-blocks, shown in figure 13.2 with different colors. In figure 13.2, the *Somatodendtritic* sub-block models the threshold variabilities and provides information about the dendritic calcium ion concentration. *Amp* is a controlled amplification stage to provide variable gain for the subsequent sub-blocks. C_{av} models the effect of the voltage-gated calcium ion channels through bursting. *Spiking Generator*, K_v, and Na_v sub-blocks are adopted from Hsu's model in which *Spiking Generator* uses gated cross-coupled inverters to model the spike initiation mechanisms, K_v models voltage-gated potassium ion channels, and Na_v models voltage-gated sodium ion channels. The *AIS Modulation* sub-block models the AIS signal processing by correlating a stimulus dynamic into specific AP patterns.

Moreover, there are seven parameters to provide a wide range of variability in modulating and shaping the APs:

- The parameter *Vsoma* models the output of the dendritic computations to be used as an input to the dynamic encoding neuronal model, while parameter *VsomaThre* models the threshold variability to dynamically control neuronal activities. Hence, the sensitivity of detecting smaller *Vsoma* potentials is inversely proportional to the value of *VsomaThre*.
- The parameter Ca++ designates the dendritic Ca^{2+} ion concentration, whereas the parameter *CaThre* models the dynamic threshold activation of Ca_v channels.

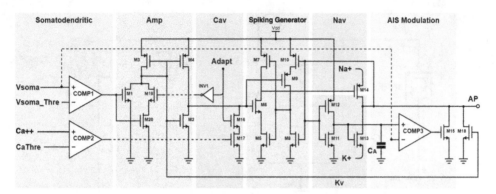

Figure 13.2. The Schematic diagram of the proposed neuron model in which *INV*1 is a single-stage CMOS inverter, and COMP1, COMP2, COMP3 are low power differential-based comparators. To enhance readability, the dashed and the solid connections are used interchangeably. Reporduced from [2]. Published by Association for Computing Machinery. Copyright 2020 Owner/Author.

- The parameter *Adapt* controls the current flow through M16 (threshold calcium current [7]) when the Ca²⁺ ion channel is opened (M17 is turned on); hence, regulating the maximum burst width. However, when the Ca²⁺ ion channel is closed (M17 is turned off), *Adapt* controls the frequency of spikes through M19. Therefore, *Adapt* regulates current flow and burst width.
- The parameters Na+ and K+ represent the sodium ion concentration and the potassium ion concentration at the AIS, respectively, whereas C_A models the AIS characteristic capacitance per unit area determining the AIS width and conduction velocity characteristics.

In addition, the model consists of three low power differential-based comparators (*COMP*1, *COMP*2, and *COMP*3). *COMP*1 models threshold variabilities by comparing *Vsoma* and *Vsoma Thre*, *COMP*2 monitors dendritic Ca²⁺ concentrations and consequently activates and deactivates Ca$_v$ channels, and *COMP*3 controls the generation of action potentials based on the voltage across C_A to allow various stimulus shapes to generate different spiking patterns. The comparators' schematic diagram is shown in figure 13.3, in which *in*+ and *in*– are the comparators' positive and negative input terminals, respectively. The output from the differential pair amplifier is followed by two cascaded inverters to digitize the output voltage swing into logic '1' for ($\Delta in > 0$) and logic '0' for ($\Delta in < 0$) where $\Delta in = (in +) - (in -)$.

In other words, *COMP*1 outputs a logic '1' when the membrane potential exceeds a certain threshold (*Vsoma > Vsoma Thre*) and outputs logic '0' when *Vsoma < Vsoma Thre*. Similarly, in modeling Ca$_v$ channels, *COMP*2 outputs a logic '1' when the dendritic Ca²⁺ concentration exceeds the Ca$_v$ threshold activation voltage (Ca ++ > *CaThre*), and outputs logic '0' when Ca ++ < *CaThre* to deactivate Ca$_v$ channels. As a result, AP patterns can be classified into bursting APs if *COMP*2 exhibits logic '1' and spiking APs otherwise. Likewise, *COMP*3 compares *Vsoma* and V_{CA} (voltage across capacitor C_A where C_A represents the biophysical capacitance per unit area of the AIS region). Consequently, *COMP*3 outputs a logic

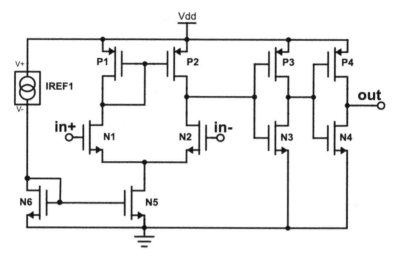

Figure 13.3. The schematic diagram of the comparators. Reproduced from [2]. Published by Association for Computing Machinery. Copyright 2020 Owner/Author.

'1' when $V_{CA} > Vsoma$, to inhibit the generation of APs by activating transistor M15, and a logic '0' when $V_{CA} < Vsoma$ to allow APs depolarization. Comparing V_{CA} and $Vsoma$ using $COMP3$ allows a direct AP modulation. In other words, the generated AP depends on the shape of $Vsoma$. Such dependency leads to continuous generation of various spiking/bursting patterns.

13.3 Various dynamic spiking and bursting patterns

In this section, we simulate the model's schematic diagram shown in figure 13.2, using Cadence Virtuoso Simulator Tools to show that various spiking patterns can be generated continuously as a function of ion channels (Na+, K+, Ca ++), *Adapt*, and dynamic *Vsoma* shapes. However, to simplify the analysis, throughout this chapter, Na+ and K+ are set to be 900 mV and 0 V, respectively. The contribution of the ion channels in shaping APs is summarized in the sketch illustration of both single and burst AP patterns shown in figure 13.4(A), in which Na+ sets the peak spike/burst amplitude, K+ sets the spike/burst resting potential, and the difference between Ca ++ and *CaThre* defines the mode of APs (bursting or spiking mode). The current states (conditions) of ion channels, *Adapt*, and *Vsoma* required for generating a specific pattern, are outlined in figure 13.4(B) for regular spikes (RS), phasic spikes (PS), tonic bursts (TB), single burst per stimulus (SB), class-1 spikes (CS1), subthreshold oscillation (OSC), depolarization after potential (DAP), integrator spikes (INT), and mixed mode (MIX) patterns.

In figure 13.4(B), when two or more patterns have the same setup conditions, such as (RS, INT, CS1, OSC) and (TB, SB) patterns, switching between patterns depends solely on the dynamic shapes of *Vsoma*. For example, the generation of both SB and TB patterns requires $Adapt > V_{dd}/2$, Ca ++ > $CaThre$, and K+ = 0, hence, the selection between SB and TB patterns depends on the dynamic shape of *Vsoma*. Similarly, the generation of RS, INT, CS1, and OSC patterns requires

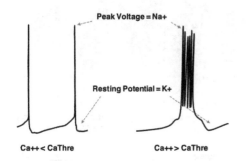

		Ca++ < CaThre	Ca++ > CaThre	
K+ > 0		PS-DAP	RS-DAP	--
K+ = 0		PS	RS INT CS1 OSC	SB TB
			MIX	
		Adapt < (Vdd / 2)	Adapt > (Vdd / 2)	

Figure 13.4. A sketch illustration of spiking and bursting APs showing the model's voltage-gated ion channels contribution in shaping APs, shown on the left. The right table shows the model's conditions associated with the generation of single burst (SB), tonic bursts (TB), regular spikes (RS), integrator spikes (INT), class-1 spikes (CS1), subthreshold oscillation (OSC), phasic spikes (PS), phasic spike with depolarization after potential (PS-DAP), regular spikes with depolarization after potentials (RS-DAP), and mixed mode (MIX). The shape of the stimulus patterns determine spiking patterns when all other parameters are the same. Reproduced from [2]. Published by Association for Computing Machinery. Copyright 2020 Owner/Author.

$Adapt > V_{dd}/2$, $Ca++ < CaThre$, and $K+ = 0$, thus, the selection between RS, INT, CS1, and OSC patterns depends on the shape of *Vsoma*.

The simulation results of the model's schematic diagram for the previously mentioned spiking/bursting patterns are shown in figure 13.5 using similar stimulus shapes of *Vsoma* presented in the Izhikevich mathematical model [12]. To discuss how each individual pattern is formed, we group the results into three groups based on the generation conditions required for each pattern.

13.3.1 Various spiking patterns using dynamic neuronal encoding circuits

The RS, INT, CS1, and OSC patterns are generated when $Ca++ < CaThre$ and $Adapt > V_{dd}/2$. The first condition is to inhibit bursting and permit spiking formation, and the second condition is to prevent current flow through transistors M19 and M20, forcing the current of M3 to flow only through M1. Since these patterns have the same conditions of generation, information about the stimuli is needed to identify which pattern the model should produce.

- The **RS** pattern shown in figure 13.5(A) is generated using a constant voltage pulse of stimulus (*Vsoma* = 300 mV). The RS pattern frequency is directly proportional to the amplitude of *Vsoma* (stimulus intensity).
- The **INT** pattern shown in figure 13.5(H) corresponds to a train of short stimulus (*Vsoma* = 150 mV, and width = 4 ns per pulse). Due to the accumulation of charges on capacitor C_A, the model is capable of detecting consecutive rapid events ($T_1 = 6$ ns). In contrast, when the time between consecutive stimulus increases ($T_2 = 26$ ns), the model becomes less excitable due to the loss of the accumulated charges on C_A.
- The **CS1** pattern shown in figure 13.5(E) resembles a ramp-like stimulus shape (*Vsoma* = 800 mV, with rising time $t_r = 60$ ns). The result is consistent

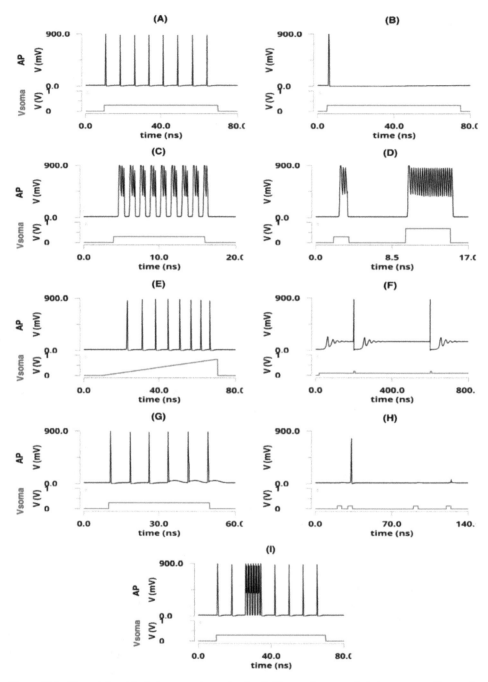

Figure 13.5. The relationship between various simulated *Vsoma* shapes and their corresponding action potentials for (A) regular spikes, (B) phasic spikes, (C) tonic bursts, (D) single burst per stimulus, (E) class-1 excitable, (F) subthreshold oscillations, (G) depolarization after potential, (H) integrator, and (I) mixed mode, following the table shown in figure 13.4. Reproduced from [2]. Published by Association for Computing Machinery. Copyright 2020 Owner/Author.

with the generated RS pattern, at which the frequency of spikes is proportional to the amplitude of *Vsoma*.

- The **OSC** pattern shown in figure 13.5(F) takes place when *Vsoma* = 100 mV at which C_A experiences multiple charging and discharging phases due to the small stimulus amplitudes. However, when introducing further stimuli (*Vsoma* = 200 mV and width = 8 ns per pulse), the model exhibits spikes. This might be important for detecting small perturbations of stimuli.

13.3.2 Various bursting patterns using dynamic neuronal encoding circuits

The TB (Figure 13.5(C)) and SB (figure 13.5(D)) patterns are formed when $Ca++ > CaThre$ and $Adapt > V_{dd}/2$. When $Ca++ > CaThre$, the output of *COMP2* sets the gate voltage of M17 to V_{dd}; Consequently, transistor M17 is switched on, allowing the current to flow from M4 through M16 and M17. Hence, reducing the gate voltage of M6 and M9 to a value near V_{th6} (the threshold voltage of M6). The current passing through M16 and M17 resembles T-current (low threshold calcium current discussed in [7]). Therefore, at each rising edge of an individual intra-burst, transistor M6 operates in the subthreshold region while M9 operates in the triode region. In contrast, at each falling edge of an individual intra-burst, M9 and M6 switch their operating regions where M9 operates in the subthreshold region, and M6 operates in the triode region. This continuous switching results in a consecutive generation of the intra-burst spikes.

Although the model relies on simulation results for extracting design parameters, the relation of the current as a function of the input gate voltage for M6 can be approximated using the drain–source current model (13.1) for the triode (linear region) and (13.2) for the subthreshold operation regions. Similarly, for M9, by using μ_p, V_{SG}, V_{SD}, $|V_{thp}|$ instead of μ_n, V_{GS}, V_{DS}, V_{thn}, respectively.

$$I_{DS} = \mu_n C_{ox} \frac{W}{L} \left[(V_{GS} - V_{th}) V_{DS} - \frac{V_{DS}^2}{2} \right] \tag{13.1}$$

$$I_{DS} = I_0 e^{\frac{V_{GS}}{n V_T}} \tag{13.2}$$

where μ_n is the mobility of electrons, μ_p is the mobility of holes, C_{ox} is the oxide capacitance, W is the diffusion width, L is the diffusion length, V_{GS} is the gate–source voltage, V_{DS} is the drain–source voltage, I_0 is the characteristic leakage current, n is the subthreshold slope factor, and V_T is the thermal voltage.

- The **SB** pattern shown in figure 13.5(D) corresponds to two single bursts per stimulus. There are two scenarios for the generation of SB pattern: (1) when the width of stimulus is shorter than the time required for *COMP3* to turn transistor M15 on (*Vsoma* = 300 mV, and width = 2 ns); (2) when the amplitude of stimulus is higher than the maximum voltage value across capacitor C_A (*Vsoma* = 700 mV, and width = 6 ns).

13.3.3 Other spiking patterns using dynamic neuronal encoding circuits

Unlike the previously mentioned spiking patterns, DAP, PS, and MIX patterns have different setup conditions and parameters.

- The **DAP** pattern requires $Ca++ < CaThre$ and $K+ > 0$. Since K+ determines the resting potential voltage, the DAP pattern is directly proportional to K+. To generate the DAP pattern, other spiking patterns are required. Therefore, **PS-DAP** and **RS-DAP** are introduced to represent PS pattern and RS pattern with the DAP effect, respectively. Figure 13.5(G) shows RS pattern without DAP (leftmost three spikes) for $K+ = 0$, and RS pattern with DAP (rightmost three spikes), at which $K+ = 900$ mV.

- The **PS** pattern requires transistors M19 and M20 to be turned on so that M3 current can flow through M1, M19, and M20 to further decrease the gate voltage of M4, M2, and M18, see figure 13.5(B). Therefore, the PS pattern requires $Ca++ < CaThre$ and $Adapt < V_{dd}/2$.

- The **MIX** pattern is generated using the dynamic activation and deactivation of Ca_v channels. In other words, the model produces bursting patterns when $Ca++ > CaThre$ and spiking patterns when $Ca++ < CaThre$, see figure 13.5(I). In both cases, the generation of mixed pattern requires $Adapt > V_{dd}/2$ to allow current flow through M16 and M17.

13.3.4 The working principles of the AIS modulation

Understanding how the AIS modulation sub-block converts dynamic stimulus into various spiking/bursting patterns requires a discussion of the relationship between $Vsoma$ and V_{CA} (the inputs of *COMP*3) is needed. Figure 13.6 represents the relationship between $Vsoma$ (red waveform) and V_{CA} (blue waveform) for all previously simulated patterns. In figure 13.6, the relationship can be described using the relative refractory period (RRP), in other words, the time between two consecutive spikes/bursts.

The ideal RRP for spikes and bursts are denoted as RRP_S (green shaded region) and RRP_B (light blue shaded region) in figure 13.6, respectively, in which both RRP_S and RRP_B represent the period at which $V_{CA} > Vsoma$. However, because switching from $V_{CA} > Vsoma$ to $V_{CA} < Vsoma$ using *COMP*3 is not ideal (spontaneous switching), COMP3 propagation delay (T_d) is added (red shaded region) as shown in figure 13.6. Thus, the actual relative refractory period can be extracted graphically from figure 13.6 as ($RRP_S + T_d$) for spikes, and ($RRP_B + T_d$) for bursts patterns. During burst formation, capacitor C_A withstands multiple fast charging and discharging phases per burst due to the formation of the intra-burst spikes, whereas during spike generation, capacitor C_A undergoes a single charging phase and a discharging phase per spike. Accordingly, RRP_B is smaller than RRP_S. However, since the value of T_d depends on the physical properties of the design, it remains the same for both spike and burst patterns.

Modeling the role of *RRP* at the AIS allows various stimulus shape patterns to result in generating different spiking patterns through which V_{CA}, the voltage across

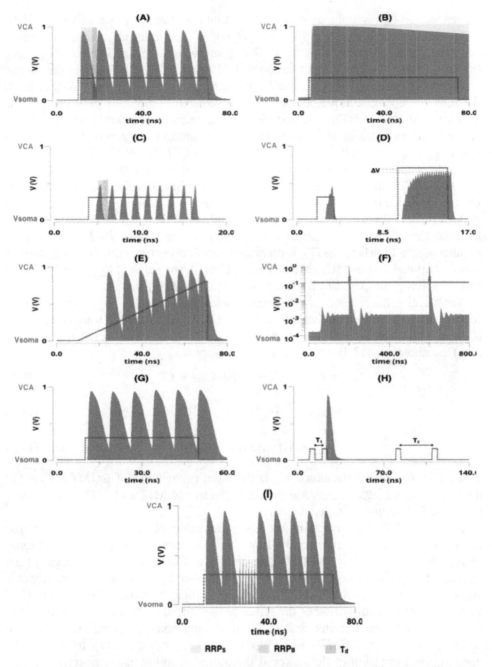

Figure 13.6. The relationship between *Vsoma* (red) and V_{CA} (blue) for all plausible patterns; (A) regular spiking; (B) phasic spiking; (C) tonic bursting; (D) single burst per stimulus; (E) class-1 excitable spikes; (F) subthreshold oscillations; (G) depolarization after potential; (H) integrator spiking; (I) mixed mode. The ideal relative refractory period for spikes and bursts is RRP_S and RRP_B, respectively. T_d represents COMP3 propagation delay. Reproduced from [2]. Published by Association for Computing Machinery. Copyright 2020 Owner/Author.

the capacitor C_A, is compared with the stimulus shape *Vsoma* using *COMP3*. Therefore, for the RS pattern (figure 13.6(A)), as the amplitude of *Vsoma* remains constant, the RRP_S remains the same for all subsequent spikes. For the PS pattern (figure 13.6(B)), due to the activation of M19 and M20, the RRP_S is the largest compared to other patterns. In the TB pattern (figure 13.6(C)), the RRP_B remains the same for all consecutive bursts due to the constant amplitude of *Vsoma*. In the SB pattern (figure 13.6(D)), the first stimulus represents the scenario where RRP_B is larger than the width of *Vsoma* and the second stimulus represents the scenario at which $\Delta V > 0$ where $\Delta V = Vsoma - V_{CA}$. For the CS1 (figure 13.6(E)), the RRP_S is inversely proportional to the amplitude of *Vsoma*; in other words, $RRP_{S1} < RRP_{S7}$. For the OSC pattern (figure 13.6(F)), the relationship between *Vsoma* and V_{CA} is plotted in the logarithmic scale to show the voltage oscillation of V_{CA}. For the DAP pattern (figure 13.6(G)), when K + >0, the rightmost three spikes compared to the leftmost three spikes, have slightly larger V_{CA}; hence, larger RRP_S. In the INT pattern (figure 13.6(H)), the V_{CA} is higher for rapid, occurring stimulus compared to slower stimulus. In the MIX pattern (figure 13.6(I)), the value of V_{CA} is higher in the case of spiking compared to bursting; thus, $RRP_S > RRP_B$.

Analytically, the relationship between *Vsoma* and V_{CA} can be approximated using the RC analysis at the positive terminal of *COMP3* in which the total capacitance (C_{tot}), the equivalent resistance for M11 (R_{11}), and the equivalent resistance for M12 (R_{12}) are shown in (13.3), (13.4), and (13.5), respectively.

$$C_{tot} = C_{g13} + C_A + C_{in} + C_{d11} + C_{d12} \tag{13.3}$$

$$R_{11} = 1/\left(\beta_{11}\left(V_{dd} - V_{thn}\right)\right) \tag{13.4}$$

$$R_{12} = 1/\left(\beta_{12}\left(V_{dd} - \left|V_{thp}\right|\right)\right) \tag{13.5}$$

where C_g is the gate capacitance; C_{in} is the input capacitance of *COMP3*; C_d is the drain capacitance; β_{12} and β_{11} are the beta effective of M12 and M11, respectively; V_{dd} is the DC supply voltage.

Using the RC time constant method, the value of V_{CA}, the voltage across capacitor C_A, can be determined using the capacitor charging and discharging equations given in (13.6) and (13.7), respectively. Therefore, the discharging time (t_{dis}) can be approximated using (13.8) because when $V_{CA} \geqslant Vsoma$, the compactor circuit at the AIS, namely *COMP3*, will output a logic '1' causing M15 to turn ON, hence shunting the formation of the spikes at the output terminal of the neuron. On the other hand, the charging time (t_{ch}) can be approximated using (13.9) because when $V_{CA} < Vsoma$, *COMP3* will output a logic '0' causing M15 to turn OFF, allowing the formation of the spikes at the output terminal of the neuron.

$$V_{CA} = Vsoma \left(1 - e^{\frac{-t}{R_{11}C_{tot}}}\right) \tag{13.6}$$

$$V_{CA} = Vsoma \ e^{\frac{-t}{R_{12}C_{tot}}} \tag{13.7}$$

$$t_{\text{dis}} = R_{11}C_{\text{tot}} \ln\left(\frac{V_{\text{CA}}(0)}{V\!soma}\right), \text{ for } V_{\text{CA}} \geqslant V\!soma \tag{13.8}$$

$$t_{\text{ch}} = R_{12}C_{\text{tot}} \ln\left(\frac{-V\!soma}{V_{\text{CA}} - V\!soma}\right), \text{ for } V_{\text{CA}} < V\!soma \tag{13.9}$$

13.4 Chapter summary

This chapter covers circuits that recognize or generate many spiking patterns reported by Izhikevich. These circuits are found in Alzahrani's dissertation [1].

Certain sections of text in this chapter have been reproduced with permission from [2]. Published by Association for Computing Machinery. Copyright 2020 Owner/Author.

The next chapter covers other neural codes and circuits.

References

[1] Alzahrani R 2022 Dynamic neuronal encoding in neuromorphic circuits *PhD Thesis* University of Southern California
[2] Alzahrani R A and Parker A C 2020 Neuromorphic circuits with neural modulation enhancing the information content of neural signaling *Int. Conf. Neuromorphic Systems 2020* 1–8
[3] Barzegarjalali S and Parker A C 2016 An analog neural network that learns Sudoku-like puzzle rules *2016 Future Technologies Conf. (FTC)* (San Francisco, CA: IEEE) 838–47
[4] Burkitt A N 2006 A review of the integrate-and-fire neuron model: I. Homogeneous synaptic input *Biol. Cybern.* **95** 1–19
[5] deCharms C and Zador A 2000 Neural representation and the cortical code *Annu. Rev. Neurosci.* **23** 613–47
[6] Hsu C-C 2014 Dendritic computation and plasticity in neuromorphic circuits *PhD Thesis* University of Southern California
[7] Huguenard J R 1996 Low-threshold calcium currents in central nervous system neurons *Annu. Rev. Physiol.* **58** 329–48
[8] Indiveri G and Liu S-C 2015 Memory and information processing in neuromorphic systems *Proc. IEEE* **103** 1379–97
[9] Indiveri G, Stefanini F and Chicca E 2010 Spike-based learning with a generalized integrate and fire silicon neuron *Proc. 2010 Int. Symp. Circuits and Systems (Paris)* (Piscataway, NJ: IEEE) 1951–4
[10] Indiveri G *et al* 2011 Neuromorphic silicon neuron circuits *Front. Neurosci.* **5** 73
[11] Irizarry-Valle Y and Parker A C 2015 An astrocyte neuromorphic circuit that influences neuronal phase synchrony *IEEE Trans. Biomed. Circuits Syst.* **9** 175–87
[12] Izhikevich E M 2003 Simple model of spiking neurons *IEEE Trans. Neural Netw.* **14** 1569–72
[13] Joshi J 2013 Plasticity in CMOS neuromorphic circuits *PhD Thesis* University of Southern California
[14] Joshi J, Parker A C and Hsu C-C 2009 A carbon nanotube cortical neuron with spike-timing-dependent plasticity *2009 Annual Int. Conf. Engineering in Medicine and Biology Society* (Minneapolis, MN: IEEE) 1651–4

[15] Lee R K and Parker A C 2019 An electronic neuron with input-specific spiking *2019 Int. Joint Conf. Neural Networks (IJCNN) (Budapest)* (Piscataway: IEEE) 1–8

[16] Mahvash M and Parker A C 2013 Synaptic variability in a cortical neuromorphic circuit *IEEE Trans. Neural Netw. Learn. Syst.* **24** 397–409

[17] de Polavieja G G 2005 Stimulus history reliably shapes action potential waveforms of cortical neurons *J Neurosci.* **25** 5657–65

[18] Polsky A, Mel B W and Schiller J 2004 Computational subunits in thin dendrites of pyramidal cells *Nat. Neurosci.* **7** 621–7

[19] Sardi S *et al* 2017 New types of experiments reveal that a neuron functions as multiple independent threshold units *Sci. Rep.* **7** 1–17

[20] Yu T, Sejnowski T J and Cauwenberghs G 2011 Biophysical neural spiking, bursting, and excitability dynamics in reconfigurable analog VLSI *IEEE Trans. Biomed. Circuits Syst.* **5** 420–9

[21] Yue K 2020 Circuit design with nano electronic devices for biomimetic neuromorphic systems *PhD Thesis* University of Southern California

[22] Yue K *et al* 2019 A brain-plausible neuromorphic on-the-fly learning system implemented with magnetic domain wall analog memristors *Sci. Adv.* **5** eaau8170

[23] Yue K *et al* 2019 Analog neurons that signal with spiking frequencies *Proc. Int. Conf. Neuromorphic Systems. ICONS'19* (Knoxville, TN: Association for Computing Machinery)

IOP Publishing

Neuromorphic Circuits
A constructive approach
Alice C Parker and Rick Cattell

Chapter 14

Other neural codes

Rebecca K Lee and Alice C Parker

Sensory information in the brain is encoded by intricate spiking patterns. Transient characteristics of individual action potentials may be used in neural encoding. This chapter covers neural coding circuits developed by Cauwenberghs and Lee; Lee implemented circuits with spike shapes from Sardi and Kantor's publication. Cauwengerghs implemented circuits exhibiting spiking patterns documented and modeled by Izhikevich, and Cauwenberghs implemented Izhikevich's mathematical models directly into analog circuits.

Inspired by behaviors found in biological neurons, Lee designed a neuromorphic circuit of a neuron that exhibits input-specific spiking. Her neuron circuit has multiple dendrites and uses properties of localized high-voltage-activated (HVA) Ca^{2+} channels to generate action potentials with distinct shapes depending on the location of stimulation received at input synapses. Through circuit simulations, we show that her neuron circuit can encode differences in spatial locations of input stimuli through precise characteristics of output spikes, and spike shapes are tuneable. We show that neuron circuits, in conjunction with astrocytes, can be used to replace damaged neurons processing sensory inputs with healthy neurons augmented to process their own sensory inputs as well as the inputs originally intended for the damaged neurons, using spiking shapes to signal input sources. Other BioRC circuits that produce and recognize spike patterns are found in [16].

14.1 Lee's dendritic morphology and plasticity

This section introduces electronic circuits that model remapping of neural connections when damage occurs by overlaying functionality onto neurons by means of different spike shapes. Remapping could occur due to other reasons as well.

14.1.1 Motivation

In the cortex, sensory stimulation information is encoded by complex neural spiking patterns. While the exact mechanisms of neural encoding and decoding are yet to be elucidated, examples of possible spiking codes have been found in cortical responses to visual, auditory, and tactile stimuli. Textures and shapes of tactile objects can be conveyed by firing rates in the S1 area of the rodent somatosensory cortex [2]. Spiking rate representations can also be used to encode rapidly-changing acoustic events in the primate auditory cortex [7]. In these examples, information encoding is performed by varying firing rates and temporal characteristics of spiking sequences such as response latency and interspike interval durations. Action potentials (APs) were modeled as all-or-nothing events and features of individual spikes were not considered.

Neurons can produce various types of APs with varying amplitudes and durations [13]. Distinct spike shapes can be generated by activation of different types of ion channels with different permeabilities and time constants. Thus it is possible for information about spiking circumstances to be encoded in precise characteristics of individual spikes emitted by a neuron, indicating, for example, the origin of the presynaptic spikes that trigger postsynaptic spiking. Biological information encoding in spiking patterns, frequencies, waveform shapes and other variations could have implications for how neuromorphic systems and artificial neural networks are constructed.

In this section, we present a CMOS neuromorphic neuron circuit that encodes spatial variations in input activity through precise postsynaptic spike shapes. The circuit emulates first-order effects of neural behaviors found in neuroscience literature. We demonstrate the circuit in HSPICE simulations. We then show a more-complex example that includes astrocytic compartments in order to demonstrate how spiking that signals multiple origins can be used to replace damaged neurons by enhancing the processing of healthy ones.

The intricate mechanisms involved in astrocytic influence on homeostasis are discussed and modeled to illustrate how the combination of astrocytic influence and spike shape variability can be used to route signals through damaged areas by overlaying multiple signals on healthy neurons. Spike shape variability and astrocytic mechanisms that use synapse strengthening to restore functionality to neurons affected by damaged synapses could provide insight and direction for neural prosthetics, and for fault-tolerant neuromorphic systems. Spike shape variability can be exploited to construct neurons that convey different signals depending on the origin of the signaling, supporting neurons that demonstrate learning of additional skills without forgetting existing skills.

14.1.2 Neuron circuit with multiple dendrites

Remapping of cortical neurons following damage has been demonstrated in rodent models of stroke [9, 15]. Tissue damage and death take place within minutes to hours of the onset of stroke. However, it has been found that functional recovery of stroke occurs in the weeks to months following brain injury. During recovery, plasticity mechanisms in surviving neurons work to strengthen remaining parts of the network and replace damaged synaptic connections.

The time course of events following stroke for the remapping of rodent contralateral forelimb sensory maps is shown in figure 14.1. Initially (pre-stroke),

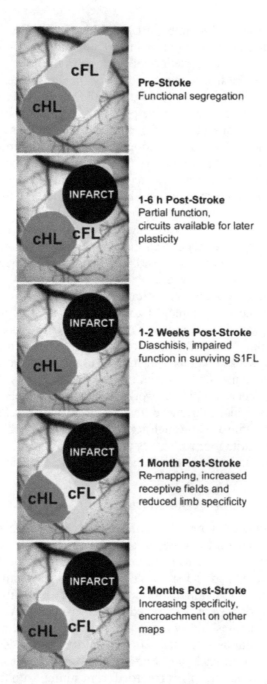

Figure 14.1. Events that occur during remapping of contralateral forelimb sensory maps after stroke damage. From [15] with permission of SAGE.

contralateral maps for the forelimb (cFL) and hindlimb (cHL) are clearly differentiable. During the first 1–6 hours of infarct injury, neurons in the stroke core (black circle) die, causing complete loss of function in the core. In this example the damage occurs in the cFL neural map. 1–2 weeks after stroke, responses to forelimb activity in the remaining cFL are reduced due to the loss of intracortical connections from neurons in the stroke core. However, the cHL area is still selective to hindlimb activity. Over the course of several weeks, plasticity mechanisms and synaptogenesis increase at the borders of the stroke core, and neural connections are rewired to compensate for reduced neural activity. One month after stroke, neurons in the remaining cFL (green region) begin to recover functionality. Receptive fields widen and some neurons at the border between the cFL and cHL (yellow region) begin to respond to stimuli from both limbs, exhibiting reduced input specificity. After two months, the network stabilizes. Now some neurons that were initially in the cHL map have been remapped to respond to the cFL, and the cHL map has reduced in size. Input specificity of neurons increases, and the number of neurons that respond to both limbs (yellow region) decreases.

In biology, reduced selectivity to stimuli may occur following recovery from stroke since neurons near the damaged zone need to respond to multiple types of stimuli in order for plasticity and repair to occur. It has been reported that 50%–85% of stroke patients exhibit reduced ability to discriminate between tactile stimuli [15].

Neuromorphic networks that repair themselves using adaptable plasticity following damage may display similar characteristics of reduced selectivity. In this section, we suggest a method for neuromorphic networks to maintain specificity. We suggest that neurons can encode specificity through differences in spike shapes. Spike shapes output from a neuron can be controlled through activation of ion channels with precise spatial locations. We use dendrite morphology as an example in our neuromorphic circuits, and we use astrocyte circuits to detect damage and initiate repair.

14.1.3 Background: dendrite-specific AP shapes

In 2017, Sardi *et al* used a new type of recording technique to accurately and consistently measure neural responses to stimulations from the same location [11]. They found that spike waveforms from a neuron vary with the spatial location of stimulation. They attributed the spike shape variability to activation of different dendrites, which act as individual threshold units for the neuron. Figure 14.2(a) illustrates how neurons were stimulated in experiments. A neuron that was stimulated with above-threshold synaptic inputs from the right activated the green dendrite (C_1). Stimulations from the left activated the pink dendrite (C_2). Spike waveforms recorded from each side were recorded and plotted in figure 14.2(b). Green waveforms plot output spikes recorded from stimuli with the setup in C_1 and pink waveforms are from stimuli as in C_2. Each of the panels are from eight different neurons, and waveforms from two recordings for each stimulus configuration were plotted to demonstrate repeatable spiking shapes.

From figure 14.2(b) it can be seen that the spike waveforms have repolarizing tails with different durations. For example, the repolarizing tail of the green waveform in

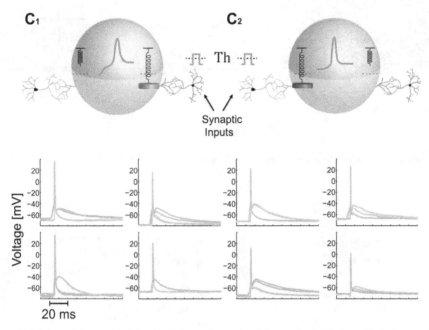

Figure 14.2. Adopted from [11] CC BY 4.0. (a) Illustration of neural stimulation. (b) Spike waveforms recorded from different neurons have shapes that depend on stimulus location.

the top left-most panel is much shorter than the pink waveform. In the bottom left-most panel, the green waveform repolarizes much slower than the pink waveform.

We suggest that the slowly-repolarizing tail may be caused by high-voltage-activated (HVA) Ca^{2+} channels that are localized at specific dendrites. As their name suggests, HVA Ca^{2+} channels require high membrane potential in order to be activated and opened. It has been shown that activation of HVA Ca^{2+} channels generate slow Ca^{2+} tail currents evoked in subicular pyramidal neurons [4]. APs evoked from a neuron activate these channels. Once activated, the channels deactivate slowly during repolarization, producing a long after-depolarization in the neuron. It has also been suggested that activation of these channels is responsible for neural bursting outputs, described earlier in chapter 13.

14.1.4 A neuron circuit with input-specific spiking

14.1.4.1 Structure of a neuron with multiple dendrites and HVA Ca^{2+} channels
The block diagram of a neuron circuit with multiple dendrites and HVA Ca^{2+} channels is shown in figure 14.3. The neuron has *n* dendritic branches, *B1-Bn*, that are connected to multiple synapses. In the figure, branch *B2* connects with *m* different synapses. Each dendritic branch sums the EPSPs it receives from its synapses to generate a dendritic potential *DENDi*, where *i* is the dendritic branch. Dendritic potentials are then summed to generate the total potential, *SOMA*, at the soma. Similar to other neuron designs, *SOMA* is fed into an axon hillock and generates a spike at *AP_POST*. Dendritic potentials *DENDi* are also used in the

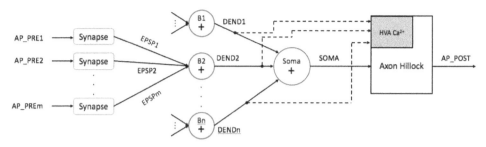

Figure 14.3. Block diagram of a neuron with multiple dendrites and HVA Ca^{2+} channels [6].

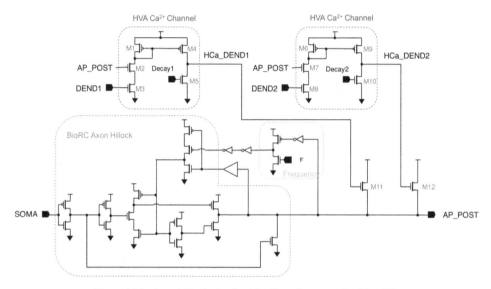

Figure 14.4. Axon hillock circuit with effects from two dendrites [6].

circuits to activate HVA Ca^{2+} channels. Activation of HVA Ca^{2+} channels affect the shape of the output AP, *AP_POST*.

14.1.4.2 Axon hillock circuit with effects from multiple dendrites

An axon hillock circuit with two dendrites is shown in figure 14.4. Different components in the design are shown in the dashed boxes. The blue box is a previous design of the axon hillock demonstrated by the BioRC group [3]. The green box is used to adjust the spiking frequency at the output. The frequency can be tuned with the control voltage *F*. Larger values of *F* increase the frequency.

The circuit compartments for the HVA Ca^{2+} channels are shown in the red boxes (*HVA Ca^{2+} channel*). They emulate the opening of channels on the postsynaptic cell following large membrane depolarization and a subsequent slow inflow of Ca^{2+} ions. In this circuit we include two dendrites with dendritic branch potentials *DEND1* and *DEND2*. We assume that each dendrite has a set of HVA Ca^{2+} channels with different densities and time constants. When the potential of a dendritic branch is large enough to cause firing, the *AP_POST* and corresponding

DEND signal briefly turn on the left side of the current mirror in the associated *HVA* Ca^{2+} *channel* module. This pulls up the output of the module, *HCa_DEND*, to VDD. *HCa_DEND* represents the Ca^{2+} that flows into the postsynaptic cell, causing it to repolarize slowly. When *HCa_DEND* is high, it pulls up the axon hillock output *AP_POST* through a resistive NMOS transistor. Here, activation through dendrite 1 pulls up *AP_POST* through M11 and activation of dendrite 2 pulls *AP_POST* through M12. *DEND1* must be high enough to turn on and generate enough current flow through M3 in order to pull up *HCa_DEND1*. Thresholds for activation can be controlled by tuning the sizes of transistors M3 and M8. The *Decay* signals represent the inactivation and closing time constants of each HVA Ca^{2+} channel. They can be tuned to generate different AP shapes for each dendrite. Although this circuit only demonstrates effects on spiking from two dendrites, it can be easily be extended to implement more dendrites by adding more *HVA* Ca^{2+} *channel* modules and pull-up transistors.

14.1.4.3 Simulation results

A neuron with two dendrites is configured using the circuits presented in this section. The structure of the neuron is shown in figure 14.5. It has two dendritic branches (*Dendritic Branch 1* and *Dendritic Branch 2*), and each branch is stimulated by input APs at two synapses. APs *AP1* and *AP2* stimulate *Dendritic Branch 1*. *Dendritic Branch 2* is stimulated by *AP3* and *AP4*. The neuron, *N*, emits spikes *AP_OUT* when it receives at least two coincident input spikes. Two coincident spikes must be received on the same dendrite in order to generate a dendritic branch potential that is large enough to activate HVA Ca^{2+} channels localized on that branch. The branch is considered to be highly active when it receives at least two coincident inputs. We configure the *HVA* Ca^{2+} *channel* modules on each dendritic branch with decay values *Decay1* = 0.22 V and *Decay2* = 0.24 V. Circuits were simulated in HSPICE using 45 nm CMOS technology and a supply voltage of 0.9 V. Transistors in the axon hillock circuit were sized so that the threshold for firing was 0.45 V. Output action potential tail durations were measured from 27% to 5% of VDD on the falling phase of the signal.

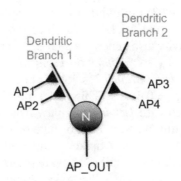

Figure 14.5. Neuron with two dendrites [6].

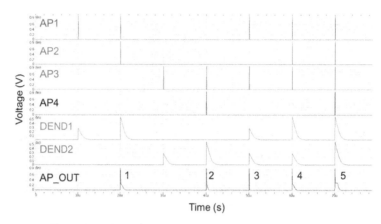

Figure 14.6. Simulation results for neuron with two dendrites [6].

Simulation results for the neuron with two dendrites are shown in figure 14.6. Input APs were triangular pulses with an amplitude of 0.9 V and duration of 0.1 μs. The input spikes, *AP1–AP4*, are shown on the top four traces, *DEND1* and *DEND2* show the dendritic branch potentials for each dendrite, and *AP_OUT* shows the spiking output on the bottom trace. At 10 μs, one action potential is given on input *AP1*, generating a small potential on *DEND1*. Since the number of active inputs is less than two, the soma potential is not greater than the firing threshold and no spike is output on *AP_OUT*. At 20 μs, two spikes are input on *AP1* and *AP2*. Since they are on the same dendritic branch, the potential on *DEND1* reaches a high value. *DEND2* stays low since its synapses have not received any input. Since the total number of spikes is at least two, a spike is emitted at *AP_OUT* (marked by the number 1). The shape of this spike is controlled by the HVA Ca^{2+} channel activated by *DEND1*. A zoom-in of the spike can be seen in figure 14.7. It exhibits a tail of duration $t_{tail} = 0.73$ μs. This spike particular spike shape is present when activity in *Dendritic Branch 1* is dominant to activity in *Dendritic Branch 2*.

At 30 μs, *Dendritic Branch 2* is stimulated with a spike on *AP3*. No other inputs are active. *DEND2* generates a small potential but it is not large enough to generate output spiking.

At 40 μs, *Dendritic Branch 2* is stimulated with two spikes on *AP3* and *AP4*. Now a spike (numbered 2) is emitted at *AP_OUT* since the soma potential is over the firing threshold. Input activity also generates a large potential on *DEND2*. It is large enough to activate the *HVA* Ca^{2+} *channel* on *Dendritic Branch 2*. The specific spike shape generated when *Dendritic Branch 2* is dominant can be seen in figure 14.7. The tail current duration is $t_{tail} = 0.33$ μs. This faster repolarization occurs since the dendrites were programmed with *Dendritic Branch 2* having a larger decay voltage.

At 50 μs, the neuron is stimulated with one spike on each branch. Enough inputs are present for the neuron to emit a spike (numbered 3). However, the *DEND* potentials at each dendrite are too small to activate the *HVA* Ca^{2+} *channel* modules, and the repolarizing tail is minimal. The spike shape for this case is shown in

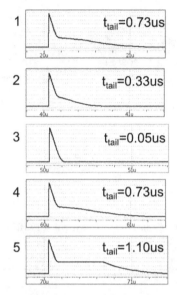

Figure 14.7. Zoom-in of AP_OUT in figure 14.6 [6].

figure 14.7. The tail duration is short at 0.05 μs. This spike shape represents the case where neither branch is highly active.

Three input spikes *AP1–AP3* stimulate the neuron at 60 μs. A spike (numbered 4) is emitted at *AP_OUT*. Since *AP1* and *AP2* were input, *Dendritic Branch 1* is highly active, as can be seen by *DEND1*. However, *DEND2* is not high since *Dendritic Branch 2* only received one input. So *Dendritic Branch 1* is dominant and the spike shape follows the one that was output at 10 μs. Figure 14.7 shows the output spike. It has a tail duration of 0.73 μs, which is the same as the duration of spike 1.

At 70 μs, the neuron is stimulated with all four inputs. Now both dendritic branches are highly active. *DEND1* and *DEND2* are high enough to turn on both HVA Ca^{2+} channels. The *AP_OUT* (numbered 5) has a longer duration tail since more HVA Ca^{2+} channels were turned on. From figure 14.7, it can be seen that the duration is 1.10 μs. This type of spike shape occurs when both dendrites are highly active.

The simulation results displayed here demonstrate that an electronic neuron circuit can output different spike shapes to encode different types of input stimulation patterns. We showed that dendritic branches could be used to generate the variations in spike shape. Next we will demonstrate how spike shape can be used in self-repairing neuronal networks.

14.1.4.4 Tunable spike shapes
Tail durations of APs output by the neuron circuit in figure 14.8 can be varied by tuning the amplitude of *Decay* control voltages in the *HVA* Ca^{2+} *channel* modules. To measure the effects of the *Decay* voltage on output spike shapes, we stimulated *Dendritic Branch 1* while leaving *Dendritic Branch 2* unstimulated. *Dendritic Branch*

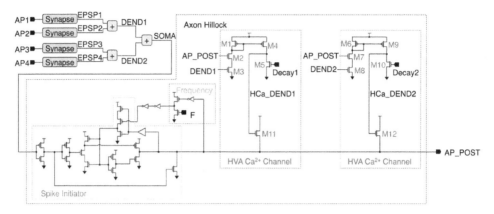

Figure 14.8. Neuron circuit for tuning spike decay. Copyright 2019 IEEE. Reprinted, with permission, from [17].

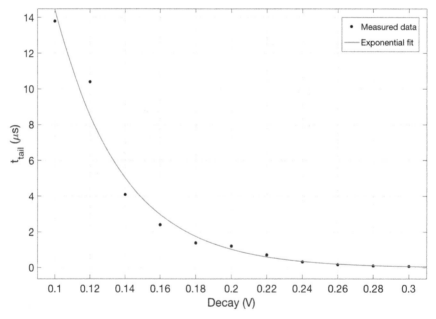

Figure 14.9. Action potential tail durations can be tuned. Copyright 2019 IEEE. Reprinted, with permission, from [17].

1 was stimulated with coincident spikes at inputs *AP1* and *AP2* in order to activate the HVA Ca^{2+} channel on that branch. The voltage of *Decay1* was varied from 0.1 V to 0.3 V and voltage spikes emitted at *AP_OUT* were recorded. Tail durations of emitted spikes were measured as the time for the signal to fall from 27% to 5% of VDD on the falling phase of the spike.

Figure 14.9 shows the dependence of spike tail duration (t_{tail}) on the *Decay* voltage. Data measured from circuit simulations are plotted as the black dots. Tail durations in the range of 0.0665 µs–13.8 µs were obtained as the *Decay* voltage was varied from 0.3 V to 0.1 V; tail duration has an inverse relationship with *Decay* voltage. The measured data was fit with an exponential curve following the function $t_{\text{tail}} = 201.1e^{-26.35 \cdot \text{Decay}}$. The exponential fit is shown as the blue trace in figure 14.9.

14.1.5 Astrocyte-mediated repair

In this section, we introduce bio-inspired circuits that emulate homeostatic behaviors found in astrocytes. These circuits will be shown to participate in rerouting signals originally processed by damaged neurons.

Astrocytes respond to neuronal activity through calcium levels. Chemical transmitters released by neurons, such as glutamate, stimulate gradual, long-lasting elevations in intracellular Ca^{2+}. The timescale of astrocyte calcium signaling (seconds to minutes) is much slower than neurotransmission (milliseconds). Due to their slow time course, astrocytes have been proposed as integrating memory elements in neuronal networks [8]. Repeated stimulation can increase the amplitude of intracellular calcium signals in an astrocyte, and astrocytes secrete gliotransmitters in response to neural activity levels.

It has been suggested that astrocytes have homeostatic roles in the brain. For example, when intracellular Ca^{2+} concentrations are high, implicating high activity levels in surrounding neurons, astrocytes have been found to inhibit neural activity by releasing ATP/adenosine [1]. Astrocytic uptake of neurotransmitters also serves to regulate ion levels in synapses [14].

The astrocyte circuits we present here have two main functions: (1) they measure the average level of neural activity over time; and (2) they determine when astrocyte-mediated homeostatic plasticity mechanisms should be implemented.

14.1.5.1 An astrocyte circuit that integrates neural activity
The circuit compartment that integrates neural activity at each astrocyte microdomain is shown in figure 14.10. APs stimulate elevations in the astrocyte's intracellular Ca^{2+} level (*AstroCa*). In the circuit, action potentials turn on transistor M2 for a brief period of time. The current mirror made by transistors M1–M3 puts charge on the gate of M5. M5 acts as a capacitor whose voltage represents the intracellular Ca^{2+} level in the astrocyte compartment. The capacitance can be varied by tuning the large transistor length and width of M5. V_{leak} is a control voltage that represents the uptake of Ca^{2+} back into the astrocyte's endoplasmic reticulum, effectively decreasing the amount of intracellular Ca^{2+}. The amplitude of V_{leak}

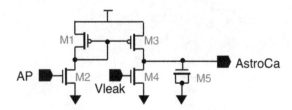

Figure 14.10. Astrocyte calcium circuit [6].

controls the time period over which the astrocyte integrates neural activity. Low values of V_{leak} increase the integration window while high values decrease it. V_{leak} should be low enough so that the integration time is 1000 times the duration of a neural action potential. We chose this factor because astrocyte Ca^{2+} signals in biology operate with time constants on the order of 1–10 s while APs have durations around 1 ms. The circuits in this chapter use a V_{leak} voltage of 0.35 V.

The astrocyte calcium circuit compartment can be used to integrate postsynaptic output activity or presynaptic activity stimulating a synapse. To use the circuit to model an astrocyte microdomain at a synapse, spikes that stimulate the synapse are used as the AP input to model neurotransmitters released from the presynaptic terminal. When the circuit is used to model an astrocyte microdomain connected to the synapse of a neuron (tripartite synapse), spikes output from the presynaptic neuron are used as the AP input to model the effect of neurotransmitters in the synapse.

14.1.5.2 Astrocyte circuit that determines when neural activity levels are in a stable range

The astrocyte thresholding circuit is shown in figure 14.11. It determines whether the average level of neural activity near an astrocyte microdomain is in a low, high, or stable operating range. It takes the *AstroCa* signal from the corresponding astrocyte calcium compartment (figure 14.10) as an input. When neural activity is below a low threshold, transistors M6–M7 pull up the signal *Low_AstroCa*. When neural activity is above a high threshold, the signal *High_AstroCa* is pulled up by transistors M1–M5. The thresholds can be controlled by tuning the sizes of the transistors. In our design, we sized M6 to be much more resistive than M7 in order to obtain a low-activity threshold closer to GND. The value of the high threshold is controlled by adjusting the resistance of the pull-down path made by transistors M2–M3. M2 acts as a resistor that can be made more resistive by increasing its channel length. We sized M2 with a large length in order to obtain a high value closer to V_{DD} for the

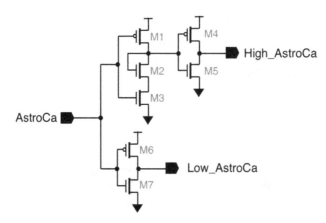

Figure 14.11. Astrocyte threshold circuit [6].

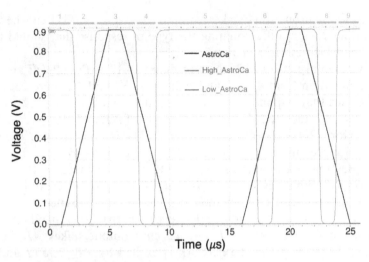

Figure 14.12. Sample output of the astrocyte threshold circuit [6].

high-activity threshold. When neither *Low_AstroCa* nor *High_AstroCa* are on, we assume that the neural activity is at a stable level.

Sample results from the astrocyte threshold circuit are shown in figure 14.12. The transistor sizes were tuned to obtain a low-activity threshold around 0.28 V and a high-activity threshold of 0.61 V. The numbered segments at the top of the figure indicate different behaviors of operation. The astrocyte Ca^{2+} level (*AstroCa*, black) starts low at 0.0 V in segment 1 (0–2.3 μs). Since it is below the low-activity threshold, *Low_AstroCa* is on at VDD and *High_AstroCa* is off at 0.0 V. In segment 2 (2.3–3.8 μs, *Astro_Ca* is above 0.28 V and below 0.61 V. Since it is between the low- and high-activity thresholds, we consider the neuron to be firing at a normal rate. Signals *Low_AstroCa* and *High_AstroCa* both remain at 0.0 V. In segment 3 (3.8–7.5 μs), *AstroCa* is above the high-activity threshold so *High_AstroCa* goes to V_{DD} while *Low_AstroCa* is at 0.0 V. *AstroCa* drops and is in a normal range again in segment 4 (7.5–8.9 μs). It goes below the low-activity threshold and *Low_AstroCa* turns on in segment 5 (8.9–17.3 μs). Segment 6 (17.3–18.8 μs) and segment 8 (22.3–23.9 μs) show cases where *AstroCa* is in the normal range. Segment 7 (18.8–22.3 μs) demonstrates another case where *AstroCa* is high, and segment 9 (23.9–25 μs) shows when *AstroCa* is in the low-activity range.

14.1.5.3 Signaling astrocyte-mediated repair in a bio-inspired ocular network
In the primary visual cortex, neurons can preferentially respond to activity in one or both eyes [12]. In this section we demonstrate plasticity mechanisms in a small neural network inspired by visual cortex neurons. We simulate damage in the network by forcing a neuron preferential to the left eye to be unresponsive. This causes the network to lose information regarding stimulation of the left eye. We show that an astrocyte-mediated homeostatic process can be used to restore functionality in the network. Following recovery, neurons that were initially preferential to the right eye now respond to stimulation from both eyes. In order to specify which eye is

stimulating, the neuron emits spikes with varying shapes. This can be useful for downstream neurons in differentiating the type of response that should be elicited depending on which eye is signaling.

The experimental network is shown in figure 14.13. APs *AP_left* and *AP_right* represent stimulation from the left and right eyes. *N1* and *N2* represent neurons in the visual cortex that respond to visual stimulation. Each neuron has two dendritic branches. *DB1_N1* and *DB2_N1* are the branches of *N1*, and *DB1_N2* and *DB2_N2* are branches for N2. Each neuron has synapses (*S1*–*S4*) to both eyes. The solid lines to *S1* and *S3* represent strong synapses. The dashed lines to *S2* and *S4* represent silent synapses that have weights too low to generate firing in their associated neurons. *AP_left* stimulates synapses *S1* and *S4* while *AP_right* stimulates *S2* and *S3*. Since *N1* is strongly excited by the left eye and weakly excited by the right eye, we say that it is preferential to the left eye. On the other hand, *N2* responds preferentially to the right eye. *N1* and *N2* emit output spikes *AP_POST1* and *AP_POST2*. An astrocyte in the network is excited by *AP_POST1* and its Ca^{2+} concentration increases when spikes are received. In response to Ca^{2+} levels that are outside of the normal range, the astrocyte secretes gliotransmitters (GTs) to synapse *S4*. With this configuration, activity in *N1* can be propagated to synapses and neurons that are not directly connected to it.

Circuits for the two-dendrite input-specific neuron were presented in the previous subsection of this section. Synapse *S4* was implemented with a previous BioRC synapse that implements modulation by an astrocyte. It is shown again in figure 14.14. The arrival of the $AstroCa^{2+}$ signal pulls up the signal *GT* to the voltage at *V(astro-glut)*. *GT* represented a concentration of gliotransmitters that the astrocyte secretes into the synaptic cleft in response to astrocyte signaling. *GT* is added to the *synaptic cleft* voltage to increase the amplitude of the output EPSP (*Out (EPSP)*). In this circuit, we used a control voltage of $V(astro - glut) = 0.3$ V. For

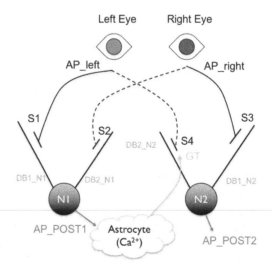

Figure 14.13. Ocular network [6].

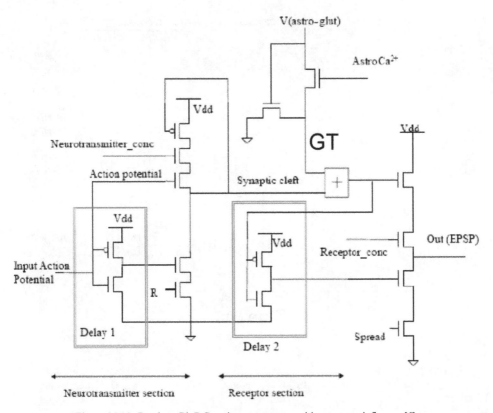

Figure 14.14. Previous BioRC excitatory synapse with astrocyte influence [6].

the astrocyte, we use the AstroCa circuit compartment presented in chapter 4 (figure 14.10) with a control voltage $V_{leak} = 0.38$V. In this network configuration, we assume that the astrocyte releases gliotransmitters in response to low intracellular Ca^{2+} as a homeostatic response that aims to increase network activity. The neural activity level is found by putting AstroCa through the AstroCa_Threshold block in figure 14.11. The Low_AstroCa signal is used to initiate homeostatic excitation by activating the AstroCa^{2+} signal (figure 14.14) on synapse *S4*.

Simulation results for the network that is repaired by enhancing spiking of surviving neurons are shown in figure 14.15(a). It is stimulated with input spikes *AP_left* and *AP_right* every 20 µs. The input APs are offset from each other by 10 µs. Neurotransmitter voltages for *S1* and *S3* were set to 0.75 V to represent strong synapses. Neurotransmitter voltages for *S2* and *S4* were set to 0.4 V to represent weak synapses. The astrocyte is initialized with an *ASTRO_CA* level of 0.5 V to simulate stable activity in *N1*.

From 0–200 µs, the network functions normally. *N1* shows preferential responses to stimulation from the left eye. When spikes are given at *AP_left*, *N1*'s dendritic branch shows large activity (*DEND1_N1*), generating spiking in *N1* (*AP_POST1*). Since synapse *S2* is weak, spikes received from *AP_right* generate small responses in *DEND2_N1*, and these are not large enough to cause spiking in *AP_POST1*. On the

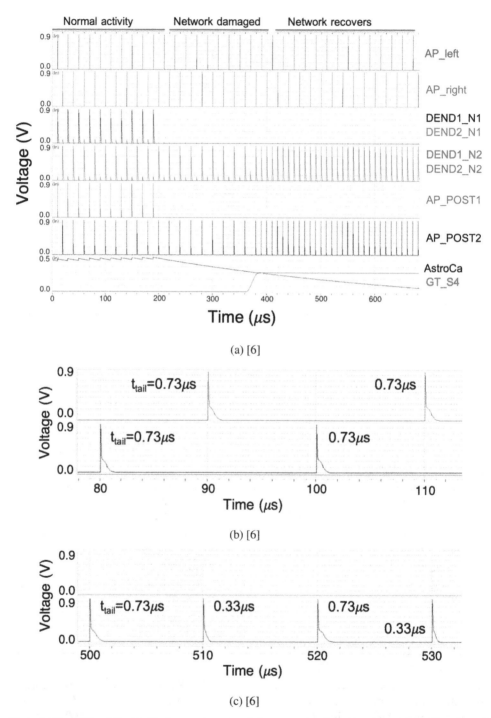

(a) [6]

(b) [6]

(c) [6]

Figure 14.15. (a) Simulation results from ocular network demonstrating that network can recover from loss of a neuron. Zoomed-in portions of the waveforms for AP_POST1 and AP_POST2 are shown from 90–120 μs (b) and 500–530 μs (c). AP_POST1 is shown in the upper, blue trace, and AP_POST2 is shown in the lower, black trace. Durations of the repolarizing tail are also shown.

other hand, *N2* shows preferential responses to the right eye. When activity is present on *AP_right*, large potentials are generated in *DEND1_N2*, generating output spiking in *AP_POST2*. Spikes given on *AP_left* generate only small potentials on *DEND2_N2*, so *AP_POST2* does not spike in response to the left eye. A zoomed-in portion of the waveforms for *AP_POST1* and *AP_POST2* from 90–120 µs is shown in figure 14.15(b). The spike shapes output from each neuron in response to the preferred eye has a repolarizing tail with duration of 0.73 µs. During the period of normal activity, *ASTRO_CA* remains at a relatively stable level (figure 14.15(a)) so the astrocyte does not need to potentiate the network and *GT_S4* remains low at 0 V.

At 200 µs we simulate the loss of neuron *N1* by forcing its dendritic branch potentials, *DEND1_N1* and *DEND2_N2*, to 0 V. This could model the death of dendrites in a neuron. Since its dendritic inputs are lost, *N1* stops firing and *AP_POST1* shows no activity. From 200–360 µs, the network is in a damaged state and it does not transmit any information regarding stimulation in the left eye. However, it still communicates information about the right eye since *N2* is intact, and *AP_POST2* continues responding to spikes from *AP_right*. During the damage period, *ASTRO_CA* decays since it is no longer receives stimulation from *AP_POST1*.

At 360 µs, *ASTRO_CA* drops below the low-activity threshold that the astrocyte considers for healthy network behavior. In order to compensate for low activity, the astrocyte begins to release gliotransmitters at synapse *S4* to promote excitability in the network. This can be seen by the rise in *GT_S4* from 360–380 µs. *GT_S4* rises maximally to the *V(astro-glut)* voltage of 0.3 V.

The network recovers functionality and begins to respond to activity in the left eye after 400 µs. The voltage at *GT_S4* provides sufficient excitation for *S4* to produce large potentials in *N2*'s dendritic branch *DEND2_N2*. Since *N1* is broken, *N2* becomes responsible for transmitting information about the left eye in addition to its regular response to the right eye. This can be seen by the increased output frequency of *AP_POST2*. *AP_POST2* fires whenever a stimulus is given in either *AP_right* or *AP_left*. A zoomed-in portion of the waveforms for *AP_POST1* and *AP_POST2* are shown in figure 14.15(c). *AP_POST2* now fires two types of spikes in response to input activity. Spikes with longer repolarizing tails of duration 0.73 µs are emitted when N2 is stimulated by the preferred right eye. Faster repolarizing spikes with tail duration of 0.33 µs are output when the neuron is stimulated by the non-preferred left eye.

The configuration of the network following damage recovery is shown in figure 14.16. *N1* is damaged (dashed circle) and no longer responds. *N2* is remapped to respond to both the right and left eye through strong synapses *S3* and *S4*. Specificity of outputs at *AP_POST2* are signaled through different spike shapes.

The original configuration of the network can be recovered if damaged neuron *N1* somehow regains functionality. Figure 14.17 simulation results extended from figure 14.15. At 700 µs, *N1*'s functionality is restored (black arrow) by reintroducing its dendritic branches. *DEND1_N1* becomes responsive to *AP_left* and spike are emitted at *AP_POST1*. From 700–920 µs, both *N1* and *N2* respond to *AP_left*. As

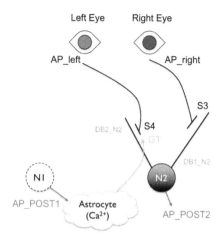

Figure 14.16. Ocular network remapping after recovery from damage in *N1* [6].

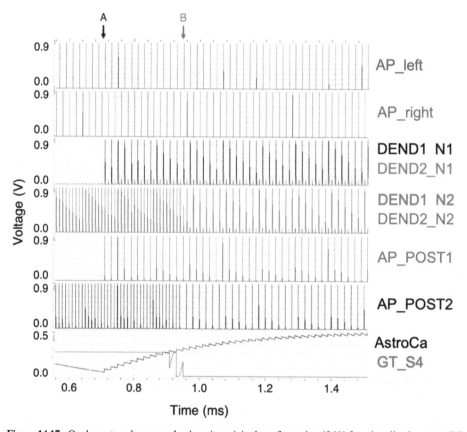

Figure 14.17. Ocular network remaps back to its original configuration if *N1* functionality is restored[6].

AP_POST1 spikes are emitted, *ASTRO_CA* begins to build up. At 920 μs (blue arrow), *ASTRO_CA* goes above the low-activity threshold and the astrocyte determines that homeostatic plasticity mechanisms can be turned off. *GT_S4* drops to 0 V and *AP_POST2* stops responding to activity in *AP_left*. At this point, the mapping of the original network is restored and each neuron responds preferentially to a single eye.

14.1.6 Summary

In this section, we introduced a neuron circuit that exhibits input-specific spiking. We believe that these types of circuits can be advantageous in signaling when a neuromorphic network has been damaged and homeostatic repair processes have been initiated. This type of signaling can help prevent reductions in selectivity in downstream neurons following synaptic restructuring. Another useful benefit could be increased communication bandwidth. For this type of specialized signaling to be functional requires neurons that can respond selectively to different spike shapes. The circuits presented here are initial designs that we believe can be useful in increasing the efficiency of neuromorphic networks.

14.2 Cauwenberghs' Izhikevich spiking circuit

Inspired by the spiking patterns that Izhikevich produced with his mathematical model, Gert Cauwenberghs implemented circuits to model the differential equations invented by Izhikevich [10]. Figure 14.18 shows the Izhikevich spiking patterns implemented in Cauwenberghs' circuit.

Research described in the paper moved variables to the upper right quadrant. The mathematics was reformulated to replace voltages v and u with currents I_v and I_u. The Iu circuit shown in figure 14.21 is a four-transistor *log domain* filter as the building block with NMOS MOSFETs biased in the subthreshold region. The drain current for this region of operation, I_d is an exponential function of the gate to source voltage V_{GS}. Log-domain circuits exploit the *trans-linear* characteristics of MOS transistors in *weak inversion* for low power applications. Weak inversion means that the transistor is not fully 'on,' and the surface of the silicon is not fully inverted in the channel. For an NMOS transistor, holes are filled with electrons, and there are other electrons in the channel but not enough (equal to number of original holes) to say the surface is 'inverted.' The transistor exhibits exponential output current as input gate voltage V_{GS} changes, hence it behaves in a trans-linear fashion. The equations implemented in Cauwenberghs' circuits include

$$\tau \dot{I}_v = a_2 I_v^2 + a_1 I_v + a_0 + I_{dc} - I_u \tag{14.1}$$

$$\tau \dot{I}_u = ab I_v - a I_u \tag{14.2}$$

where τ is 1 mS.

The differential equations are by nature unstable once the membrane voltage exceeds a threshold. This condition results in a sudden increase in the membrane voltage similar to that experienced by the biological equivalent. The potassium

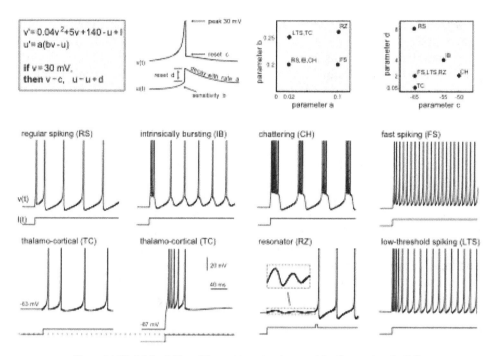

Figure 14.18. Izhikevich's spiking patterns implemented by Cauwenberghs [10].

influx is modeled by a reset term following the detection of a spike. The equations achieve this effect by forcing the membrane voltage to a reset value and also to 'increment' the accommodation variable.

The circuit in figure 14.21 implements the differential equation for I_u (equation (14.2)) and contains two current mirrors, and addition/subtraction of currents in the middle block. Thus, I_v is mirrored in I_2, and I_3 is mirrored in I_u. The current mirrors are shown in the red dashed boxes, and the current addition/subtraction in the blue dashed box. The middle block could act as a differential pair since, if we hold I_5 constant, and inject current with I_d using switch S_u, the total current is still I_5 and the output current I_3 drops. I_u, mirroring I_3, drops as well. Understanding the details of this circuit is not important here: what is important is that the circuit fairly directly models the differential equation for I_u and not the biology of the axon initial segment.

The circuit in figure 14.19 implements the differential equation for I_v (equation (14.1)). Note that there are two current mirrors, and a differential pair in the middle. V_v increases as I_u decreases, since, once again the total current, I_5 is held constant. M_6 and M_7 are biasing transistors, and there is positive feedback in the circuit.

Finally, there is a membrane voltage reset circuit, shown in figure 14.20, so that the membrane voltage is reset after the spike. For transistor M_3, $V_{ds} = 0.0$ V and V_v is the membrane voltage.

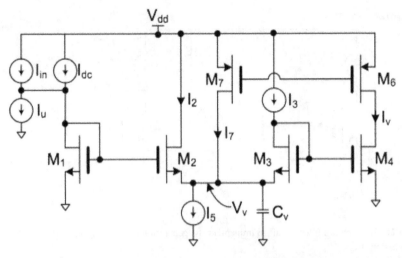

Figure 14.19. Membrane voltage circuit. Copyright 2010 IEEE. Reprinted, with permission, from [10].

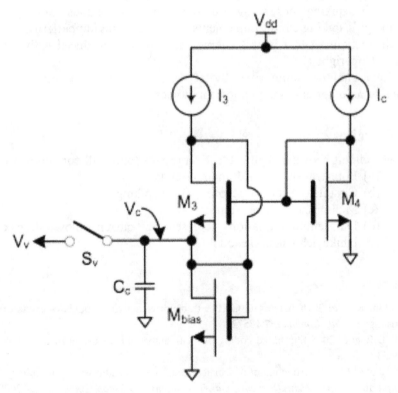

Figure 14.20. The membrane voltage reset circuit. Copyright 2010 IEEE. Reprinted, with permission, from [10].

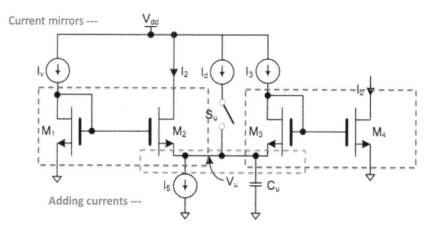

Figure 14.21. Log domain filter circuit to implement the generation of *Iu*. Copyright 2010 IEEE. Reprinted, with permission, from [10].

14.3 Chapter summary

This chapter covered other neural codes implemented in circuits. Lee's circuit shows variations in spiking depending on the origin of signals causing spiking. Cauwenbergh's spiking circuit implements Izhikevich' spiking patterns.

Certain sections of text in this chapter have been reproduced with permission from [17]. Copyright IEEE.

The next chapter summarizes BioRC circuits using nanotechnologies, and mentions some other emerging nanotechnologies.

14.4 Exercises

1. The circuit shown in figure 14.21 represents (mark all correct answers):
   (a) Four-transistor log domain circuit;
   (b) Circuit to calculate recovery from spiking;
   (c) Membrane voltage circuit;
   (d) Differential equation representing current flow derived from Izhikevich's neural model.

References

[1] Boddum K *et al* 2016 Astrocytic GABA transporter activity modulates excitatory neurotransmission *Nat. Commun.* **7** 13572

[2] Isett B R *et al* 2018 Slip-based coding of local shape and texture in mouse S1 *Neuron* **97** 418–33

[3] Joshi J *et al* 2009 A carbon nanotube cortical neuron with excitatory and inhibitory dendritic computations *Life Science Systems and Applications Workshop, 2009. LiSSA 2009. IEEE/NIH* 133–6

[4] Jung H-Y, Staff N P and Spruston N 2001 Action potential bursting in subicular pyramidal neurons is driven by a calcium tail current *J. Neurosci.* **21** 3312–21

[5] Lee R K and Parker A C 2019 An electronic neuron with input-specific spiking *2019 Int. Joint Conf. Neural Networks (IJCNN)* 1–8

[6] Kim Lee R 2018 Astrocyte-mediated plasticity and repair in CMOS neuromorphic circuits *PhD Thesis* (University of Southern California)

[7] Lu T, Liang L and Wang X 2001 Temporal and rate representations of time-varying signals in the auditory cortex of awake primates *Nat. Neurosci.* **4** 1131–8

[8] Min R and Nevian T 2012 Astrocyte signaling controls spike timing dependent depression at neocortical synapses *Nat. Neurosci.* **15** 746–53

[9] Murphy T H and Corbett D 2009 Plasticity during stroke recovery: from synapse to behaviour *Nat. Rev.* **10** 861–72

[10] Rangan V *et al* 2010 A subthreshold aVLSI implementation of the Izhikevich simple neuron model *2010 Annual Int. Conf. of the Engineering in Medicine and Biology* (Piscataway, NJ: IEEE) 4164–7

[11] Sardi S *et al* 2017 New types of experiments reveal that a neuron functions as multiple independent threshold units *Sci. Rep.* **7** 18036

[12] Scholl B, Burge J and Priebe N J 2013 Binocular integration and disparity selectivity in mouse primary visual cortex *J. Neurophysiol.* **109** 3013–24

[13] Sengupta B *et al* 2010 *PLoS Comput. Biol.* **6** e1000840

[14] Somjen G G 2002 Ion regulation in the brain: implications for pathophysiology *The Neuroscientist* **8** 254–67

[15] Winship I R and Murphy T H 2009 Remapping the somatosensory cortex after stroke: insight from imaging the synapse to network *Neuroscientist* **15** 507–24

[16] Yue K *et al* 2019 Analog neurons that signal with spiking frequencies *Proc. Int. Conf. Neuromorphic Systems* 1–8

[17] Lee R K and Parker A C 2019 An electronic neuron with input-specific spiking *2019 International Joint Conference on Neural Networks (IJCNN) (Budapest)* 1–8

IOP Publishing

Neuromorphic Circuits
A constructive approach
Alice C Parker and Rick Cattell

Chapter 15

Circuits with nanotechnologies

Kun Yue, Jon Joshi, Chih-Chieh Hsu, Rebecca K Lee and Alice C Parker

This chapter first covers BioRC nanotechnologies that have been fabricated, along with conventional CMOS circuits, to create neuromorphic circuits. Then the chapter covers future designs of some nanotechnological circuits that combine with CMOS circuits to create neuromorphic designs. Finally the chapter surveys nanotechnologies that have a future use in neuromorphic circuits due to their traits that meet one of more needs of neuromorphic circuits.

15.1 Introduction

Complex neuromorphic circuits that exhibit advanced learning and memory are believed to depend on the dense interconnectivity, scale and interactions of biological neural circuits with other brain cells, including astrocytes. Analog circuits are a leading candidate for implementation to compress the hardware required per neuron by exploiting the ability to 'compute' using charge, current and voltage. Even so, constructing these circuits at scale (10 000 synapses per neuron, fan out of 10 000 to adjacent neurons, and billions of neurons in the artificial brain) will probably require innovations in nanoelectronics, including layers of nanomaterial in addition to 3D CMOS connectivity. Memristor neuromorphic circuits have been widely researched and will not be covered here, beyond the devices intended for use in BioRC circuits since the most common memristor device discussed in the literature is a two-terminal device, and does not support the more-complex synaptic control that BioRC circuits require. Multiple memristor devices are required in some neuromorphic implementations [10]. An early neuromorphic memristor implementation is found in [16]. A neuromorphic circuit with memristors implementing synaptic and intrinsic plasticity is found in [35].

15.2 Carbon nanotube (CNT) neuromorphic circuits

From its inception, the BioRC project aimed at implementation with some form of nanotechnology. A simulation of a CNT synapse was presented ([13]) using SPICE circuit models of the nanotube [20, 21], and many BioRC circuits were constructed using this model, including entire neural networks [16]. A few years after the first BioRC CNT synapse was designed as an analog circuit, a nanotube synapse was constructed and tested in the laboratory [23]. The waveforms input to the synapse and output from the synapse resemble biological waveforms in shape and relative amplitudes and durations. This circuit is believed to be the first use of CNTs in a neural circuit that has been physically implemented, and only the second analog circuit being constructed using nanotubes, the nanotube radio circuit being the first [26]. The text presents here the circuit, the laboratory configuration, and the test waveforms the BioRC group obtained. At USC, Chongwu Zhou and his team had proposed a technique to design CNT circuits immune to misalignment and mispositioning that could guarantee the correct function being implemented [30]. Liu, Han and Zhou had demonstrated directional growth of high-density CNTs on a- and r-plane sapphire substrates. They had developed a novel nanotube-on-insulator (NOI) approach, and a way to transfer these nanotube arrays to flexible substrates [28]. Zhou and his team made two significant achievements. First, they synthesized massively aligned nanotubes with uniform and high density (over 10 tubes per µm) on 4 inch full sapphire/quartz substrate for large-scale integration of devices. The as-grown nanotubes were then transferred onto a Si/SiO$_2$ substrate using Zhou's facile transfer imprinting method. Second, based on transferred nanotubes, they fabricated advanced aligned nanotube circuits such as NAND, and NOR logic gates which consisted of p-type pull-up transistors and n-type pull-down transistors. The major difficulty in achieving n-type nanotube transistors was solved by using a potassium doping technique [38].

The aligned nanotubes were grown on a 4 in. quartz wafer and then transferred onto a Si substrate with 50 nm SiO$_2$ using a facile transfer printing method [19, 32]. For the device fabrication process, 50 nm SiO$_2$ was used to act as the back-gate dielectric. The source and drain electrodes were patterned by photo-lithography, and 5 Å Ti and 70 nm Pd were deposited followed by the lift-off process to form the source and drain metal contacts. Finally, since the nanotubes covered the entire wafer, in order to achieve accurate channel length and width and to remove the possible leakage in the devices, one more step of photo-lithography plus O$_2$ plasma was used to remove unwanted nanotubes outside the device channel region. Figure 15.1 shows the schematic diagram of a back-gated CNTFET (carbon nanotube field-effect transistor) built on aligned nanotubes with Ti/Pd (5 Å/70 nm) contacts and SiO$_2$ (50 nm) gate dielectric on the left. The parallel nanotubes forming the CNTFET are shown in figure 15.1 on the right.

After the device fabrication, they performed electrical breakdown to these devices to remove the metallic nanotubes. Electrical performance of the device was measured and typical curves ($L = 4$ mm, and $W = 200$ mm) are shown here. Figure 15.2 shows the transfer ($I_D - V_G$) characteristics with different drain voltages (VD). Figure 15.3 shows the output ($I_D - V_D$) characteristics.

Figure 15.4 shows the schematic design for the implemented synapse circuit. From the transfer ($I_D - V_D$) and output ($I_D - V_D$) characteristics (straight line in figures 15.2 and 15.3, respectively) they obtained the CNT device information like

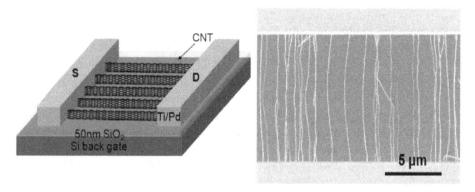

Figure 15.1. Back-gated CNTFET Schematic shown on the left and parallel nanotubes forming the CNTFET are shown on the right for all nanotube figures shown in this section. Copyright 2011 IEEE. Reprinted, with permission, from [25].

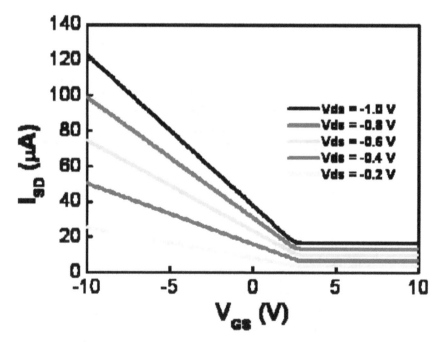

Figure 15.2. I_D–V_G characteristics for the nanotube device used in the synapse. Copyright 2011 IEEE. Reprinted, with permission, from [25].

the on/off ratio, threshold voltage and transconductance. Using these parameters, they built an HSPICE model for their CNTFET device and, using this model they simulated their single-transistor synapse circuit. The circuit used a P-type CNTFET so that associated input (presynaptic action potential (AP)) and output (postsynaptic potential—PSP) are negative voltages. The AP turns on the CNTFET and current

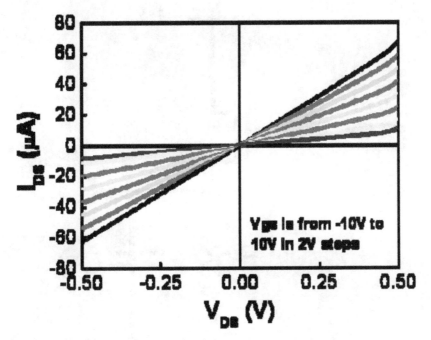

Figure 15.3. I_D–V_D characteristics for the nanotube device used in the synapse. Copyright 2011 IEEE. Reprinted, with permission, from [25].

flows, causing the output voltage (the excitatory EPSP (EPSP)) to decrease below 0.0 V. When the AP returns to zero, the synapse returns slowly to its resting potential of 0.0 V. Figure 15.5 shows the input AP (yellow trace, V_{AP}) and the resulting postsynaptic potential (green trace, V_{PSP}). The input AP to test the synapse during simulation was 3 ms in time period with amplitude of −0.9 V. The resulting PSP was observed to be 10 ms in time period with amplitude of −0.06 V, as shown in figure 15.5. The actual time period of the PSP is about 20 ms as the complete decay time for the PSP is not available on the image, due to the APs impinging in succession. Figure 15.6 shows the synapse response for changes in resistor values. The fabricated synapse circuit follows the schematic shown in figure 15.4. For this first experiment as shown in figure 15.5, the amplitude of the AP (black trace) was −10 V and the resultant PSP (blue trace) was about −0.2 V. The AP duration was 3 ms, and the PSP duration about 10 ms. They observed that the ratio between the corresponding amplitudes and time periods of the AP and PSP are in line with biological ratios.

They varied the resistor values to test for changes in synaptic strength. Figure 15.6 shows the waveforms for the variations and table 15.1 shows the observed changes. The results demonstrate synaptic strength change, a key neural behavior that is commonly observed in biological neurons and is believed to play a role in learning. CNT transistors have since been used in more extensive circuits, but rarely in neuromorphic analog circuits.

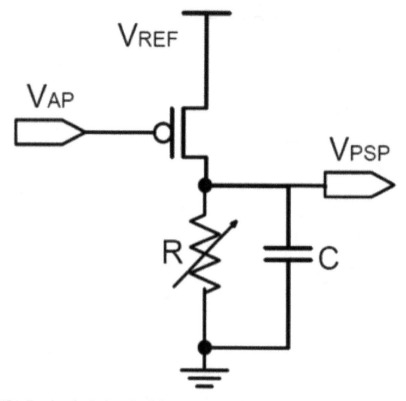

Figure 15.4. Transistor-level schematic of the synapse. Copyright 2011 IEEE. Reprinted, with permission, from [25].

15.3 Molybdenum disulfide neuromorphic circuits

Kun Yue, Han Wang and Alice Parker showed that molybdenum disulfide (MoS_2) transistors can be used in neuromorphic circuits and the results are in Yue's thesis [42]. The advantage of MoS_2 transistors is the presence of a second gate, a back gate, that allows astrocytes to modulate transistors, strengthening or weakening synapses in neuromorphic circuits.

15.3.1 Introduction and background

A particular nanotechnology, the MoS_2 transistor, possesses a dual-gate structure that supports tight integration of astrocytic circuits with neural circuits by exploiting the back gates of the MoS_2 transistors to incorporate astrocytic control of the neural circuits. This innovation removes the need for an explicit adder that incorporates astrocyte intervention into the PSP of the target neurons, possibly saving a dozen transistors for each synapse implemented.

Based on successful demonstrations of flexible MoS_2 FET instances and circuits fabricated with flexible MoS_2 FETs [39], the BioRC group designed a SPICE model for neuromorphic circuit simulation. The group then designed and simulated a

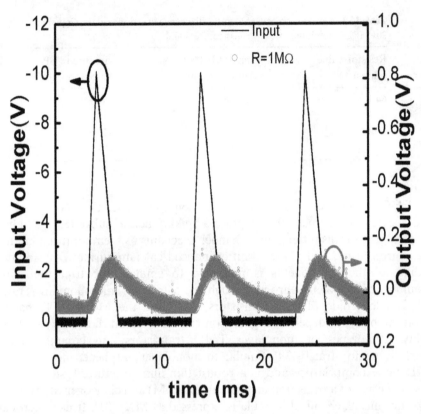

Figure 15.5. Waveforms of the synapse. Copyright 2011 IEEE. Reprinted, with permission, from [25].

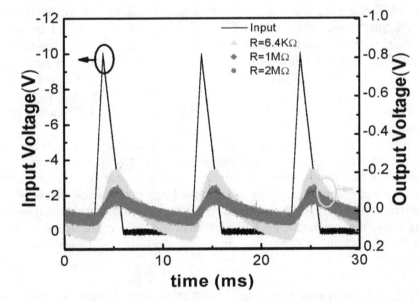

Figure 15.6. Waveforms of the synapse varying resistances. Copyright 2011 IEEE. Reprinted, with permission, from [25].

Table 15.1. Synaptic strength variation with change in resistor values. Copyright 2011 IEEE. Reprinted, with permission, from [23].

Resistor value (ohms)	Simulated PSP Amplitude (mV)	Measured PSP Amplitude (mV)
64 k	−63.461	−200
94 k	−49.688	−180
1 M	−6.5295	−120
2 M	−3.3184	−80

MoS_2 FET analog circuit model of a neural synapse, dendritic arbor, axon hillock and astrocyte microdomain that capture a spiking neural subsystem including the actions of neurotransmitters, ion channel mechanisms, temporal summation of PSPs, neuron firing, and gliotransmitter-induced calcium current. An architecture including all the components is presented to emulate the tripartite synapses' communication between neurons through the astrocytes microdomain. Transition metal dichalcogenide (TMD) transistors, including the MoS_2 FET, have high electron mobility, independent gate control, and strain flexibility that affects mobility. Prototypes of monolayer TMD transistors and circuits have been successfully demonstrated [39]. Similar to monolayer graphene, monolayer TMD is a 2D honeycomb lattice and is a robust thin-film structure. Instead of carbon atoms, it consists of a transition metal (denoted as M) and chalcogen atoms (denoted as X), and thus its chemical formula is expressed as MX_2 [31]. It has electrical and physical properties like graphene and it has an intrinsic band gap that limits the short-circuit current better than graphene FETs. In this work, MoS_2, the most well-studied TMD material, was chosen to implement synapses and astrocyte circuits. Circuits implemented with MoS_2 FETs will have low short-circuit current and supply voltage. MoS_2 can be deformed with strain, making it a semiconductor and interesting for dual-gated electronics applications. A simulation was performed to study the strain effect on the dual-gated MoS_2 FET [15]. Furthermore, [11] presented a 1 nm gate length transistor fabricated with MoS_2 and CNTs, which raises the possibility of making neuromorphic circuits closer to the human brain in size, number and density of synapses and neurons[1].

The astrocyte plays an important role for information processing in the human brain [37], including neuronal communication. An astrocyte monitors synaptic activity in an autonomous manner through individual regions, known as microdomains. Astrocytic microdomains are activated according to the release of neurotransmitters from synapses in close proximity. Activation of microdomains induces calcium waves that propagate into different microdomains of the astrocyte. It is the dynamics of calcium waves that evoke the release of transmitters, called

---

[1] Working CNT synapses were demonstrated early by the BioRC group in conjunction with Zhou's Nanolab [22] and many circuit models of CNT neurons were simulated with CNT device models beginning with [29].

gliotransmitters, from the microdomain. This endows the astrocyte with the ability to modulate synaptic information. Their capability to synchronize neuronal activity by inducing slow inward currents (SICs) on adjacent dendrites with a high degree of temporal correlation is currently a subject of interest due to its possible role in neural processing [12]. The BioRC project introduced astrocytes into neuromorphic circuits beginning in 2010 [18, 24] presented an astrocyte microdomain circuit implemented using CMOS 0.18 μm technology including a 10-transistor analog voltage adder. In this chapter, the adder combining the effects of neurotransmitters and gliotransmitters is replaced by one dual-gated MoS_2 FET and the circuit implemented achieves similar circuit behavior with 90% less transistors in the circuit combining astrocyte and neural signaling.

15.3.2 The molybdenum disulfide FET

A long channel drift-diffusion compact SPICE model for MoS_2 FET was designed to model a device with more than 100 nm gate length and was validated by experimental results [36]. When the transistor is further scaled down to sub-20 nm gate length, a ballistic transport model is more suitable for describing the current since the channel length becomes comparable or even less than the mean free path of TMDFET (15 nm). However, the ballistic transport model requires numerical integration and is not directly SPICE-compatible, making it difficult to perform circuit-level simulations. Gholipour [15] introduced the ballistic enhancement factor (BEF) to the original drift-diffusion model, so that they obtained an approximated ballistic transportation for the SPICE compact model. Based on these two models, the BioRC group designed their dual-gated MoS_2 SPICE model. In figure 15.7, their model simulations show the drain-to-source voltage is fixed at 0.5 V, back gate is

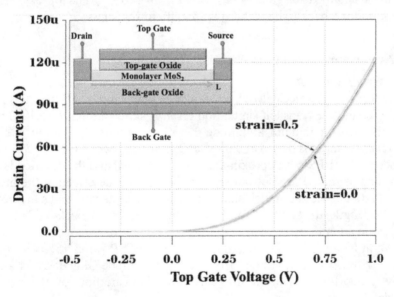

Figure 15.7. $I-V$ curve of MoS_2 FET [42].

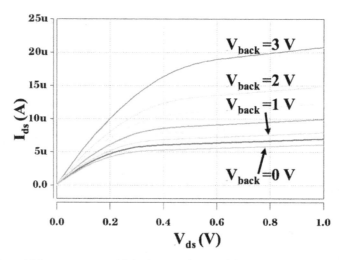

Figure 15.8. I_{ds} versus V_{ds} with back-gate voltage and fixed top-gate voltage [42].

rounded, x-axis is top gate voltage, y-axis is the current flowing through the materials, and 0, 10%, and 50% strains are plotted. The geometry of the monolayer MoS$_2$ is 32 nm wide, and 16 nm long. The gate metal material is not considered in this model; the source and drain metal material is idealized as a resistor with value 0.1 Ω.

Due to the difference between top-gate oxide and back-gate oxide in material and geometry, the current through drain and source will respond to the gate voltages differently. In figure 15.8, our initial device simulations show the top gate voltage fixed at 0.3 V and the back gate voltage varies from 0 to 3 V. The top-oxide is 2.8 nm thickness, and the back-oxide is SiO$_2$ with 100 nm thickness.

15.3.3 Neuromorphic circuit models

15.3.3.1 Synapse circuit

Figure 15.9 shows a BioRC CMOS excitatory synapse circuit. All the transistors are MoS$_2$ FETs, and the transient simulation result is shown in figure 15.10. The input AP is spikes with maximum amplitude 0.7 V; *neurotransmitter* input is biased at 0.15 V; *reuptake* input is biased at 0.05 V; *RR* input is biased at 0.1 V; *gliotransmitter* is grounded. The (EPSP) is approximately 14% of the AP and the duration is about 4 times as long as the AP, somewhat shorter than EPSPs described in the literature.

To validate this circuit model, simulations with process variations are necessary. The width, length, thickness of top-oxide, and thickness of back-oxide are varied within 10% in a Gaussian distribution, then 10^4 simulations were run and the results are shown in figure 15.11. The maximum value of EPSP varies 15% with the delay varying 7%, but the correlation between the amplitude and delay is −0.6. An inversely proportional relationship constrains the variation of the product of amplitude and delay.

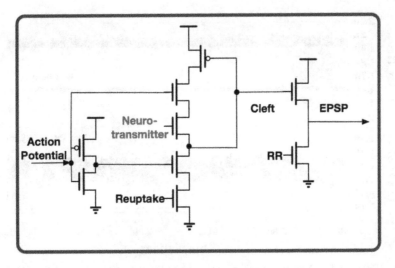

Figure 15.9. BioRC excitatory synapse circuit [29].

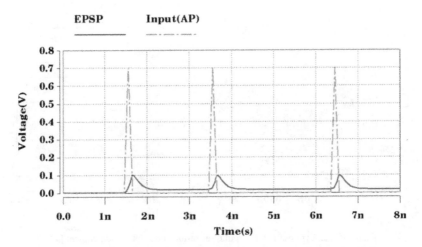

Figure 15.10. The action potential and EPSP under normal operation [42].

15.3.3.2 The astrocyte/synapse circuit

Astrocytes can increase the complexity of neural networks in another dimension of variability. The compartmentalized construction of our neuromorphic circuits and the ability to control neural parameters directly by means of specific control voltages allow us to insert additional mechanisms intuitively. Irizarry-Valle [17] uses this compartmentalized approach to insert the uptake of glutamate by astrocytes and the synapse inactivation mechanism, along with the astrocytic calcium ions release causing glutamate release into the neurotransmitter section of our synapses. However, overhead in the form of an explicit voltage adder is introduced to sum the transmitters and a more complicated synapse circuit design is used to implement

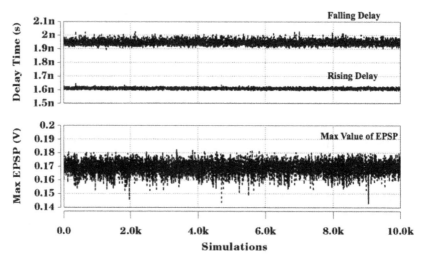

Figure 15.11. Delay and maximum value of the EPSP under process variation [42].

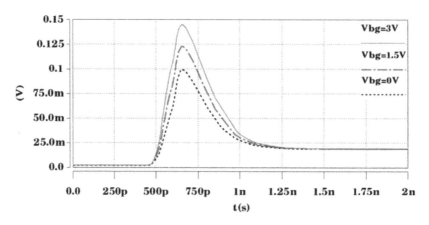

Figure 15.12. Synapse EPSP simulation result under back-gate control [42].

that model. Considering the number of synapses in the human brain is in the trillions and 60% of the synapses are tripartite, connecting with glial cells, reducing the overhead significantly is necessary for mimicking this feature in neuromorphic systems. In this section, by exploiting the back gate control of an MoS_2 FET (labeled *'Gliotransmitter'* in figure 15.9), the explicit adder is not required and they can use the simple synapse design presented above. The simulation result is shown in figure 15.12 with the input spike omitted to illustrate the details of the EPSP. The input of this simulation is a 20 ns spike with maximum 0.7 V and neurotransmitter control is fixed at 0.15 V. The *gliotransmitter* control is set from 0 to 3 V, and the EPSP response to the back gate voltage changes gradually. By applying different oxide materials and geometries, the response factor can be changed.

15.3.3.3 *Astrocyte microdomain circuit*

Figure 15.13 shows several compartments of an astrocyte analog circuit. It is a distributed resistive (pass transistor) network that takes inputs from the voltages representing synaptic cleft neurotransmitter concentrations of different synapse circuits. A voltage representing effects of neurotransmitter concentration from each synapse is fed into a non-inverting delay circuit whose output voltage representing released neurotransmitters is summed in the astrocyte with delayed effects of neurotransmitter voltages from other synapses. This distributed sum represents calcium waves in the astrocyte process. In previous BioRC neural designs [29], an adder was used to sum the effects of synapse neurotransmitters, increasing complexity and power consumption. In this experiment, a single MoS_2 FET replaces each adder to vastly simplify the design.

15.3.4 Network with astrocytes

The network shown in figure 15.14 illustrates the configuration we used for this experiment. In a network of neurons with spiking inputs, an astrocyte spans several synapses to create the neural-astrocyte interactions. In this experiment, five synapse PSPs connect to the astrocytic microdomain. The input of the synapses is sequential spikes applied to each of the synapses. The calcium wave in the astrocyte is translated to the calcium induced gliotransmitter releasing and connected with the glotransmitter control of synapse *S6*. To show the modulation effect of the astrocytic mechanisms on synapse *S6*, we ran simulations of the circuit network. For comparison, the synapse *S7* has the same input AP as the synapse *S6*, while without the modulation from the astrocyte. In figure 15.15, the propagation and correlation of the calcium ion signal is shown with respect to the independent synaptic cleft signals. In figure 15.16, the PSP of synapse *S6* is modulated in

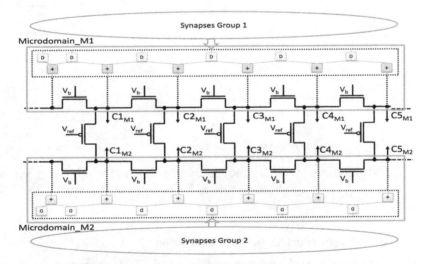

Figure 15.13. Several compartments of an astrocyte analog circuit.

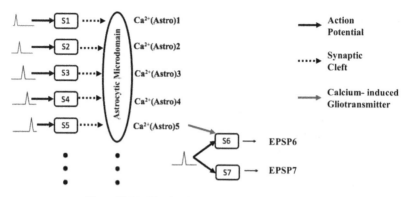

Figure 15.14. Sketch of astrocyte neural network [42].

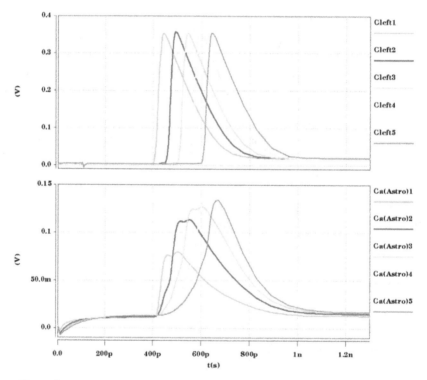

Figure 15.15. Simulation results of astrocytic Ca+ signals with synaptic cleft signals [42].

amplitude and duration by the astrocytic microdomain through the calcium ion signal $Ca(Astro)5$, causing gliotransmitters to be released increasing the PSP of synapse 6.

15.3.5 MoS$_2$ FET neuromorphic network conclusion

The BioRC group proposed and designed an MoS$_2$ FET neuromorphic network with astrocytic modulation. Through the dual-gate MoS$_2$ FET, this advanced

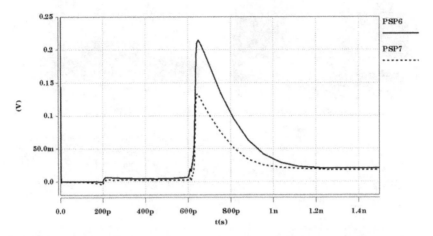

Figure 15.16. Simulation results of astrocytic modulation to synapse 6 and no modulation to synapse 7 [42].

astrocyte feature is more easily implemented in a neuromorphic system. Moreover, the small network they designed shows the importance of astrocytic processes to the synapse. The results show that the MoS$_2$ FET can be used to reduce complexity in neuron-astrocyte circuits and is of use in implementing astrocytic mechanisms.

15.4 Other BioRC nanotechnological neuromorphic circuits

15.4.1 Hybrid carbon nanotube/silicon neuromorphic circuits

Barzegarjalali, in his thesis [2], incorporated MOS and CNT models in his circuit simulations. The CNT models formed the synapses, and the MOS models formed the neurons. Circuits using these models were widely published in conference papers [3–8]. The basic idea was to use planar MOS transistors in dies to form the neural structure, and use thin-film CNT sheets of transistors over the top of the silicon dies to form the synapses. Other researchers had integrated CNT and MOS technologies in the past, but not to form neural structures [1].

In a later investigation, the BioRC team explored using CNTs to model astrocytes, as shown in figure 15.17 but the ideas were not published.

15.4.2 Magnetic analog memristor/silicon neuromorphic circuits

Kun Yue and others described the use of a novel technology, magnetic analog memristors (MAMs), that provide persistent memory, and demonstrated its use in neuromorphic circuits [43]. The MAMs demonstrate variable resistance, and persistence of resistance value when programmed. Yue used them to model memory persistence in neurons that have been infused with dopamine, a neurotransmitter that has several functions, including memory persistence.

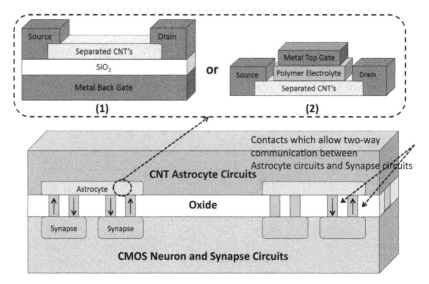

Figure 15.17. Astrocyte compartments with thin-film CNT transistors, one version with a metal back gate and another with a metal top gate.

15.5 Future neuromorphic nanotechnologies

Other nanotechological neuromorphic circuits are described in the literature, including the widespread use of memristors spurred by the DARPA SyNAPSE and DARPA FRANC funding in the United States. Narayan Srinivasa from the HRL (formerly Hughes Aircraft research lab) Center for Neural and Emergent Systems led a memristor-based project funded by DARPA SyNAPSE that started in 2011 [40].

FinFETS are replacing planar MOS technologies in commercial applications and could soon be replaced by *nanosheets*. A double-gate FinFET is shown in figure 15.18. Scaling (making FINFETs smaller) seems to be very difficult, and nanosheets are believed to be the best replacement technology. In nanosheets, stacks of silicon form the channel and the stacks are surrounded by the metal transistor gate, separated from the channel by an insulating dielectric. A basic tutorial for nanosheet transistor structures can be found in *IEEE Spectrum* [41].

In a nanotechnology breakthrough in Sweden, there is an organic transistor that can act as a synapse, and can form new connections. The channel in the transistor consists of an electropolymerised conducting polymer. The channel can be formed, grown or shrunk, or completely eliminated during operation. It uses a polymer of a newly-developed monomer, ETE-S. 'An evolvable organic electrochemical transistor (OECT), operating in the hybrid accumulation–depletion mode is reported, which exhibits short-term and long-term memory functionalities. The transistor channel, formed by an electropolymerized conducting polymer, can be formed, modulated, and obliterated *in situ* and under operation. Enduring changes in channel conductance, analogous to long-term potentiation and depression, are attained by electropolymerization and electrochemical overoxidation of the channel

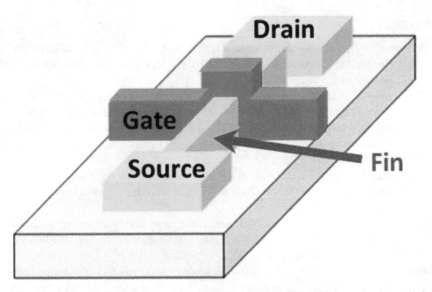

Figure 15.18. A double-gate FinFET device. This File:Doublegate FinFET.PNG image has been obtained by the authors from the Wikimedia website https://commons.wikimedia.org/w/index.php?curid=3833512 where it was made available under a CC BY-SA 3.0 licence. It is included within this book on that basis. It is attributed to Irene Ringworm.

material, respectively. Transient changes in channel conductance, analogous to short-term potentiation and depression, are accomplished by inducing nonequilibrium doping states within the transistor channel. By manipulating the input signal, the strength of the transistor response to a given stimulus can be modulated within a range that spans several orders of magnitude, producing behavior that is directly comparable to short- and long-term neuroplasticity. The evolvable transistor is further incorporated into a simple circuit that mimics classical conditioning. It is forecast that OECTs that can be physically and electronically modulated under operation will bring about a new paradigm of machine learning based on evolvable organic electronics [14].'

Rzeszut *et al* [33] presented an analog magnetic tunnel circuit where serially-connected magnetic tunnel junctions form a multi-state memory cell in a neuromorphic circuit modeling a neuron. The circuit was tested on hand-written digit recognition [27] described a carbon based system for a robot, as summarized in [9]. Another publication describes the use of a honey-based memristor in a synapse [34].

15.6 Chapter summary

This chapter focused on neuromorphic circuits implemented with nanotechnologies.

Certain sections of text in this chapter have been reproduced with permission from [23]. Copyright IEEE.

The next chapter covers some advanced topics in neuromorphic circuits covered in the BioRC group.

References

[1] Akinwande D *et al* 2008 Monolithic integration of CMOS VLSI and CNT for hybrid nanotechnology applications *ESSDERC 2008—38th European Solid-State Device Research Conf.* (Piscataway, NJ: IEEE) 91–4

[2] Barzegarjalali S 2016 Demonstrating the role of multiple memory mechanisms in learning patterns using neuromorphic circuits *PhD Thesis* University of Southern California

[3] Barzegarjalali S and Parker A C 2016 A bio-inspired electronic mechanism for unsupervised learning using structural plasticity *2016 Future Technologies Conf. (FTC)* (Piscataway, NJ: IEEE) 806–15

[4] Barzegarjalali S and Parker A C 2015 A hybrid neuromorphic circuit demonstrating schizophrenic symptoms *2015 Biomedical Circuits and Systems Conf. (BioCAS)* (Piscataway, NJ: IEEE) 1–4

[5] Barzegarjalali S and Parker A C 2016 A neuromorphic circuit mimicking biological short-term memory *2016 38th Annual Int. Conf. of the Engineering in Medicine and Biology Society (EMBC)* (Piscataway, NJ: IEEE) 1401–4

[6] Barzegarjalali S and Parker A C 2016 An analog neural network that learns Sudoku-like puzzle rules *2016 Future Technologies Conf. (FTC)* (Piscataway, NJ: IEEE) pp 838–47

[7] Barzegarjalali S and Parker A C 2016 Neuromorphic circuit modeling directional selectivity in the visual cortex *2016 38th Annual Int. Conf. of the Engineering in Medicine and Biology Society (EMBC)* (Piscataway, NJ: IEEE) 6130–3

[8] Barzegarjalali S, Yue K and Parker A C 2016 Noisy neuromorphic circuit modeling obsessive compulsive disorder *2016 29th Int. System-on-Chip Conf. (SOCC)* (Piscataway, NJ: IEEE) 327–32

[9] Bolakhe S 2022 Lego robot with an organic 'brain' learns to navigate a maze *Sci. Am.* https://www.scientificamerican.com/article/lego-robot-with-an-organic-brain-learns-to-navigate-a-maze

[10] Boybat I *et al* 2018 Neuromorphic computing with multi-memristive synapses *Nat. Commun.* **9** 1–12

[11] Desai S B *et al* 2016 MoS$_2$ transistors with 1-nanometer gate lengths *Science* **354** 99–102

[12] Fellin T *et al* 2004 Neuronal synchrony mediated by astrocytic glutamate through activation of extrasynaptic NMDA receptors *Neuron* **43** 729–43

[13] Friesz A K *et al* 2007 A biomimetic carbon nanotube synapse circuit *Biomedical Engineering Society Annual Fall Meeting*

[14] Gerasimov J Y *et al* 2019 An evolvable organic electrochemical transistor for neuromorphic applications *Adv. Sci.* **6** 1801339

[15] Gholipour M, Chen Y-Y and Chen D 2016 Flexible transition metal dichalcogenide field-effect transistor (TMDFET) HSPICE model
Hsu C-C 2014 Dendritic computation and plasticity in neuromorphic circuits *PhD Thesis* University of Southern California

[16] Hu M *et al* 2014 Memristor crossbar-based neuromorphic computing system: a case study *IEEE Trans. Neural Netw. Learn. Syst.* **25** 1864–78

[17] Irizarry-Valle Y, Parker A C and Joshi J 2013 A neuromorphic approach to emulate neuro-astrocyte interactions *The 2013 Int. Joint Conf. Neural Networks (IJCNN)* (Piscataway, NJ: IEEE) 1–7

[18] Irizarry-Valle Y and Parker A C 2015 An astrocyte neuromorphic circuit that influences neuronal phase synchrony *IEEE Trans. Biomed. Circuits Syst.* **9** 175–87

[19] Ishikawa F N *et al* 2009 Transparent electronics based on transfer printed aligned carbon nanotubes on rigid and flexible substrates *ACS Nano* **3** 73–9

[20] Wong H-S P and Deng J 2007 A compact SPICE model for carbon-nanotube field-effect transistors including nonidealities and its application—Part I: model of the intrinsic channel region *IEEE Trans. Electron Devices* **54** 3186–94

[21] Wong H-S P and Deng J 2007 A compact SPICE model for carbon-nanotube field-effect transistors including nonidealities and its application—Part II: full device model and circuit performance benchmarking *IEEE Trans. Electron Devices* **54** 3195–205

[22] Joshi J *et al* 2011 A biomimetic fabricated carbon nanotube synapse for prosthetic applications *IEEE/NIH 2011 LIfe Science Systems and Applications Workshop*

[23] Joshi J *et al* 2011 A biomimetic fabricated carbon nanotube synapse for prosthetic applications *2011 IEEE/NIH Life Science Systems and Applications Workshop (LiSSA)* 139–42

[24] Joshi J, Parker A and Tseng K-C 2011 *In-silico* Glial Microdomain to Invoke Excitability in Cortical Neural Networks *2011 IEEE Int. Symp. Circuits and Systems (ISCAS)* 681–4

[25] Joshi J *et al* 2009 A carbon nanotube cortical neuron with excitatory and inhibitory dendritic computations *2009 IEEE/NIH Life Science Systems and Applications Workshop* (Bethesda, MD: IEEE) 133–6

[26] Kocabas C 2008 Radio frequency analog electronics based on carbon nanotube transistors *Proc. Natl Acad. Sci.* **105** 1405–9

[27] Krauhausen I *et al* 2021 Organic neuromorphic electronics for sensorimotor integration and learning in robotics *Sci. Adv.* **7** eabl5068

[28] Liu X, Han S and Zhou C 2006 Novel nanotube-on-insulator (NOI) approach toward single-walled carbon nanotube devices *Nano Lett.* **6** 34–9

[29] Parker A C *et al* 2008 A carbon nanotube implementation of temporal and spatial dendritic computations *Circuits and Systems, 2008. MWSCAS 2008. 51st Midwest Symp.* (Piscataway, NJ: IEEE) 818–21

[30] Patil N *et al* 2008 Design methods for misaligned and mispositioned carbon-nanotube immune circuits *IEEE Trans. Comput.-Aided Des. Integr. Circuits Syst.* **27** 1725–36

[31] Radisavljevic B *et al* 2011 Single-layer MoS2 transistors *Nat. Nanotechnol.* **6** 147–50

[32] Ryu K *et al* 2009 CMOS-analogous wafer-scale nanotube-on-insulator approach for submicrometer devices and integrated circuits using aligned nanotubes *Nano Lett.* **9** 189–97

[33] Rzeszut P *et al* 2021 Multi-state MRAM cells for hardware neuromorphic computing *arXiv preprint* arXiv:2102.03415

[34] Sueoka B and Zhao F 2022 Memristive synaptic device based on a natural organic material —honey for spiking neural network in biodegradable neuromorphic systems *J. Phys. D: Appl. Phys.* **55** 225105

[35] Sung S H *et al* 2022 Simultaneous emulation of synaptic and intrinsic plasticity using a memristive synapse *Nat. Commun.* **13** 1–12

[36] Suryavanshi S V and Pop E 2015 Physics-based compact model for circuit simulations of 2-dimensional semiconductor devices *Device Research Conf. (DRC), 2015 73rd Annual* (Piscataway, NJ: IEEE) 235–6

[37] Volterra A, Liaudet N and Savtchouk I 2014 Astrocyte Ca^{2+} signalling: an unexpected complexity *Nat. Rev. Neurosci.* **15** 327–35

[38] Wang C *et al* 2008 Device study, chemical doping, and logic circuits based on transferred aligned single-walled carbon nanotubes *Appl. Phys. Lett.* **93** 033101

[39] Wang H *et al* 2012 Integrated circuits based on bilayer MoS_2 transistors *Nano Lett.* **12** 4674–80

[40] Wheeler D *et al* 2011 CMOS-integrated memristors for neuromorphic architectures *2011 Int. Semiconductor Device Research Symp. (ISDRS)* 1–2

[41] Ye P, Ernest T and Khare M V 2019 The nanosheet transistor is the next (and maybe last) step in Moore's law *IEEE Spectr.*

[42] Yue K 2021 Circuit design with nano electronic devices for biomimetic neuromorphic systems *PhD Thesis* University of Southern California

[43] Yue K *et al* 2019 A brain-plausible neuromorphic on-the-fly learning system implemented with magnetic domain wall analog memristors *Sci. Adv.* **5** eaau8170

IOP Publishing

Neuromorphic Circuits
A constructive approach
Alice C Parker and Rick Cattell

Chapter 16

Advanced topics

Chih-Chieh Hsu, Yilda Irizarry-Valle, Ko-Chung Tseng, Pezhman Mamdouh and Alice C Parker

This chapter surveys some advanced neuromorphic circuits, including sound localization in birds and burst potentiation in the neuron. A depressive synapse neuromorphic circuit is then presented. The chapter includes description of a complex pair of neuromorphic neurons that exhibit border-ownership (BO) using dendritic processing. Ultra-low power dendritic computations are summarized in the chapter.

16.1 Sound localization in birds

Coincidence detection in birds' sound localization systems is a good example in Hsu's thesis [6] and all figures in this section are found in the thesis, providing strong evidence for dendritic computation as a key component to neural information processing. Results from Agmon-Snir *et al* in computational neuroscience have shown that the unique dendritic structure of the bipolar neuron improves auditory coincidence detection [1]. Coincident inputs from both ears arriving at the two dendrites are summed superlinearly at the soma causing the neuron to fire, while the inputs from the same ear are summed sub-linearly, causing the neuron to remain silent.

A *bipolar* neuron model[1] is presented in figure 16.1(a), where each dendrite receives inputs from one ear (right or left), the top synapses originate at neurons sensing sound from the front direction, and the bottom synapses originate at neurons sensing sound from the rear direction. Two input patterns are shown in figure 16.1(b) and (c): *Case 1* for sound coming from the same side and *Case 2* for sound coming from both sides in the same direction, for example, the front side.

When the clustered synapses on the same branch are activated, a large amount of potential is built up locally but limited by the reduction of the depolarizing current

---

[1] A neuron with short dendritic arbor and single axon, processing visual and aural sensory signals.

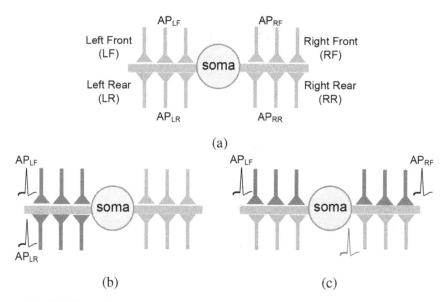

Figure 16.1. Coincidence detection: sound localization in auditory bipolar neuron [6]. (a) Bipolar neuron model setup. Six synapses on each dendritic branch which consists of front and rear directions. (b) Case 1: all inputs come from the same ear, therefore no action potential initiates at the soma. (c) Case 2: inputs come from both ears, therefore the soma is firing an action potential. Synapses highlighted in red represent the ones being activated by the sound inputs.

which is often referred to as the saturation effect in the literature. Hsu used the sub-linear adder (amplifier pair) that inherently limits the amount of current that can be drawn into the dendritic compartment to mimic this nonlinear saturation biophysical mechanism. On the other hand, when the activated synapses are segregated onto two different branches, more depolarization current can be generated at the soma. In this case, Hsu uses the superlinear adder (amplifier pair) which inherently has the capability to draw more current through the multiple carbon nanotubes per transistor in comparison to the linear adder[2].

The circuit implementation is shown in figure 16.2 where the synaptic inputs coming from the same branch are integrated sub-linearly and the synaptic inputs coming from different branches are integrated superlinearly to achieve coincidence detection when a sound wave arrives at both sides. The circuit algorithm works as follows. A *coincidence detection* module is used to generate signals indicating whether action potential (AP) inputs come from both sides or one side only. The signal CD is 1 when inputs from both sides are concurrently present, and is 0 when they are not. The signal, $RIGHT$ is 1 when inputs are from the right side, and is 0 when they are from the left side. When inputs arrive to both sides, PSP_L and PSP_R should sum superlinearly and the overall somatic potential, V_{SOMA}, would be passed through $MUX2$ ($CD = 1$) to the *axon hillock* module. When inputs arrive to one side

---

[2] The superlinear addition could be seen as a dendritic spike, and implemented differently.

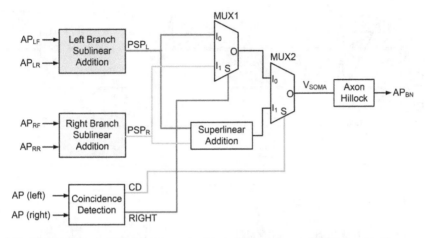

Figure 16.2. Bipolar neuron circuit implementation block diagram. Inputs from the same side are summed sub-linearly and inputs from different sides are summed superlinearly. The coincidence detection module generates an output, *CD*, which indicates whether AP inputs from both sides are present concurrently. The *CD* signal determines the inputs going to the *superlinear addition* module or bypassing to the *axon hillock* module, selected by the multiplexer [6].

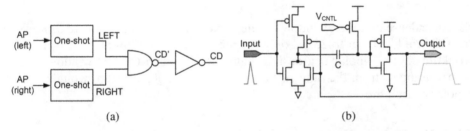

Figure 16.3. (a) *Coincidence detection* module at the gate level. When both *LEFT* and *RIGHT* are 1, *CD* is 1 indicating that coincident inputs are detected. (b) *One-shot* module at the transistor level. The voltage input V_{CNTL} control the duration of the output [6].

only, either PSP_L ($RIGHT = 0$) or PSP_R ($RIGHT = 1$) would be passed through *MUX1* and *MUX2* ($CD = 0$) to the *axon hillock* module. Figure 16.3 shows the gate level and the transistor-level implementations of Hsu's *coincidence detection* module presented in figure 16.2. The *one-shot* module is used to generate a time window within which the inputs' arrival from both sides are considered coincident. This time window can be controlled by the voltage V_{CNTL}.

The simulation results of Case 1 (inputs from same side) and Case 2 (inputs from both sides) are presented here. Hsu demonstrates that, with the point neuron model, the neuron cannot distinguish whether the sound is coming from one side or both sides. The output fires in both cases, as seen in figure 16.4. In figure 16.5, at $t = 50$ ps, the only inputs arriving are at the left side, so the bipolar neuron is silent (Case 1) and at $t = 200$ ps, inputs are arriving at both sides, therefore the bipolar neuron fires (Case 2). Hsu varied the delay of the input coming from one side, Δt, to demonstrate

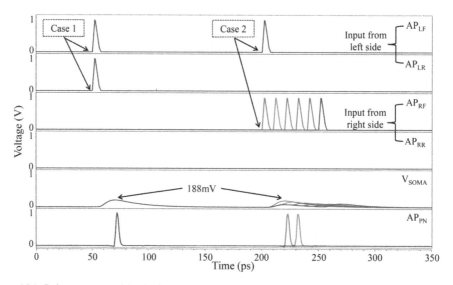

Figure 16.4. Point neuron model. The first four panels represent the AP inputs arriving at left (AP_{FL}, AP_{RL}) and right (AP_{FR}, AP_{RR}) sides. The overall somatic potential (V_{SOMA}) is shown in the 5th panel and the first and second V_{SOMA} are the same because at both times four synapses are activated causing enough depolarization at the soma to make the point neuron fire (AP_{PN}, last panel) [6].

the coincidence detection window is adjustable in her circuit implementation. When the CD window is set to 25 ps, only the inputs from the right at $\Delta t = 0, 10, 20$ ps would make the bipolar neuron fire (figure 16.5). When the CD window is set to 65 ps, all inputs from the right side at $\Delta t = 0, 10, 20, 30, 40, 50$ ps would make the bipolar neuron fire.

16.2 Burst potentiation possibilities

In addition to regular spiking, burst is another axonal firing mechanism that has been observed in a variety of cortical pyramidal neurons [10, 12, 23]. Bursts usually appear as multiple spikes riding on top of a DC potential.

The burst of APs possesses important neuronal information and enhances the synchronization among cortical neurons. Bursts are more reliable than single spikes, because they facilitate the neurotransmitter release process [14]. Bursts carry more temporal information such as burst duration, and inter-spike intervals encoded within a burst than single spikes do. Bursting mechanism in the cortical pyramidal neurons has a close relationship to the calcium signal. Kampa and Stuartdiscovered that AP bursts can evoke calcium spikes in basal dendrites [11]. More evidence supports the theory that a burst can evoke long-term potentiation because it triggers regenerative interaction between back-propagating action potentials (bAPs)and dendritic calcium spikes. Williams and Stuart suggested that back-propagating action potentials reduce the threshold to generate dendritic calcium spikes, which leads to increasing dendritic depolarization and therefore the likelihood of successful bAP increases [23]. Larkum and Zhu also suggested that calcium spikes function as a

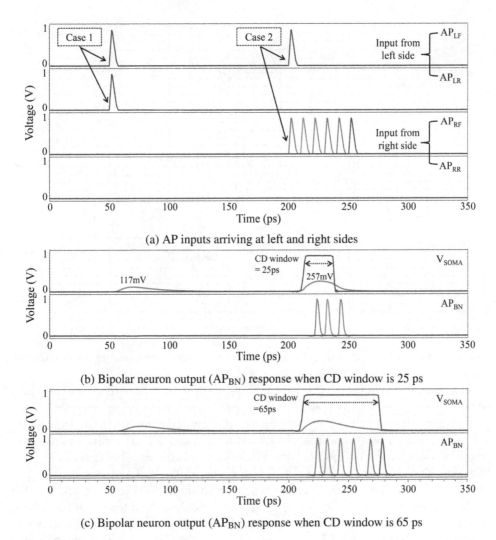

(a) AP inputs arriving at left and right sides

(b) Bipolar neuron output (AP$_{BN}$) response when CD window is 25 ps

(c) Bipolar neuron output (AP$_{BN}$) response when CD window is 65 ps

Figure 16.5. Bipolar auditory neuron coincidence detection simulation with various time windows. (a) The AP inputs arriving at left and right sides. (b) The top panel shows the coincidence detection time window and overall somatic potential (V_{SOMA}) in red. The first V_{SOMA} is smaller than the second one because the former results from sounds from the same side. The bottom panel represents the output of the bipolar neuron AP_{BN}. If the inputs arriving at the right (AP_{FR}) are less than 25 ps apart from inputs arriving at left (AP_{FL}), the bipolar neuron fires. If the inputs arriving at the right are more than 25 ps apart from those at the left (the 4th to 6th AP$_{RF}$), the neuron is silent. (c) Bipolar neuron output response when the CD time window is set to 65 ps [6].

switch to convert the regular firing behavior to bursting in cortical pyramidal neurons [12]. More recently, Bender *et al* found that the axon initial segment contains calcium channels that are down-regulated by dopamine neurotransmitter and this calcium influx can cause the neuron to burst [3]. In addition, Jensen *et al* concluded that the burst firing pattern is modulated by the extracellular potassium

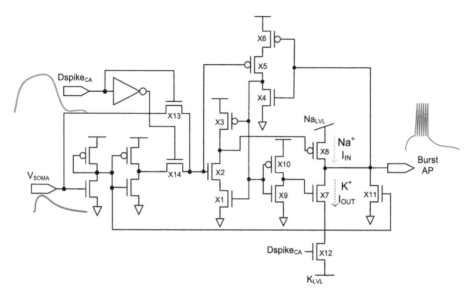

Figure 16.6. Bursting *axon hillock* circuit at the transistor level [6].

concentration. Elevated extracellular K^+ concentration increases the depolarization potential the burst spikes ride on [10].

Hsu includes additional control circuitry such as the dendritic calcium spike signal, and extracellular potassium level in her original *axon hillock* module, shown in figure 16.6 This figure, along with figures 16.7 and 16.8 are found in Hsu's thesis, [6]. The principle is to make both transistors X2 and X5 partially turned on to produce a continuously firing output. When Ca^{2+} spikes are generated at the distal dendrite, they trigger the burst firing at the axon hillock. The potential V_{SOMA} is directly fed into the Na^+/K^+ section when dendritic Ca^{2+} spikes are present. We characterizes the circuit by varying $Dspike_{CA}$ to modulate the intensity of burst firing and hence the duration between two spikes. The circuit simulation result is shown in figure 16.7. Then we varied K_{LVL} to modulate the depolarized membrane potential the burst spikes residing on. The circuit simulation result is shown in figure 16.8.

A capacitor, judiciously placed, could result in burst potentiation in the synapse by delaying the fall time of the synaptic response, as shown in figure 16.9. It should be noted that the synaptic cleft voltage could (and should) be mirrored before the large capacitor, to isolate the synapse's presynaptic response to the input action potential from the capacitance. The receptor concentration is controlled by two transistors, one that raises receptor concentration voltage when syn_cleft voltage is raised, and one that lowers receptor concentration voltage over the long term, as burst potentiation effects are reduced, and the receptor concentration voltage is divided between the two transistors. There are other locations proposed for burst potentiation, including the axon initial segment, and other possible causes for the potentiation, including lowered thresholds for calcium spikes due to AP back propagation.

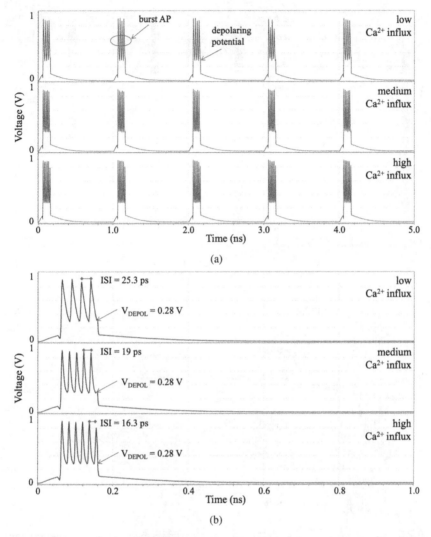

Figure 16.7. Burst firing characterization: modulated by calcium influx. Increase in the Ca^{2+} influx results in more burst spikes per activation and decreased inter-spike interval. (a) The burst AP is firing at a lower frequency, 40 GHz, when Ca^{2+} influx is low. The burst AP frequency increases to 61 GHz when Ca^{2+} influx is high. (b) Zoom-in to 1 ns of the entire simulation time to further examine the inter-spike interval (ISI). In all three scenarios, the depolarizing potential, V_{DEPOL}, remains the same [6].

16.3 A depressing synapse

In this section we present a circuit that captures the adaptability of a synapse, from the Irizarry-Valle thesis [9]. This circuit demonstrates short-term synaptic depression and also captures an important behavior, the Weber–Fechner relationship. We show that a synapse subjected to a change in spike rates at high and low frequencies has a similar contribution in terms of the updated synaptic strength. Our circuit is

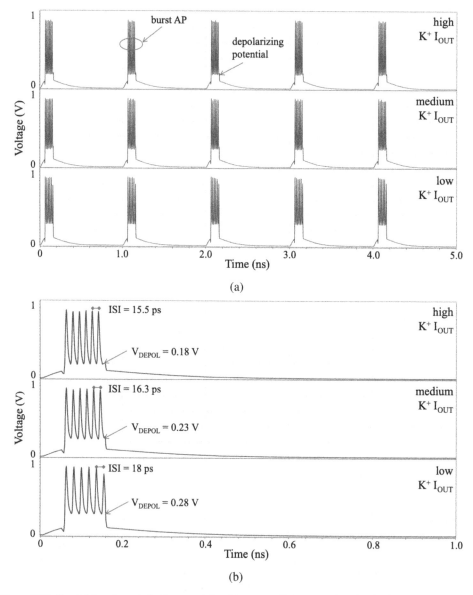

Figure 16.8. Burst firing characterization: modulated by extracellular potassium level. Elevated extracellular K^+ concentration can limit the outward K^+ current, and therefore the depolarizing potential increases. (a) The burst AP rides on a larger depolarizing potential when the extracellular K^+ concentration is higher. (b) zoomed-in to 1 ns of the entire simulation time. There is less impact on the inter-spike interval of the burst spikes, however, the depolarizing potential, V_{DEPOL}, changes due to the K^+ concentration [6].

designed such that we can capture time between spikes. By detecting the time between spikes we can detect when changes in spike rates occur, shown in figure 16.10. This is a complex circuit that is discussed in greater detail in Irizarry-Valle's thesis [8] and the related publication [9].

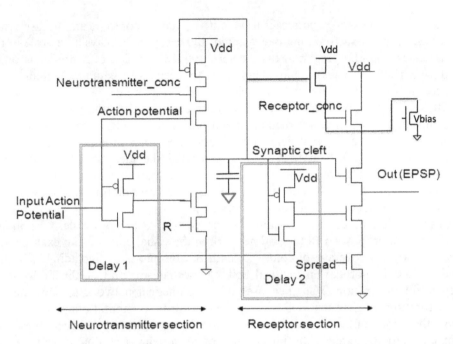

Figure 16.9. Implementation of burst potentiation with a large capacitor.

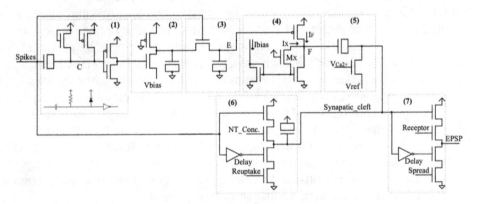

Figure 16.10. Depressing synapse. Copyright 2014 IEEE. Reprinted, with permission, from [9].

16.4 Border ownership

BO is a task performed by the human visual system to determine whether an object or background is to the right or left of a border. Chih-Chieh Hsu modeled this in an intricate example in her thesis [6] and in a conference paper [9]. All figures not specifically cited in this section come from Hsu's thesis [6] or are original or derived from the thesis.

Humans perceive a huge amount of visual input every second their eyes are open and their brains must process the massive amount of information efficiently. One of the early human visual processes is to identify occluding contours and to distinguish an object from its surrounding background. BO assignment plays a key role in this figure–background segregation task, determining which side of a border is object and which side is background. Therefore, to accurately emulate human visual cortical neurons, it is important to include the BO function.

Biological cortical neurons are much more complex than the integrate-and-fire neurons that are widely implemented in neuromorphic circuits. A recent study from Smith *et al* have shown that dendritic spikes can enhance orientation selectivity in cortical neurons [20]. This has further supported the idea that active dendritic spiking enriches the computational capacity, e.g., spatio-temporal pattern recognition, within individual neurons, increasing their computational efficiency, e.g., same result achieved with fewer numbers of neurons. Therefore, it has motivated Hsu's inclusion of dendritic spiking in the cortical neurons we describe in this chapter. Hsu proposes a BO neural network in the visual cortex as an example that provides a good coverage of complex dendritic computations, including excitation and inhibition modulation, a local spiking mechanism, and nonlinear location-dependent integration. Hsu then uses this hypothetical network to simulate two configurations of neurons; one has complex dendritic computational capacity and the other does not[3]. The difference in the BO assignment between these two implementations signifies the importance of intra-neuron computation in neuromorphic circuit emulation.

Employing the complex dendritic structures (nonlinear integration among dendrites at different locations) and spiking mechanisms (nonlinear computation), Hsu proposed that contour detection based on the Gestalt convexity principle, relying on convex borders forming the foreground object, can be carried out in individual BO neurons. With each dendritic branch being a computational unit, Hsu reduces the complexity of connections between neurons and make more local connections within an individual neuron. Her hypothetical neuron can detect different types of contours, then integrate this information along with stereo-depth (disparity) cues, helpful when object contours are concave, to perform BO assignment. Hsu demonstrates that both dendritic properties, the active spiking and the passive location-dependent attenuation and integration, together with the disparity can perform BO assignment. Further, we demonstrate that nonlinear dendritic computation and lateral inhibition can enhance BO assignment.

16.4.1 Border-ownership background

There have been a few studies on the BO mechanism in the mammalian visual cortex; some assume it is achieved by the lateral propagation of signals in V2, and some propose it is done by feedback from a higher visual cortex region. Zhou *et al* proposed that for each orientation and position in the visual field there are two types of neurons to represent the two possible contrast borders [24]. For instance, a light-to-dark border can be interpreted as a light object or light background seen through

---

[3] i.e. it contains integrate-and-fire neurons.

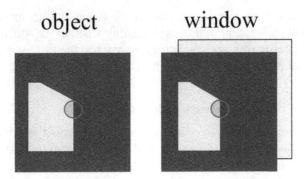

Figure 16.11. Object and window image representation [6]. Left: border belongs to the light object. Right: border belongs to the window on a dark screen. Circle represents the receptive field.

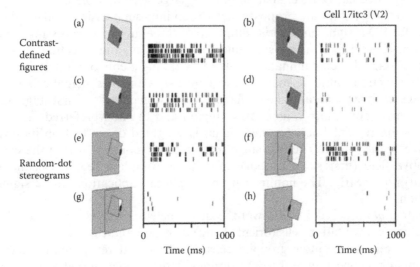

Figure 16.12. Biological BO neuron response. Responses of a biological V2 neuron tuned to fire at a dark object on the left, to contrast-defined figures (a, b, c, d) and to disparity-defined figures (e, f, g, h) presented as random-dot stereograms. Reprinted from [18], copyright (2005), with permission from Elsevier. In the absence of disparity cues, the neuron assumes the square (convexity) is the object hence it fires more vigorously when the object is on the left. In the random-dot stereograms, the neuron fires more robustly when the front object is on the left.

a window on dark screen (shown in figure 16.11). Hence two types of BO-selective neurons would respond to this particular visual stimulus at each orientation and position, one responding to a light object on the left and the other to a dark object on the right. It is shown in figure 16.12(a) and (b) that the contrast edges to the receptive fields in the ellipses are locally identical and those in (c) and (d) are as well.

In [5] von der Heydt *et al* found that the stereoscopic edge-selective cells are only found in V2. Qiu *et al* argued that V2 cells combine the disparity cue with the Gestalt principles to segregate foreground and background [18]. In figure 16.12, responses of a V2 cell, which is selective for left side of BO, to contrast-defined figures (a, b, c, and d) show that this neuron assumes the square is the object due to its convexity. When disparity is present (e, f, g, and h) it does not matter whether the square appears on the left or right, this neuron distinguishably fires more when the front surface is on the left. Hsu implements this behavior in her BO neurons at the circuit level.

16.4.2 Discussion of border-ownership algorithms

BO-selective neuron models using inter-neuron feedforward and feedback connections have been proposed in [4, 21, 22], and a model using lateral facilitation and inhibition has been proposed in [13]. However, in these models, the intra-neuron dendritic computation was not utilized. Furthermore, these research efforts focus on computational modeling in the software algorithms, while our proposed neural network is implemented at the circuit level, which has the advantage of smaller size and accelerated hardware emulation time for large-scale networks.

Sakai and Nishimura proposed a surrounding suppression and facilitation model for BO assignment that is composed of three stages of processing: contrast detection and normalization, surrounding modulation, and detection of BO [21]. The first stage detects luminance contrast by taking a convolution with oriented Gabor functions and normalizes the contrast within its neighborhood. The second stage then separates the preferred orientation contrasts (first stage output) in the surrounding into a facilitation region and the non-preferred ones into a suppression region. Each contrast signal is weighted dependent on its position relative to the center. The last stage integrates the contrast within the classical receptive field (first stage output) and the surrounding region (second stage output) nonlinearly. The nonlinearity is simply multiplication, and a sigmoidal function.

Craft *et al* proposed a feedforward/feedback network that is composed of layers of feature representation cells (oriented-edge detection and edge-termination detection), BO cells, and contour grouping cells [4]. The feature representation cells form an excitatory connection to the BO neuron with the same preferred orientation and an inhibitory connection to the neuron with the opposite preferred orientation. The mutual inhibitory connection is modeled between a pair of BO neurons. The contour grouping cells with larger receptive fields reside at higher level of the hierarchy and inhibit the BO neuron which preferred the opposite direction.

Our bio-inspired (or neuro-inspired) approach utilizes an intra-neuron dendritic computation, including the active dendritic spiking and passive dendritic attenuation mechanisms, and location-dependent integration to perform contour detection, convexity detection, and BO assignment within one neuron. Our biomimetic BO neuron combines a Gestalt visual convexity rule with the disparity cue to determine side of ownership as the biological BO-selective neuron does, even though the exact mechanism or connection between neurons in different visual cortex regions remains unclear. In our proposed BO neuron, the excitatory connection from a disparity cue is assigned the highest weight by configuring an axosomatic excitatory synaptic connection. Each BO neuron also mutually inhibits its opposite BO neuron. Contour detection is computed by each dendritic branch receiving inputs from a group of nearby edge-selective (edge-detection, ED) neurons and convexity detection is computed by the location of each dendritic branch in our proposed model. Since each building block is one neuron, a computational unit, our approach has the flexibility to scale up to a larger network harboring more edge-selective neurons, BO neurons, and depth-selective neurons with a pre-defined (hardwired) intra-network connection.

16.4.3 The proposed border-ownership neuron

The basic idea behind our hypothetical BO neuron is that it is postsynaptic to ED neurons such as the simple cells found in V1, and it responds preferentially in individual dendrites to convex contours that represent object borders. It also responds to concave contours, with attenuation due to distance from the soma. It will determine BO if the response is superlinear due to dendritic spiking in response to the convex contour or if disparity information is present even though the contour is concave.

16.4.3.1 Edge detection and border-ownership assignment

An ED neuron (*simple cell*, often called 'edge-selective cell', in the visual cortex) responds most vigorously to an edge at a preferred orientation (vertical, horizontal, or diagonal) as well as a preferred contrast polarity (dark-to-light or light-to-dark). In our proposed neural network for BO assignment, there are eight types of ED neurons for each receptive field (RF) shown in figure 16.15(a), each with an axonal projection presynaptic to the BO neuron. These eight θ-oriented edges are 0°, 45°, 90°, 135°, 180°, 225°, 270°, and 315° respectively. θ represents the angle between a preferred edge orientation/contrast polarity and the horizontal baseline. An ED neuron is shown in figure 16.13.

A hypothetical BO neuron responds selectively to a preferred orientation, a preferred contrast polarity, and a preferred side of ownership. It receives information from a collection of ED neurons surrounding the center of a BO neuron's receptive field. Because neurons responding to similar visual features are believed to

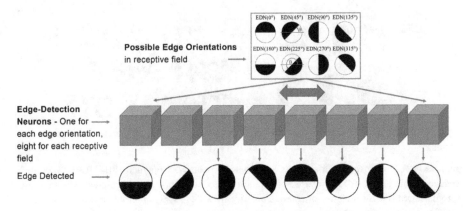

Figure 16.13. ED neurons with eight possible edge orientations [6].

be preferentially connected based on activity-dependent mechanisms, we propose the idea that neural processing that identifies the formation of a contour can be performed by a nonlinear computation within a dendritic branch. With several different dendritic branches, we propose that a BO neuron can therefore detect several types of contours. Figure 16.14 shows contour detection in a single dendrite of a BO neuron. The detailed implementation will be discussed in the next two sections.

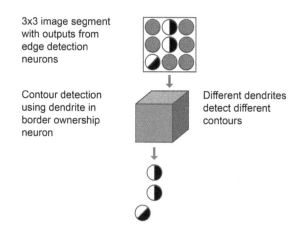

3x3 image segment with outputs from edge detection neurons

Contour detection using dendrite in border ownership neuron

Different dendrites detect different contours

Figure 16.14. Contour detection by a dendrite in a BO neuron.

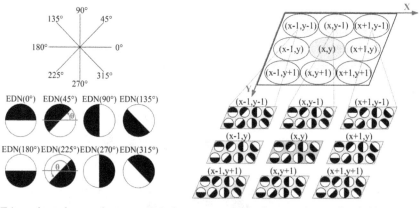

(a) Edge orientations and contrast polarities

(b) 3×3 array of receptive fields

Figure 16.15. EDN preferred orientation and contrast polarity. Copyright 2014 IEEE, reprinted, with permission, from [7]: (a) EDN preferred orientation and contrast polarity. θ represents the angle from the horizontal baseline to the preferred orientation/polarity. (b) A 3×3 array of RFs with coordinates labeled. For each RF, there are eight ED neurons, each only responding to its preferred visual stimulus.

Table 16.1. Types of BO neurons. Reproduced from [6].

Type	Edge orientation	Contrast polarity	Side of ownership
BON_{DL}	Vertical	Dark-to-light	Left
BON_{LR}			Right
BON_{LL}		Light-to-dark	Left
BON_{DR}			Right
BON_{DL}	Horizontal	Dark-to-light	Top
BON_{LR}			Bottom
BON_{LT}		Light-to-dark	Top
BON_{DB}			Bottom

In our example, we choose an array of 3×3 RFs as the minimal visual space, shown in figure 16.15(b), where each circle represents a non-overlapping RF of an ED neuron. Each RF is labeled with a coordinate, for example, for the center RF and $(x - 1, y - 1)$ for the top-left RF. There are eight ED neurons each of which responds to each RF in our proposed implementation and each ED neuron is assigned with its location coordinate and the preferred orientation. For instance, the eight ED neurons responding to different visual stimuli at center RF are labeled $EDN(x, y, 0°)$, $EDN(x, y, 45°)$, $EDN(x, y, 90°)$, $EDN(x, y, 135°)$, $EDN(x, y, 180°)$, $EDN(x, y, 225°)$, $EDN(x, y, 270°)$, and $EDN(x, y, 315°)$.

We categorize the BO neurons into eight types based on their preferred edge orientations, contrast polarities, and sides of ownership (table 16.1). The edge orientation can be either vertical (90°, 270°) or horizontal (0°, 180°). The contrast polarity can be either dark-to-light or light-to-dark. The side of ownership (the object in foreground) can be either left, right, top, or bottom. For example, BON_{DL} fires more robustly if the border belongs to the dark object on the left side of the receptive field while BON_{LR} fires more if the border belongs to the light object on the right side of the RF. For simplicity we do not specify BO neurons that identify top left and lower right, for example. Those could be included in a practical system without modifying our approach.

16.4.4 Contour detection using nonlinear dendritic computation

The representation of contour plays a fundamental role in BO assignment. Aside from disparity, convexity is another clue to segregate the object from the background. In the absence of stereo-depth information, convexity becomes the key feature to determine which side owns the border. The Gestalt visual convexity principle suggests that the region that is convex (protrusion) rather than concave (notch) is more likely to be perceived as an object [2]. We propose that contour detection can be implemented using nonlinear dendritic computation that includes active and passive properties. Our approach is to utilize (1) the active dendritic spiking property to detect any form of contours, and (2) the passive location-dependent attenuation property to distinguish the convex contours from the concave

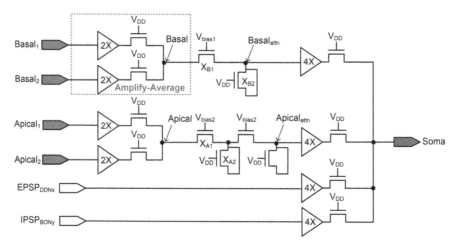

Figure 16.16. BO neuron passive dendritic arbors integration. Circuit modeling of passive nonlinear dendritic computation [6].

ones. Therefore, for each type of BO neuron, the dendritic branches that detect convex contours are arranged closer to the soma while those detecting concave contours are further from the soma, and become significantly more attenuated at the soma. The active dendrite circuit (figure 8.6) is introduced and discussed in chapter 5. We use dendritic spikes that are initiated with spatiotemporally synchronous synaptic inputs to indicate whether a contour is presented to the BON.

The passive dendritic cable is modeled with transistors (e.g. X_{B1}, X_{B2}, etc) as shown in figure 16.16. The overall dendritic potential from basal and apical dendrites are integrated using *amplify-average* circuits. The attenuated basal and apical potential ($V_{Basal,attn}$ and $V_{Apical,attn}$) are described in equations (16.1) and (16.2), where V_{Basal} and V_{Apical} represent the basal and apical dendritic arbor potentials (assuming they are step responses). The delay time constant can be approximated using an Elmore delay model, as described in equations (16.3) and (16.4). R_B is the effective resistance of transistor X_{B1}, and C_B is the lumped diffusion capacitance of transistor X_{B2} in the *Basal* RC circuit shown in figure 16.16. Similarly, R_A is the effective resistance of transistor X_{A1}, and C_A is the lumped diffusion capacitance of transistor X_{A2} in the *Apical* RC circuit. The diffusion capacitance of transistors X_{A1} and X_{B1} is negligible compared to that of transistors X_{A2} and X_{B2}, respectively. C_{AMP} represents the input capacitance of the 4X amplifier and it is approximately 0.1 fF. R_A and R_B are configured to be approximately 100 kΩ, and C_A and C_B to be 0.8 fF. Therefore, based on equation (16.3) and equation (16.4), the RC time constant is 90 ps for the basal dendritic cable and 260 ps for the apical dendritic cable.

$$V_{Basal,attn} = V_{Basal} \cdot (1 - e^{-t/\tau_B}) \tag{16.1}$$

$$V_{Apical,attn} = V_{Apical} \cdot (1 - e^{-t/\tau_A}) \tag{16.2}$$

$$\tau_B = R_B \cdot (C_B + C_{AMP}) \tag{16.3}$$

$$\begin{aligned} \tau_A &= R_A \cdot (C_A + C_A + C_{AMP}) + R_A \cdot (C_A + C_{AMP}) \\ &= R_A \cdot (3 \cdot C_A + 2 \cdot C_{AMP}) \end{aligned} \tag{16.4}$$

16.4.4.1 Contour representation

The dendritic arbor in our BO neurons can detect two groups of contours: vertical and horizontal, shown in figure 16.17. Because neurons with similar properties such as close RF or stimuli preference tend to cluster together, we propose the idea that collinear (located on a straight line) or cocircular (located on a circle) ED neurons with similar preferred contrast and orientation form excitatory connections onto the same dendritic branch in a BO neuron. Therefore, we assume that each center ED neuron (tagged in blue circle) and two adjacent ED neurons in the 3×3 RF array can form seven shapes of contour (e.g. a, b, ..., g), shown in figure 16.17(a) for vertical contours. Among those seven shapes of contours, we further expand them into two opposite contrast polarities: dark-to-light (default) and light-to-dark (denoted with $*$), e.g. a_V and a_V^*, two complementary contours. Each contour has two representations, for example, if there is a dark object on the left side, patterns b_V, c_V, d_V are considered convex and patterns e_V, f_V, g_V are considered concave for BON_{DL}. Conversely, if there is a light object on the right side, these patterns' convexity and concavity are reverse for BON_{LR}. The representation horizontal contours (figure 16.17(b)) share the similar characteristics of the vertical contours except they are the 90°-shifted version of the vertical ones.

16.4.4.2 Dendritic branch assignment and implementation

ED neurons whose RFs are in proximity and share similar preference are clustered together and form synapses onto the same dendritic branch in a BO neuron. Each contour is formed by three collinear or cocircular ED neurons, including the center ED neuron, $EDN(x, y, \theta)$. The assignments of the ED neurons for each form of vertical contour and horizontal contour are tabulated in tables 16.2 and 16.3 respectively.

The dendritic branches of a BO neuron are configured in the way that each branch can detect two patterns of contours (either vertical or horizontal depending on the type of the BO neuron). For example, in BON_{DL}, one of the apical dendritic branches can detect a_V and e_V contours. Contour a_V is composed of $EDN(x, y - 1, 90°)$, $EDN(x, y, 90°)$, and $EDN(x, y + 1, 90°)$, while contour e_V is composed of $EDN(x + 1, y - 1, 45°)$, $EDN(x, y, 90°)$, and $EDN(x, y + 1, 90°)$. Hence, each of $EDN(x, y, 90°)$ and $EDN(x, y + 1, 90°)$ forms two synapses on that branch. Because of this design methodology, when there is a contour presented, it activates five synapses on a specific dendritic branch at the same time. The dendritic spike threshold is therefore adjusted to five times of the excitatory synaptic potential (EPSP). The initiation of the dendritic spike indicates a vertical contour is detected. Because the attenuated apical dendritic potential is less than the attenuated basal dendritic potential, we configure the apical dendritic arbor to detect concave

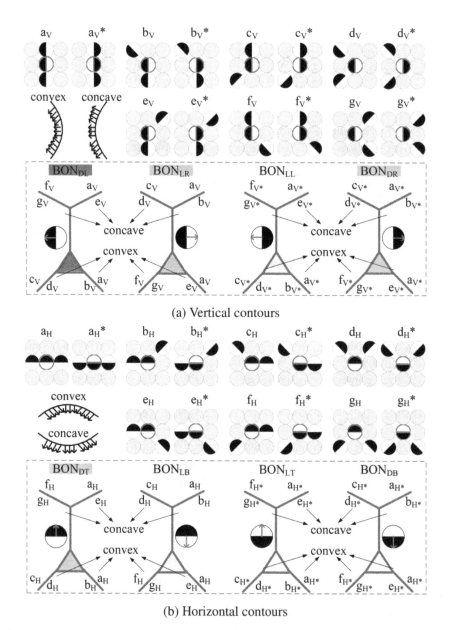

Figure 16.17. Forms of vertical and horizontal contours [6]. (a) The representation of vertical contours in a 3×3 RF array. Fourteen contour patterns: half in dark-to-light contrast polarity (e.g. a_V, ..., g_V) and half in light-to-dark contrast polarity (e.g. a_V^*, ..., g_V^*). In the dashed box: the dendritic arbor configurations for the four BONs prefer different sides of ownership (indicated by the red arrow). Each dendritic branch is labeled by the patterns it can detect. BON_{DL}: dark object on the left. BON_{LR}: light object on the right. BON_{LL}: light object on the left. BON_{DR}: dark object on the right. (b) The representation of horizontal contours. Similar notation used here. BON_{DT}: dark object on the top. BON_{LB}: light object on the bottom. BON_{LT}: light object on the top. BON_{DB}: dark object on the bottom.

Table 16.2. EDN assignment for vertical contour. Reproduced from [6].

Dark-to-light

Contour	**Edge-detection neurons (EDNs)**		
a_V	$(x, y - 1, 90°)$	$(x, y, 90°)$	$(x, y + 1, 90°)$
b_V	$(x - 1, y - 1, 135°)$	$(x, y, 90°)$	$(x, y + 1, 90°)$
c_V	$(x, y - 1, 90°)$	$(x, y, 90°)$	$(x - 1, y + 1, 45°)$
d_V	$(x - 1, y - 1, 135°)$	$(x, y, 90°)$	$(x - 1, y + 1, 45°)$
e_V	$(x + 1, y - 1, 45°)$	$(x, y, 90°)$	$(x, y + 1, 90°)$
f_V	$(x, y - 1, 90°)$	$(x, y, 90°)$	$(x + 1, y + 1, 135°)$
g_V	$(x + 1, y - 1, 45°)$	$(x, y, 90°)$	$(x + 1, y + 1, 135°)$

Light-to-dark

Contour	**Edge-detection neurons (EDNs)**		
a_V^*	$(x, y - 1, 270°)$	$(x, y, 270°)$	$(x, y + 1, 270°)$
b_V^*	$(x - 1, y - 1, 315°)$	$(x, y, 270°)$	$(x, y + 1, 270°)$
c_V^*	$(x, y - 1, 270°)$	$(x, y, 270°)$	$(x - 1, y + 1, 225°)$
d_V^*	$(x - 1, y - 1, 315°)$	$(x, y, 270°)$	$(x - 1, y + 1, 225°)$
e_V^*	$(x + 1, y - 1, 225°)$	$(x, y, 270°)$	$(x, y + 1, 270°)$
f_V^*	$(x, y - 1, 270°)$	$(x, y, 270°)$	$(x + 1, y + 1, 315°)$
g_V^*	$(x + 1, y - 1, 225°)$	$(x, y, 270°)$	$(x + 1, y + 1, 315°)$

Table 16.3. ED neuron assignment for horizontal contour. Reproduced from [6].

Dark-to-light

Contour	**Edge-detection neurons (EDNs)**		
a_H	$(x - 1, y, 0°)$	$(x, y, 0°)$	$(x + 1, y, 0°)$
b_H	$(x - 1, y, 0°)$	$(x, y, 0°)$	$(x + 1, y - 1, 45°)$
c_H	$(x - 1, y - 1, 315°)$	$(x, y, 0°)$	$(x + 1, y, 0°)$
d_H	$(x - 1, y - 1, 315°)$	$(x, y, 0°)$	$(x + 1, y - 1, 45°)$
e_H	$(x - 1, y, 0°)$	$(x, y, 0°)$	$(x + 1, y + 1, 315°)$
f_H	$(x - 1, y + 1, 45°)$	$(x, y, 0°)$	$(x + 1, y, 0°)$
g_H	$(x - 1, y + 1, 45°)$	$(x, y, 0°)$	$(x + 1, y + 1, 315°)$

Light-to-dark

Contour	**Edge-detection neurons (EDNs)**		
a_H^*	$(x - 1, y, 180°)$	$(x, y, 180°)$	$(x + 1, y, 180°)$
b_H^*	$(x - 1, y, 180°)$	$(x, y, 180°)$	$(x + 1, y - 1, 225°)$
c_H^*	$(x - 1, y - 1, 135°)$	$(x, y, 180°)$	$(x + 1, y, 180°)$
d_H^*	$(x - 1, y - 1, 135°)$	$(x, y, 180°)$	$(x + 1, y - 1, 225°)$
e_H^*	$(x - 1, y, 180°)$	$(x, y, 180°)$	$(x + 1, y + 1, 135°)$
f_H^*	$(x - 1, y + 1, 225°)$	$(x, y, 180°)$	$(x + 1, y, 180°)$
g_H^*	$(x - 1, y + 1, 225°)$	$(x, y, 180°)$	$(x + 1, y + 1, 135°)$

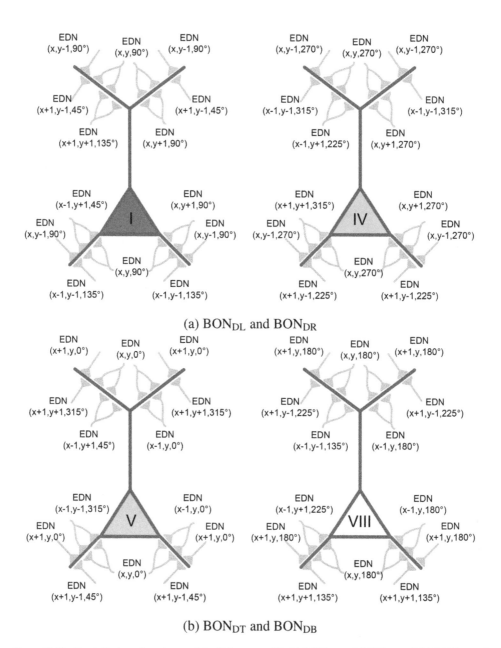

(a) BON$_{DL}$ and BON$_{DR}$

(b) BON$_{DT}$ and BON$_{DB}$

Figure 16.18. Dendritic branch assignment for BO neurons [6]. (a) BON$_{DL}$ and BON$_{DR}$ and (b) BON$_{DT}$ and BON$_{DB}$. The presynaptic inputs come from the EDN associated with each synapse on the dendritic branches.

contours and the basal dendritic arbor to detect convex contours. This configuration fulfills the Gestalt convexity principle which proposes that a concave surface is less likely to be the shape of an object. Figure 16.18 represents the dendritic branch assignment of BON$_{DL}$, BON$_{DR}$, BON$_{DT}$, and BON$_{DB}$, respectively.

16.4.5 Proposed border-ownership neural network

In this section, we describe our proposed neural network to implement the BO assignment. It is noted that contour information alone may not be sufficient to segregate the object from the background; therefore it is necessary to have the disparity (stereo-depth) component included in the BO neural network [18]. The exact connections among the visual cortical neurons are not well understood. Studies have shown there exist stereoscopic edge-selective cells in V2 that respond to discontinuity in depth (disparity) for a certain orientation. For instance, some stereoscopic edge-selective neurons respond to depth changing from near (left) to far (right) while some respond to the opposite. Some respond to depth changing from near (top) to far (bottom) while some respond to the opposite. Figure 16.19 illustrates our proposed hypothetical neural network for BO assignment in the

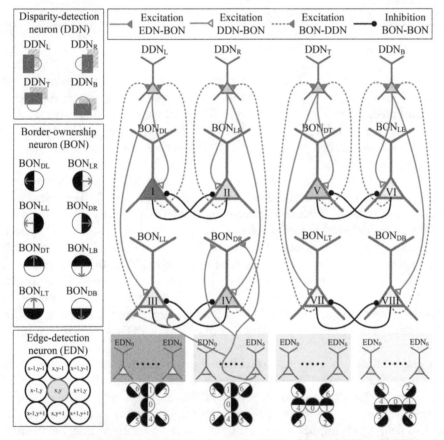

Figure 16.19. Hierarchical view of the BO neural network. DDN_L, DDN_R, DDN_T, and DDN_B are the stereoscopic edge-selective cells. The solid grey rectangle represents the object in foreground and the hatched region represents the object's shade. Four different subsets of EDNs (color-coded: red, green, blue, and yellow) feed local contrast polarity information to the corresponding four pairs of BONs (same color-coded). Only one EDN's (EDN_6) synaptic connection to one pair of BON is shown. The representations of the notation used here are explained in table 16.4 [6].

Table 16.4. Definition of the neurons in the hypothetical BO neural network. Reproduced from [6].

Neuron type	Representation
DDN_L	responds to near-to-far vertical edge sweeping from left to right
DDN_R	responds to far-to-near vertical edge sweeping from left to right
DDN_T	responds to near-to-far horizontal edge sweeping from top to bottom
DDN_B	responds to far-to-near horizontal edge sweeping from top to bottom
BON_{DL}	responds to dark object on the left side
BON_{LR}	responds to light object on the right side
BON_{LL}	responds to light object on the left side
BON_{DR}	responds to dark object on the right side
BON_{DT}	responds to dark object on the top side
BON_{LB}	responds to light object on the bottom side
BON_{LT}	responds to light object on the top side
BON_{DB}	responds to dark object on the bottom side

visual cortex. In this proposed network, there are four types of disparity-detection neurons (DDN), namely DDN_L, DDN_R, DDN_T and DDN_B which represent the stereoscopic edge-selective neuron along with eight types of BO neurons (BON, explained earlier in table 16.1), and twenty-eight types of edge-detection neurons (EDN, illustrated earlier in figure 16.15). The representation of these neurons is summarized in table 16.4.

Evidence suggests that there exist connections from BON to DDN which either enhance or null the disparity-selective neuron response [19]. The focus of our current work is on BO neuron implementation; the disparity-detection neurons function as the external input spikes to the corresponding BO neurons. Therefore, the excitatory synaptic connections from BON to DDN (dotted line) will be implemented in the future work. Excitation from EDN to BON carries contour information while excitation from DDN to BON conveys disparity information about the visual stimulus. For instance, DDN_L represents a neuron that responds to depth changing from near (left) to far (right) suggesting the object is on the left and hence it forms excitatory synaptic connection to BON_{DL} which has preferred left side of ownership.

Lateral inhibition is included to facilitate the convergence of a pair of BON firing states. The BO neuron that prefers one side of ownership forms an inhibitory connection to the BO neuron that prefers the opposite side of ownership. For instance, BON_{DL} fires more robustly if a dark object on the left is presented in the receptive field which implies it is not a light object on the right side; therefore there exists lateral inhibition between (BON_{DL} and BON_{LR}). The same concept applies to (BON_{LL} and BON_{DR}), (BON_{DT} and BON_{LB}), and (BON_{LT} and BON_{DB}).

More details and simulation results for the BO neurons are found in the Hsu thesis and conference paper.

16.5 Ultra-low-power dendritic computations

In his thesis [15], Pezhman Mamdouh described some low-power and ultra-low-power methods for dendritic computation circuits. These methods were introduced in conference papers [16] and [17]. In his thesis, Mamdouh also modeled the lactate shuttle that moves energy where needed in the biological brain.

16.6 Chapter summary

This chapter covered some advanced topics in neuromorphic circuits found in the BioRC project.

Certain sections of text in this chapter have been reproduced with permission from [7]. Copyright IEEE.

The final chapter covers neuromorphic systems.

References

[1] Agmon-Snir H, Carr C E and Rinzel J 1998 The role of dendrites in auditory coincidence detection *Nature* **393** 268–72

[2] Wagemans J *et al* 2012 A century of Gestalt psychology in visual perception: I. Perceptual grouping and figure-ground organization *Psychol. Bull.* **138** 1172–217

[3] Bender K J, Ford C P and Trussell L O 2010 Dopaminergic modulation of axon initial segment calcium channels regulates action potential initiation *Neuron.* **68** 500–11

[4] Craft E, Schütze H, Niebur E and von der Heydt R 2007 A neural model of figure–ground organization *J. Neurophysiol.* **97** 4310–26

[5] von der Heydt R, Zhou H and Friedman H S 2000 Representation of stereoscopic edges in monkey visual cortex *Vis. Res.* **40** 1955–67

[6] Hsu C-C 2014 Dendritic Computation and Plasticity in Neuromorphic Circuits *PhD thesis* University of Southern California

[7] Hsu C-C and Parker A C 2014 Border ownership in a nano-neuromorphic circuit using nonlinear dendritic computations *2014 Int. Joint Conf. Neural Networks (IJCNN)* (Piscataway, NJ: IEEE) 3442–9

[8] Irizarry-Valle Y 2016 Modeling astrocyte-neural interactions in CMOS neuromorphic circuits *PhD Thesis* University of Southern California

[9] Irizarry-Valle Y, Parker A C and Grzywacz N M 2014 An adaptable CMOS depressing synapse with detection of changes in input spike rate *2014 IEEE 5th Latin American Symp. Circuits and Systems* (Piscataway, NJ: IEEE) 1–4

[10] Jensen M S, Azouz R and Yaari Y 1994 Variant firing patterns in rat hippocampal pyramidal cells modulated by extracellular potassium *J. Neurophysiol.* **71** 831–9

[11] Kampa B M and Stuart G J 2006 Calcium spikes in basal dendrites of layer 5 pyramidal neurons during action potential bursts *J. Neurosci.* **26** 7424–32

[12] Larkum M E and Zhu J J 2002 Signaling of layer 1 and whisker-evoked Ca and Na action potentials in distal and terminal dendrites of rat neocortical pyramidal neurons *in vitro* and *in vivo J. Neurosci.* **22** 6991–7005

[13] Zhaoping L 2005 Border ownership from intracortical interactions in visual area V2 *Neuron* **47** 143–53

[14] Lisman J E 1997 Bursts as a unit of neural information: making unreliable synapses reliable *Trends Neurosci.* **20** 38–43

[15] Mamdouh P 2019 Power-efficient biomimetic neural circuits *PhD Thesis* University of Southern California

[16] Mamdouh P and Parker A C 2017 A power-efficient biomimetic intra-branch dendritic adder *2017 Int. Joint Conf. Neural Networks (IJCNN)* (Piscataway, NJ: IEEE) 3946–52

[17] Mamdouh P and Parker A C 2017 A switched-capacitor dendritic arbor for low-power neuromorphic applications *2017 Int. Symp. Circuits and Systems (ISCAS)IEEE* (Piscataway, NJ: IEEE) 1–4

[18] Qiu F T and von der Heydt R 2005 Figure and ground in the visual cortex: V2 combines stereoscopic cues with Gestalt rules *Neuron* **47** 155–66

[19] Raskob B L 2012 Frequency-based mathematical model of binocular complex cell responses *PhD Thesis* University of Southern California

[20] Smith S L, Smith I T, Branco T and Häusser M 2013 Dendritic spikes enhance stimulus selectivity in cortical neurons *in vivo Nature* **503** 115–20

[21] Sakai K and Nishimura H 2006 Surrounding suppression and facilitation in the determination of border ownership *J. Cogn. Neurosci.* **18** 562–79

[22] Supèr H, Romeo A and Keil M 2010 Feed-forward segmentation of figure-ground and assignment of border-ownership *PLoS One* **5** e10705

[23] Williams S R and Stuart G J 1999 Mechanisms and consequences of action potential burst firing in rat neocortical pyramidal neurons *J. Physiol.* **521** 467–82

[24] Zhou H, Friedman H S and Von Der Heydt R 2000 Coding of border ownership in monkey visual cortex *J. Neurosci.* **20** 6594–611

Chapter 17

Neuromorphic systems

Rick Cattell, Michael Boemler-Rudolph Mercury and Alice C Parker

In this chapter, we look at five projects to build 'artificial brains,' based on many of the ideas discussed in this book. We cover Intel's Loihi, IBM's TrueNorth, Manchester University's SpiNNaker, EPFL's BrainScaleS and BrainChip's Akida. Note that almost all of the projects this chapter discusses are moving targets; we apologize where these descriptions may be out of date; we used the latest descriptions we could find at the time of this writing. Wikipedia has discussion of most of these systems under the heading *Cognitive Computer*.

17.1 Introduction

A number of neuromorphic brain projects have made progress in the past decade toward large-scale networks of emulated neurons. This chapter looks at several of those projects, along with pros and cons to each approach.

Some of these and other neuromorphic chip projects can be simulated using *Nengo*, a Python-based tool. Another Python package for neuronal network simulators is PyNN. A number of other software packages exist that can be used to simulate spiking neural networks. A comprehensive list can be found at https://github.com/norse/norse. In terms of accelerating spiking neural networks on neuromorphic hardware, the Lava toolkit[1] has plans to become the go-to open-source software library for this, providing an interface between different existing software toolkits and different neuromorphic and non-neuromorphic hardware.

The first three projects, IBM's TrueNorth [3], Intel's Loihi [1, 2] and Brainchip's Akida [8] have produced digital neuromorphic hardware based on custom-fabricated chips. In all three of these cases, these chips can be combined to construct successively more sophisticated multi-processors. The fourth project, SpiNNaker [3] at Manchester University in the UK, has produced a massively parallel digital multiprocessor, and in 2020 the group embarked on the SpiNNaker2 project, scaling

---

[1] https://github.com/lava-nc/lava

up a factor of about 50 from their existing system with a new custom-fabricated chip. The fifth project, BrainScaleS [6] at the École Polytechnique Fédérale de Lausanne (EPFL) in Geneva Switzerland, differs from the others in using an analog neuron model. A BrainScaleS 2 project is now in the works as a follow-on to BrainScaleS, as part of the European Brain Project. The web page reference provides a list of several hundred publications.

A short discussion of each follows.

17.2 IBM's true north

IBM's neuromorphic computing project, TrueNorth, is led by Dharmendra Modha at IBM's Almaden Research Center in San Jose, California. TrueNorth utilizes completely digital neural emulation; it was funded as a DARPA SyNAPSE research project. The TrueNorth chip was the largest integrated circuit ever produced by IBM at the time of its fabrication.

The fundamental building block for TrueNorth is a neurosynaptic core with 256 outputs (i.e., up to 256 neurons), and 256 inputs connected via 256×256 programmable connections. In order to reduce network traffic, a single axon spike packet 'message' can be sent from a simulated neuron to a destination core, and the message can then 'fan-out' to multiple neurons at the destination core as required. If more than 256 destination cores are called for, intermediate neurons can be used to increase fan-out. Neuron operations are discretized into 1 ms time steps by a 1 kHz clock. Neurons on a chip as well as cores on a chip and chips on a board are tiled in a two-dimensional grid for communication purposes.

Various configurations of systems are envisioned by the TrueNorth team:

- The largest configuration at the time of this writing is based on a 28 nm chip manufacturing process, with 16 chips encompassing a simulation of 16 million neurons and 4 billion synapses.
- Multiple smaller configurations of TrueNorth are being produced to allow use of the hardware by development partners.
- Eventually the team hopes to scale to 10 billion neurons and 100 trillion synapses.

17.3 Intel's Loihi

The Loihi project at Mike Davies' Neuromorphic Computing Laboratory at Intel Labs bears many similarities to TrueNorth, but is built on a fundamentally different architecture: asynchronous versus synchronous[2]. Loihi's asynchronous architecture enables significant power efficiencies compared to synchronous designs, as much of the power draw of an integrated circuit is in clock management [7] and an async network-on-a-chip runs much faster in the average case as the full network does not need to wait for worst case spike activity.

---

[2] https://download.intel.com/newsroom/2021/new-technologies/neuromorphic-computing-loihi-2-brief.pdf

Intel's second generation Loihi2 is a custom SoC with spiking neural network chips (a.k.a. neural cores) that are configured in a two-dimensional (four neighbor) mesh for routing of spikes and several general-purpose coprocessors. As with other systems we discuss, destination spikes must exceed a threshold sum before a simulated neuron generates an output spike. This chip supports a wide variety of custom neuron models using a proprietary 'microcode' language for their implementation. Loihi2 can be programmed using an open-source software framework designed by Intel called Lava. As of the time of this writing, Lava includes the basic Leaky Integrate and Fire (LIF) model and plans to release more soon. A single Loihi2 chip has 128 neural cores that can be time multiplexed by 8192x to provide 1,048,576 neurons. Each chip also contains 120 million synapses. Three factor learning rules are possible.

Loihi appeared earlier as well [2]. Loihi1 had 1/10th the number of neurons and 1.1x the number of synapses. Loihi1 also had 1/2 the number of embedded microprocessors (three versus six).

Loihi chips are utilized in a variety of deployments:

- Kapoho Bay: one or two chips are utilized in a USB deployment.
- Wolf Mountain: four chips are utilized on a board, emulating a total of 524 K neurons.
- Nahuku: 8–32 chips are utilized in a FPGA expansion card.
- Pohoiki Beach: in a multi-board system, 64 chips are utilized to emulate 8 million neurons.
- Pohoiki Springs: in a many-board system, up to 768 chips are utilized to emulate up to 100 million neurons.

Loihi2 chips are implemented in two new form factors:

- Oheo Gulch: a single chip system for early evaluation and cloud use.
- Kapoho Point: $4'' \times 4''$ stackable 8 chip system with high-throughput interfaces.

One significant improvement from the Loihi1 to Loihi2 systems is improved networking across chips. The new Radix-6 mesh routing allows efficient connections across a three- dimensional set of networked chips.

17.4 BrainChip's Akida

BrainChip, a company started out of Australia and now in Europe and the USA has created a neural accelerator system on a chip. Their Akida AKD1000 chip has 1.2 million neurons implemented on 80 neural processing units (NPUs). 10 billion synapses can connect these neurons. They include a machine learning software package called Meta TF for training models. The Akida AKD1000 offers incremental learning after online training. Up to 64 Akida AKD1000 devices can be wired together into a larger network[3].

17.5 Manchester's SpiNNaker

The SpiNNaker1 project was led by professor Steve Furber at Manchester University in the UK. The SpiNNaker1 system, comprising 1 million CPU cores intended to emulate 1 billion neurons, was 'switched on' at the end of 2018. SpiNNaker1 as designed should scale to 1 percent of the size of the human brain in neuron count. It is based on Acorn RISC Machine (ARM) processors, a 1985 computer architecture predating the project. An array of ARM processors on each chip share memory.

Many experiments have already been performed on SpiNNaker1, as outlined in Furber's book [3]. For example, the team implemented online sound processing with a 'SpiNNakEar' project modeled after mammalian auditory recognition. SpiNNakEar operates in three stages:

1. The first stage module models the outer and middle ear;
2. The second stage mimics the sound stimulus frequency separation; and
3. The third stage implements the functionality of the inner hair cells and auditory nerves.

The algorithm SpiNNakEar used is based on a MATLAB auditory periphery model [4, 5]. The outer and middle ear model is triggered by auditory input in real time, after that a non-linear inner ear hair cell model runs asynchronously, driven by events from the auditory nerve output stage.

For SpiNNaker2, Furber has passed the baton to Christian Mayr of the Technische Universität Dresden in Dresden, Germany. SpiNNaker2, like SpiNNaker1, is based on ARM processors, but uses 10 million cores and additional efficiency improvements, including a higher clock rate, numerical accelerators, and dynamic scaling. SpiNNaker2 also addresses I/O performance and memory sharing bottlenecks in the SpiNNaker1 design, supporting 100 Mbit Ethernet I/O supporting Ethernet is up to 1 Gbit s^{-1} on chip-level, a larger routing table, access to shared SDRAM between processor cores, and a Globally Asynchronous Locally Synchronous (GALS) architecture allowing independent scaling of individual components. With six parallel bi-directional network ports, SpiNNaker2 can route 2.4 billion packets per second. In contrast, SpiNNaker1 could route only 100 000 packets per second, and with less routing efficiency than SpiNNaker2.

SpiNNaker2 incorporates 152 processing elements (PEs) per chip. Each PE, an ARM Cortex-M4 with floating point unit, incorporates 128 KBytes of local SRAM accessable as both data and instruction memory by the processors through a crossbar. Four cores share memory in quad processing elements (QPEs). All PEs are connected in a two-dimensional mesh network for better scalability.

---

[3] https://brainchip.com/akida-neural-processor-soc/

A communications controller with DMA is the bridge between the ARM M4 and the network-on-a-chip, providing a method to access remote registers and SRAM.

A seventh SpiNNaker link (in addition to the six of the existing SpiNNaker1 mesh) provides an optional hyper-connection to any other PE in the system, avoiding the need to route through intermediate nodes and significantly reducing latency for long-distance routing in simulations.

As a result of all these improvements, SpiNNaker2 achieves a projected scale of 50 billion simulated neurons, roughly the neuron population of the human cerebral cortex, or about 50 percent of that of the entire human brain. Each SpiNNaker2 chip yields roughly the simulation capacity of an entire 48 processor board in SpiNNaker1. As such, SpiNNaker2's scale far exceeds that of all the other systems we examine in this chapter. SpiNNaker's full brain system is expected to be up and running in Dresden, Germany by late 2023.

17.6 BrainScaleS

Professor Johannes Schemmel at Heidelberg University in Germany leads the BrainScaleS project, conducted as part of the European Human Brain Project (HBP). The latest instantiation at the time of this writing is BrainScaleS 2.0, the latest release of which was implemented in 2022. To avoid confusion, note that the European HBP includes the SpiNNaker work as well as BrainScaleS as sub projects. The HBP is an umbrella organization for the European projects, however, SpiNNaker and BrainScaleS both started before HBP.

In contrast to SpiNNaker and the other projects we discuss in this chapter, the BrainScaleS work has focused more on biological realism in brain emulation, including analog functionality. By emulating analog neurons, BrainScaleS's approach provides a different frame of reference for understanding the brain than digital implementations.

The first generation BrainscaleS-1 and associated HICANN (High Input Count Analog Neural Network) application-specific integrated circuit (ASIC) was based on 180 nm chip technology. Rather than conventional integrated circuit chips, BrainScaleS is constructed from 20 uncut 8 inch silicon wafers.

The current generation BrainScales-2 is based on 65 nm technology, allowing for a 'digital plasticity processing unit', a highly parallel microprocessor specifically designed for learning.

BrainScaleS's analog circuits for continuous-time modeling of neurons and synapses are designed for fast emulation of spike-based dynamics of neurons. Compared to biological real-time, the emulation is accelerated by orders of magnitude. The analog circuits are attached to built-in digital compute cores used to simulate the higher-level biological processes happening on slower time scales such as learning.

17.7 Further reading

TrueNorth (Dharmendra Modha) https://en.wikipedia.org/wiki/Cognitive_compute r#IBM_TrueNorth_chip and a video on TrueNorth: 'IBM's Incredible TrueNorth

Chip' is found at https://www.youtube.com/watch?v=X2TYAcr36r0. Loihi is discussed more in depth on wikichip at https://en.wikichip.org/wiki/intel/loihi and in a video by its chief architect, Mike Davies at: https://www.youtube.com/watch?v=GN3eSMoJcM8. Akida is discussed more in depth on wikichip: https://en.wikichip.org/wiki/brainchip/akida SpiNNaker is written about at https://en.wikipedia.org/wiki/SpiNNaker.

17.8 Conclusions

At a fundamental level, there are more similarities than differences between TrueNorth, Loihi, Akida, and SpiNNaker: all four represent a similar approach: a digital network of integrate-and fire digital neurons that exchange weighted digital spike messages via an any direction network. All four use similar algorithms to communicate spikes on a network and to decide when a neuron fires. In contrast, BrainScaleS differs in that the neurons are analog, so simulated neurons send a waveform rather than a simple digital spike message to connected neurons.

TrueNorth, Loihi, SpiNNaker, Akida, and BrainScaleS differ in scale, but all five are moving targets. At the time of this writing, SpiNNaker2 appeared to scale the furthest by far, in terms of neuron count.

17.9 Exercises

1. Which of the following uses an analog neural model?
    (a) Brainscales;
    (b) Loihi;
    (c) Spinnaker;
    (d) TrueNorth.
2. What are the similarities between TrueNorth, Loihi and Spinnaker?
3. Among the five models, which is based on an X86 core, and which is based on ARM processors?
4. Give some reasons BrainScales is different from the others.
5. If you were going to build a neural simulation at the scale of a human brain, which system would you pick and why? What would be your second choice, and why?

References

[1] Davies M *et al* 2021 Advancing neuromorphic computing with Loihi: a survey of results and outlook *Proc. IEEE* **109** 911–34

[2] Davies M *et al* 2018 Loihi: a neuromorphic manycore processor with on-chip learning *IEEE Micro* **38** 82–99

[3] Furber S and Bogdan P 2020 *A Spiking Neural Network Architecture* (Boston, MA: now Publishers) http://dx.doi.org/10.1561/9781680836523

[4] James R 2020 *Spikes from sound: a model of the human auditory periphery on SpiNNaker* (Manchester: The University of Manchester)

[5] Meddis R *et al* 2013 A computer model of the auditory periphery and its application to the study of hearing *Basic Aspects of Hearing* ed B Moore, R Patterson, I Winter, R Carlyon and H Gockel (New York: Springer) pp 11–20

[6] Meier K *et al* 2020 *Brainscales Project Overview* http://brainscales.kip.uni-heidelberg.de
[7] Myers C J 2001 *Asynchronous Circuit Design* (New York: Wiley)
[8] Vanarse A *et al* 2019 A hardware-deployable neuromorphic solution for encoding and classification of electronic nose data *Sensors* **19** 4831

Chapter 18

Epilogue

Alice C Parker and Rick Cattell

Advances in neuromorphic circuits and advances in artificial intelligence (AI) are emerging at an increasingly rapid pace. An AI tool, GPT-3, writes articles, including one written by GPT-3 about itself [8]. Another AI tool, DALL-E, draws images, often fanciful, like dolphins lounging in chairs [5]. One paper describes a probabilistic relational database that implements consciousness in AI tools [9]. In neuromorphic hardware advances, Cerebras technology, already boasting the world's largest computer chip [6], can implement a neural network with 120 trillion connections—several orders of magnitude greater than current systems [4]. Carbon nanotubes are envisioned to provide connectivity in biological brains [1, 7]. Other materials, like graphene (the basic fabric of carbon nanotubes), are envisioned as synaptic material [2].

Almost science fiction, future organic neuromorphic circuits will be able to connect biological neurons with neuromorphic circuits [3]. The explosion of AI and neuromorphic hardware is leading to increased levels of machine intelligence, and the technologies described in this book are just a tiny stepping stone along the way.

References

[1] Fabbro A *et al* 2012 Carbon nanotubes: artificial nanomaterials to engineer single neurons and neuronal networks *ACS Chem. Neurosci.* **3.8** 611–8
[2] Kireev D *et al* 2022 Metaplastic and energy-efficient biocompatible graphene artificial synaptic transistors for enhanced accuracy neuromorphic computing *Nat. Commun.* **13** 1–11
[3] Kleiner K 2022 Making computer chips act more like brain cells *Knowable Mag.* https://knowablemagazine.org/article/technology/2022/making-computer-chips-act-more-like-brain-cells
[4] Knight W 2021 A new chip cluster will make massive AI models possible *Wired* https://www.wired.com/story/cerebras-chip-cluster-neural-networks-ai/
[5] Ramesh A *et al* 2022 Hierarchical text-conditional image generation with clip latents *arXiv preprint* arXiv:2204.06125

[6] Spicer D 2022 The Biggest Chip in the World *Computer History Museum Blog* https://computerhistory.org/blog/the-biggest-chip-in-the-world/

[7] Sucapane A *et al* 2009 Interactions between cultured neurons and carbon nanotubes: a nanoneuroscience vignette *J. Nanoneurosci.* **1** 10–6

[8] Osmanovic Thunströmm A 2022 We asked GPT-3 to write an academic paper about itself—then we tried to get it published *Sci. Am.* https://www.scientificamerican.com/article/we-asked-gpt-3-to-write-an-academic-paper-about-itself-mdash-then-we-tried-to-get-it-published/

[9] Wolfson O 2021 A relational-database methodology for incorporating consciousness into AI agents *J. Artif. Intell. Conscious* **8** 67–80

Printed in the USA
CPSIA information can be obtained
at www.ICGtesting.com
JSHW061341241223
54197JS00004B/73